Adolescent Psychiatry

Current Reviews in Psychiatry

Series Editors

Eugene S. Paykel MB ChB FRCP FRCPsych DPM
Professor of Psychiatry, Department of Psychiatry, University of Cambridge,
Addenbrooke's Hospital, Cambridge

H. Gethin Morgan MD FRCP FRCPsych DPM
Norah Cooke Hurle Professor of Mental Health, University of Bristol

Volumes already published

Alcoholism and Drug Addiction *D. S. Raistrick and R. J. Davidson*
Mental Handicap *O. Russell*

Peter Hill
MRCP FRCPsych

Senior Lecturer in Child and Adolescent Psychiatry,
St. George's Hospital Medical School;
Honorary Consultant Psychiatrist,
St. George's Hospital, London

Adolescent Psychiatry

Series Editors
EUGENE S. PAYKEL AND H. GETHIN MORGAN

Churchill Livingstone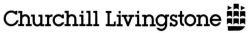

EDINBURGH LONDON MELBOURNE AND NEW YORK 1989

CHURCHILL LIVINGSTONE
Medical Division of Longman Group UK Limited

Distributed in the United States of America by Churchill
Livingstone Inc., 1560 Broadway, New York, N.Y. 10036,
and by associated companies, branches and representatives
throughout the world.

© Longman Group UK Limited 1989

First published 1989

ISBN 0-443-02774-9

British Library Cataloguing in Publication Data
Hill, Peter
    Adolescent psychiatry. — (Current reviews
    in psychiatry, ISBN 0266–5026).
    1. Adolescents. Psychiatry
    I. Title   II. Series
    616.89′022

    ISBN 0-443-02774-9

Library of Congress Cataloging-in-Publication Data
Hill, P. D. (Peter David)
    Adolescent psychiatry.
    (Current reviews in psychiatry, ISSN 0266-5026; 3)
    1. Adolescent psychiatry. I. Title.   II. Series.
[DNLM: 1. Adolescent Psychiatry. W1 CU8093MF v.3/
WS 463 H647a]
RJ503.H55   1989   616.89′022   88-7250
ISBN 0-443-02774-9

Produced by Longman Singapore Publishers (Pte) Ltd.
Printed in Singapore

Preface

A specialty of psychiatry which applies itself to adolescents has yet to establish a secure identity for itself, bridging as it does the two fields of child psychiatry and adult psychiatry without being clearly separate from either. It mirrors the status of adolescents themselves. The consequence has been a neglect of service and research pertinent to this developmental phase and age group. There have been a few books on adolescent psychiatry but they have either been written from the standpoint of psychiatrists in charge of in-patient units or concerned only with psychoanalytic approaches. I believe this to be the first book to be influenced and inspired principally by mainstream out-patient experience. Far more adolescents will be seen by psychiatrists in out-patient clinics than in adolescent units. I have endeavoured to reflect the *Zeitgeist* by placing an emphasis on normal development and how the psychopathology of various conditions relates to this. In doing so, a debt to the conceptual approaches taken by Michael Rutter, Lionel Hersov and Arthur Crisp is apparent. Such influences may be evident but what is probably less obvious is the continuing effect of working clinically with Mike Berger, a man courteously intolerant of loose thinking.

I hope that the end result will prove useful to postgraduate trainees and to established psychiatrists who wish to bring their knowledge of the field up to date. It is essentially about psychiatry but I intend that psychologists, social workers, teachers and therapists of all denominations who work with adolescents should find it useful. I make an assumption that readers will have a working knowledge of both child and adult psychiatry and have tried not to duplicate knowledge specific to each of those fields. Indeed, some of the conditions and problems familiar to psychiatrists who see adolescents are much more typical of childhood, have arisen then and present late. This is particularly true of enuresis and faecal soiling; their appraisal and treatment differ but little from how they are managed in middle and late childhood so I have not dealt with them here.

It has taken a long time to write and the patience of my family has been sorely tried. I am grateful for their support. The same should also be said of the editorial staff at Churchill Livingstone to whom I am equally indebted for their forbearance. A number of people have provided helpful criticism, particularly Ian Berg, Joan Bicknell, Alan McClelland, the two series editors and the Senior Registrars on the St. George's higher training schemes. I have not accepted all of it so they are not to blame for errors and shortcomings.

London, 1989   Peter Hill

Contents

Contents

1
Introduction

Adolescence is the period of growth which starts with puberty and ends with adulthood or maturity; vague end-points given the amount of variation between individuals. Many people clearly equate adolescence with the teenage years yet covert (and often overt) pubertal changes can be detected before the age of 13, and legal maturity is technically achieved at age 18 though this is not always evident in psychological terms. Certainly adolescence cannot easily be defined by mere chronological age, yet it is often necessary to do so for administrative purposes or to bring the subject into conceptual focus. For practical purposes it can reasonably be assumed to occupy the years between the 13th and 18th birthdays, though close study of human development reveals this to be a considerable simplification (see Ch. 3.)

With such procrustean surgery in mind, it is nevertheless usual to consider adolescence to be a developmental phase. It spans the final years of compulsory education and the time during which young people are expected to seek employment. During this period a number of challenges are set which adolescents have to face and which arise from social expectations and biological maturation. Although attempts to meet such challenges may be maladaptive and can result in psychopathology, it would be wrong to see adolescent psychiatric disorder entirely in terms of developmental tasks specific to adolescence. Most adolescent psychopathology has its roots in childhood disturbance and long-standing family dysfunction: to treat adolescence as if it were divorced from earlier development is mistaken. The effects of distorted attachments in infancy, deficient socialisation in childhood, earlier educational failure or incoherent parenting may present clinically in the teenage years but have their origins in an earlier phase of development.

Specialisation, such as it is, in adolescent psychiatry is unusual. Because psychiatric resources specifically for teenagers are sparse, only the most disturbed are seen. The result of this is that the professional literature reflects assumptions that normal adolescence can be understood by extension from the abnormal. There are good grounds for thinking that this is unsound practice, particularly in terms of generalisations about identity crises and the nature of so-called adolescent turmoil. A further complication is that psychiatrists commonly use their memories of their own adolescence when attempting to understand their young patients. The same caveats apply: doctors are unusual people in terms of their intelligence and education (to say the least) and generalisations based upon their own personal experience are suspect.

Specialist adolescent psychiatry has also tended to be focussed upon in-patients, yet most psychologically disturbed adolescents will either not be seen at all by psychiatrists or be assessed and treated as out-patients by departments of child or adult psychiatry. This book tries to redress this imbalance by giving due weight to the psychiatric problems of adolescents as these may be dealt with on an out-patient basis. At the same time, there is an attempt to link adolescent psychopathology with what is known about normal adolescent psychosocial development.

There are no psychiatric conditions specific to adolescence though some, such as eating disorders, link closely to the adolescent developmental process. Similarly, antisocial behaviour outside the home (although not usually a psychiatric problem) is remarkably prominent in the mid-teens and may attract psychiatric involvement. It follows that there are no treatment procedures which are specific to adolescent psychiatry, and a range of techniques derived from child psychiatry on one hand and adult psychiatry on the other are employed. Treatment techniques are therefore discussed somewhat briefly since these are well described in other texts. Apart from the major mental illnesses, most interventions in adolescent psychiatry use psychological methods: psychotherapy in its widest sense.

Most teenagers live at home and their families are crucial in promoting their development, their welfare, and their care generally. No attempt to deal with adolescent psychopathology can do other than reflect this fact. The interactive impact of adolescent distress upon the family as a whole and the power of the family to harm or heal the disturbed adolescent is taken as axiomatic.

Adolescents are, as a crude generalisation, difficult patients. They commonly find it difficult to communicate verbally and openly with their medical advisers. They can misunderstand the attempts to help them and may retreat into a position where all therapeutic activity is seen as part of a general conspiracy to constrain them. Strong feelings may be elicited in parents and professionals and these feelings, like those of the adolescents themselves, may be expressed in actions rather than words. The management of treatment has to acknowledge this but it is best learned clinically through experience and supervision rather than through the pages of a book. It will often involve liaison with a host of agencies, medical and otherwise, but the extent and nature of such agencies will vary according to local provision, the clinical problem in question, and the age of the teenager.

With respect to the last point it is obvious that an 18-year-old is very different from a 13-year-old. General statements about "adolescence" are accordingly weakened by this fact and the common observation that the rate of developmental progress through adolescence will vary between girls and boys and between individuals of either sex. Added to this is the way in which the psychiatric services for children and those for adults are organised separately, have differing assumptions and practices, and contain different people. Adolescence extends beyond the age at which many child psychiatric services bow out of the therapeutic arena (usually around 16), yet it will be evident that some older teenagers would benefit from the developmental bias of child psychiatrists. Conversely, the presentation of serious mental illness, to which adult psychiatry services are orientated, may be met with diffidence by child psychiatrists when it presents in the early teenage years.

The recent publication of a report by the Health Advisory Service (1986), *Bridges Over Troubled Waters* (summarised by Horrocks 1987), is an attempt to grapple with this difficulty in delivering a coherent psychiatric service for adolescents as a whole. It makes a number of recommendations including: a broader and more eclectic service for adolescents, the extension of child psychiatric activity to include older adolescents, the establishment in each Health Service District of a designated Consultant Psychiatrist who will have responsibility for planning and coordinating psychiatric services for adolescents but who will not treat all psychiatrically disordered adolescents themselves. Such a post will be additional to the specialist adolescent teams which already exist in most Health Service Regions and which are commonly based on in-patient adolescent units. There is an emphasis within the report on the provision of local services which will utilise out-patient clinics, day-units and consultative work.

In a text of this length it is impossible to provide adequate detail on the organisation of services and the delivery of day-to-day treatment. Many readers will want to pursue additional reading elsewhere and on occasion this is specified, though there are books, journals and articles which are useful in this respect yet are too numerous to cite. One exception is the *Journal of Adolescence* (Academic Press) which is the journal of the Association for the Psychiatric Study of Adolescents and which contains a wealth of articles, many of which are descriptive, reflecting the broad compass of adolescent psychiatry in Britain.

Within this book there is an acknowledged bias towards the use of the male pronoun. This reflects the fact that most adolescent patients are male (and so, too, are most of their psychiatrists). Where this is patently not so, as for example in anorexia nervosa, the female pronoun is used.

REFERENCES

Health Advisory Service 1986 Bridges over Troubled Waters. HMSO, London
Horrocks P 1987 Bridges over troubled waters — services for disturbed
    adolescents. Health Trends 19: 15–17

2

Assessment

The assessment process in adolescent psychiatry is complex. The multifactorial causation of much adolescent psychopathology means that treatment interventions will likewise often be plural and interactive. To obtain a satisfactory formulation, information must be gathered from a variety of sources: referral agent, patient, other family members, school or employer, general practitioner, nursing staff, social services and so forth. The mode of data collection will also be various: verbal and written report, interview, observation, interviewer's subjective response, and formal testing or examination. Integration of all this information depends upon exactly what the purpose of assessment is: does psychopathology exist, how may it be treated, would admission to hospital be appropriate? Assessment is not a standard procedure to be undertaken in all circumstances; it must answer specific questions and these need to be framed at the outset.

Steinberg (1983) has written a critique of the referral process which is a helpful guide to those beginning work in an adolescent unit. He draws a distinction between:

1. Those problems which disappear between referral and assessment, probably for a variety of reasons including the resolution of a crisis, and the perception of a situation as problematic when it is not

2. Problems which, on clarification, are more appropriately dealt with by a non-psychiatric agency (e.g. social services, special educational resources)

3. Problems which can be dealt with equally effectively by a psychiatric team or by another agency (e.g. when family therapy or counselling are indicated)

4. Problems that can only be effectively managed by a psychiatric team.

This underlines the advisability of seeking information about the case when referral information is sparse (as in the classic urgent telephone call). It would be inappropriate to process all referrals automatically through a complex and protracted assessment, since a large proportion are going to fall into Groups 1–3 (Steinberg et al 1981). Caution in entering referrals automatically for a full assessment is also suggested, e.g., when a family presents a teenager as a patient and there is a history of multiple previous psychiatric contacts from which the boy or girl has been prematurely withdrawn, or when psychiatry is perceived as supplying control over a wayward (but not necessarily psychiatrically disordered) young person. There may be other unstated reasons for an assessment being requested, such as the use that may be made of psychiatric opinion in legal battles, whether arising out of an offence, a claim for compensation or a contested custody case. Assessment cannot take place in a vacuum and the reasons for a referrer requesting an assessment need clarification. In order to answer some specific questions, assessment can be suitably brief.

Interviewing

Obtaining information from the individual adolescent and his caretakers, most usually his parents, is central to assessment. This information must include verbal report of past and present functioning and experience. It needs to be coupled with direct observation and examination so that a composite picture of psychosocial and mental functioning is established. Strengths as well as deviance and pathology have to be identified and construed within a developmental and social framework. This should include special reference to family, peer relationships and school or job environment as appropriate. The adolescent's own account of his situation and experience is always valuable and becomes crucial when major intrapsychic pathology is suspected, just as it is essential to evaluate neurological functioning when intracranial pathology is suspected.

There are various frames of reference within which suffering or deviance may be placed: family therapy models such as a structural approach, intrapsychic metaphors such as Kleinian psychoanalysis, ideas derived from developmental psychopathology, notions of mental illness and so forth. The most obvious statement to make about such attempts to understand adolescent psychological problems is that no single scheme offers a useful conceptualisation of all psychological difficulties experienced or created by teenagers. Clinics or psychiatrists may elect to develop expertise in one conceptual mode but appear foolish when they choose to translate all psychopathology, suffering or deviance into one language of explanation and intervention: their sources of referral learn to use them selectively.

Accordingly it is unwise to spurn individual interviews on the grounds that only a whole-family therapy model is applicable in the psychiatric management of adolescent disorder, just as it is nonsense always to avoid a family interview because of possible future adverse effects on transference or confidentiality. Nor should psychiatrists with six or more years expensive training in physical medicine (and a salary commensurate with this) evade their responsibilities by not physically examining their patients. Given that there is no evidence for the superiority of any one mode of thought about adolescent psychopathology and its treatment, this book is eclectic and thus reflects what seems to be a mainstream in British psychiatric thought about adolescent psychiatry. Interviewing the individual patient, his parents (or other caretakers) and possibly his siblings, and observing and testing the interactions and mutual assumptions of family members in order to characterise the family system — all have a place in assessment.

The general principles of diagnostic interviewing are reviewed elsewhere, from an academic viewpoint (Cox & Rutter 1985, Hill 1985) or described in terms of practical guidance (Bebbington & Hill 1985). Some points are particularly important and are repeated here.

Initial diagnostic interviewing needs to engage the teenager and his family in the process of clinical assessment and possible future treatment. Either (or all of them) may have been sent to a psychiatric service by a third party such as a school or social services department without their wholehearted agreement, and in consequence they are likely to be somewhat dubious about the whole business. The implications for the interviewer are that he or she should be courteous, reasonably well groomed and explain the nature, purpose and duration of each assessment interview.

The interviewer needs to consider whom to see when. Many clinicians consider it good practice to see the patient and both his parents together initially to agree on what the problems are

that need appraisal. This can be followed by an individual interview with the adolescent, followed by an interview with his
parents. Alternatively, a conjoint interview of adolescent patient
together with his parents (with or without siblings present) may
be pursued as a continuation of the initial problem-definition
phase if it appears to the clinician that the problem requires
exploring in whole-family terms. In such circumstances it is
sensible to preserve a low threshold for supplementary individual
interviews, particularly when it is likely that the adolescent has
information which he or she will not readily divulge in the
hearing of his or her parents. Thus the advisability of separate
interviews is greater with certain symptoms (depression, schizophrenia, obsessions, antisocial behaviour outside the home,
sexual problems, drug taking etc.) and where there appears to
be a particularly important issue arising from developmental
individuation which can be acknowledged metaphorically by
granting a separate interview.

Many of the difficulties that young children have in understanding how a psychiatric service might help them with their
psychological problems will also apply to teenagers. It is not
obvious to the average teenager that talk can be helpful; some
will say that it is not. Many will assume that if they disclose their
inner world, they will be thought mad, or that the process of
discussion with a psychiatrist will make them mad. Besides, they
may say, as all psychiatrists are mad themselves, you cannot
afford to take them seriously. They may have fears of forcible
admission to hospital, automatic breach of confidentiality, brain
surgery, or being hypnotised. Fantasies about the functions of
tape- and video-recorders, of what is being written down in notes
and what is said to parents, schools or employers are likely to
be both colourful and inhibitory.

In order to compensate for all this, the temptation is for the
interviewer to be ingratiating, over-nice, or even to join sides
with the adolescent against perceived authority. Factors in the
interviewer's own personality or personal history may encourage
this as well. The risks are those of inaccuracy because the interviewer concentrates too much on creating a positive relationship
(see Shapiro 1979), or suppression of disclosure because the
interviewee jumps to an assumption that the interviewer already
understands or knows about the topic (Heller, 1968). As far as
adolescents and their parents are concerned it is best to be

straightforward, to inform rather than seduce, and to concentrate on collecting information.

Cox and his colleagues, in a series of studies conveniently summarised in Cox & Rutter (1985), demonstrated that optimal disclosure of both information and emotion rested upon an interviewing style that used systematic probing for detail and example but which was not rigid and allowed the interviewees to use their own words to describe their problems at the start of an interview. At this initial stage, open questions are used with little cross-examination. Later, systematic questioning across a range of topics and areas allows coverage of relevant areas with examples being sought of particular behaviours or emotions. A reasonably standard format allows an interviewer to make comparisons between interviews and to become familiar with the range of normality in terms of information obtained and interview behaviour observed. Encouraging adequate emotional expression and gathering facts are not at all mutually exclusive; both are facilitated by direct questioning and empathic reflection within a flexible yet managed interview.

The above general findings may be expected to hold true for both teenagers and parents. There are some specific elements which pertain to adolescents which represent a modification of standard interviewing practice with adults. Multiple-choice questions appear to facilitate self-disclosure with young adolescents, perhaps because they give an indication as to the sort of replies sought (see Hill 1985). They should always include a branch which itself is open and are probably best left until open questioning has failed. The following is taken from an interview with a girl whose sister was killed when a lorry crashed into a bus queue, and indicates how the branch "some rather different feeling" was important.

Interviewer	I wonder how that left you feeling; can you tell me what it was like, how you felt?
Subject	(Shrugs silently)
Interviewer	Was it bad?
Subject	(Further silence)
Interviewer	Some people would have been sad if that had happened to them, others would have become very bitter, or angry or *had some rather different feeling*. How was it for you?
Subject	I think it was more, sort of angry but it took a long time before I felt anything.

Interviewer	A long time before you had much in the way of feelings?
Subject	Yeah, a week or two. Numb, spaced out, know what I mean? I thought I was really weird because I wasn't crying and things. I thought I was really mean and I felt really ashamed, like I wasn't a real person, not human. When I first cried about her, I was really pleased I could feel sad, it was funny.

Silence is, indeed, the bugbear of interviewing adolescents, as is the "don't know" response. As above it may indicate that the adolescent really doesn't know how to answer the question, doesn't know what is expected of them, or is wary of making a fool of themselves because they don't know the unspoken rules of clinical interviewing. To avoid such traps it is sensible to spell out how an interview works: who the interviewer is and how long the interview will take, what the interviewer wants to ask about and why, what happens to the information gained and who will hear about it. The adolescent's trust and cooperation cannot be taken for granted and there is no point in interviewers complaining that they are "only trying to help"; little ice is cut thereby. Apart from the adolescent who is clearly resentful at being thought mad by being dragged off to see a psychiatrist (which the interviewer should acknowledge openly, perhaps by a question: "Are you here under protest?" or less directly: "Whose idea was it that you come here?"), the commonest reason for silence is probably not understanding what the interviewer is driving at because he is using abstract concepts beyond the adolescent's cognitive capacity. The ability to conceptualise in the abstract and manipulate competing hypotheses in thought is not usually acquired before the mid-teens at the earliest, whereas psychiatrists, as well as being more intelligent and having a larger vocabulary than most of their patients, are so well used to abstract conceptualisation that they have difficulty abandoning it in interviewing. Cross-checking ("Do you know what I mean?") is invaluable. When silence arises out of anxious inhibition, the use of indirect techniques such as drawing a family tree or the squiggle game can be helpful. The topic is discussed further in Hill (1985).

Even when silence does not impede an interview, the sensitive interviewer will appreciate when an emotionally laden topic is inhibiting disclosure. It is wise to back off the subject of discussion at that point, perhaps with an open acknowledgement of how difficult it is to talk about, and return to it later. There is no point in rubbing a young person's nose in emotional discomfort for the sake of "catharsis" at a first interview, if indeed ever. Conversely, it may be wise not to prolong a first interview that seems to be going well since the adolescent may end up exhausted, even resentful, at being drained of private information and feel there is no point in further discussion. As a rough guide, many young adolescents find an individual interview lasting three-quarters of an hour quite long enough.

During such an interview, the adolescent's view of the problem and any further private information about it should be sought. An account of leisure activities, peer group and family relationships, and the general situation at work or school provides a framework for the early part of the interview and allows relevant issues to be taken up in detail as necessary. There should be an enquiry into emotional life, abnormal perceptions, thoughts and beliefs, an evaluation of self-concept and cognitive capacity along the lines of a conventional mental state though it is often not possible to cover all this at a single session.

The interview with the parents is more likely to resemble the pattern established in child psychiatry than the model of interviewing relatives in adult psychiatry, since developmental data is important in formulation, and detailed information about family life is vital if the teenager lives at home or has just left it. The content and form of such an interview is described in a number of texts (e.g. Bebbington & Hill 1985, Steinberg 1983).

Carrying out a whole-family interview for assessment purposes is comparatively easy compared with family interviews for treatment purposes. Adolescents are quite often the most revealing commentators on family relationships so long as they feel supported by the interviewer. They are not, however, particularly likely to be forthcoming about sexual matters or delinquent behaviour outside the home in their parents' hearing, nor will some be willing to express powerful affect openly, because they wish to protect their parents and siblings from the knowledge that, for example, they are suicidal. Nevertheless, so long as an opportunity for also being seen on their own can be provided, such caveats are not very important. The interviewer will want to obtain a picture of how the family functions as a unit and what the valence of the adolescent's problematic behaviour or emotional state is within the system of interactions and relationships that constitute family life. In order to do this, the interviewer must be active in probing assumptions and promoting interactions within the session that are between family members and not allowing matters to degenerate into a series of individual interviews held in the presence of others. This is well described in a number of family therapy texts (e.g. Gorell Barnes 1982, Haley 1976, Will & Wrate 1985). Young children may well be present if the designated patient has younger siblings and they will require involvement using communication techniques that recognise their special developmental status (Dare & Lindsey 1979, Bebbington & Hill 1985).

Assessment in particular settings
Reports for criminal courts

If the purpose of referral is to obtain a court report, then the role of the psychiatrist and the principles of confidentiality are different from ordinary clinical work. It needs to be explained to the teenager and his family that the purpose of any interview or examination is to provide such a report. If the report is asked for by the court, then the contents are covered by "absolute privilege" and the author cannot be sued for libel. Magistrates are obliged to tell adolescents what is in a report and although common practice is to summarise verbally, there is a chance that they may be shown the whole report, which means that it is unwise to put anything in the report which cannot be revealed to the adolescent directly (such as his illegitimacy if he is unaware of it). A report prepared at the request of the adolescent's legal advisors is not immune from libel and will certainly be seen by the family. Because of this, it is wise to discuss the contents of such a report with the adolescent and his parents before it is completed. Once again, it is wise to be discreet about confidential information unless this is central.

Avoid protracted discussion of the offence in the report unless it is highly relevant to psychiatric status. Guidance on the content of reports for criminal courts is provided in Bebbington & Hill (1985).

Reports in compensation claims

Psychiatric opinion may be requested when brain injury or psychological harm is thought to have been caused by someone other than the affected adolescent. Assessment in such cases is difficult because of the vested interest of the adolescent and his or her family. It is important to find ways of checking allegations of altered behaviour or loss of skills and to be cautious about estimating the degree of suffering. Reports from sources outside the family of the adolescent's status before and after the incident are vital. The issue is discussed in the book by the Royal College of Psychiatrists (1988).

Delays in such cases must be avoided because of the risk of enhancing compensation "neurosis" and both family and legal advisors should be urged to press for early settlement in order to avoid the enquiry causing more psychological invalidism than was originally present.

Reports in cases of sexual abuse

Sexual abuse within the family is not infrequently directed at an adolescent girl. Many such cases will need to come to court and the necessary involvement of the police and social services means that the victim is at risk of having to undergo multiple interviews by various persons. Guidance as to the veracity of claims by an apparently abused adolescent is discussed by Bentovim (1987), Green (1986) and Topper & Aldridge (1981). In crude summary, this amounts to assuming the claim is true when there is substantial detail in a spontaneous, consistent account, strong affect is expressed at disclosure, corroboration by witnesses, physical findings, or other suggestive evidence such as hypersexualisation, unusual behaviour by the perpetrator and altered roles and boundaries in the family system of relationships (see Ch. 4).

A combination of individual, marital and family interviews will be needed; care must be taken that all of this does not constitute further abuse and cause avoidable suffering. It is good practice to maintain continuity of interviewer between interviews, and between assessment and any required treatment. Although it is often assumed that abused girls should be interviewed by a female professional, the gender of the interviewer should not take precedence over competence. In the instance of a girl abused by a father (or father substitute), a preliminary interview with both girl and mother allows the latter to give sanction for the girl to disclose family events to a stranger. The limits of confidentiality and the purpose of each interview need open explanation.

Within the interview, several issues need to be addressed. In addition to an account of the abuse, it will be necessary to assess the degree of coercion involved, the presence of psychiatric symptomatology, the girl's feelings towards her abuser and the capacity of the girl to use an interview setting therapeutically.

Formulation

A statement about the elements which combine to cause a particular psychiatric problem: gives them relative weight, and includes information about treatment and prognosis will carry more information about the case than diagnostic label alone. There is ambiguity about the term "formulation" and its content will vary according to whether it is used in the context of a professional examination or a working clinic. In the latter setting, the subject is well discussed by Steinberg (1983). A minimal framework should include:

1. A statement of the problem including the source of referral, e.g.

A 16-year-old girl, the elder of two sisters living at home, referred by her general practitioner because of a two-month history of apparent unhappiness coupled with a decline in her schoolwork and a withdrawal from social activities.

2. Findings on assessment, e.g.

Depressed mood with irritability, inappropriate feelings of guilt, occasional suicidal ideation, self-reproach and reported poor concentration. Above-average intelligence and normal physical health.

3. Significant aetiological factors. These can conveniently be entered into a grid with a + or − added to indicate strengths and adversities accordingly; for example:

	Individual	Family	Social
Predisposing	good previous personality +	good family relationships + family history of depression −	
Precipitating	error in exam resulting in a failed subject − (acute onset) +		
Perpetuating		somewhat dismissive attitude of father − effortless academic success of sister −	social withdrawal

4. Management plan, e.g.

She should be given lofepramine 70 mg at night for three days followed by 70 mg twice daily for a further four weeks. She and her parents will be seen by me at weekly intervals to monitor her clinical response and offer supportive counselling. Her school must be contacted and in the meantime she should attend there. Admission to hospital is not required at present but will need continual review. A total appraisal must take place in six weeks' time.

5. Prognosis, e.g.

Bearing in mind her excellent previous personality, good family relationships, clear precipitant, and moderate severity of her condition, the response to treatment should be good.

REFERENCES

Bebbington P E, Hill P D 1985 Manual of Practical Psychiatry. Blackwell Scientific, Oxford

Bentovim A 1987 The diagnosis of child sexual abuse. Bulletin of the Royal College of Psychiatrists 11: 295–299

Cox A, Rutter M 1985 Diagnostic appraisal and interviewing In: Rutter M, Hersov L (eds) Child and Adolescent Psychiatry: Modern Approaches. Blackwell Scientific, Oxford

Dare C, Lindsey C 1979 Children in family therapy. Journal of Family Therapy 1: 253–270

Gorell Barnes G 1982 Initial work with the family. In: Bentovim A, Gorell
Barnes G, Cooklin A (eds) Family Therapy. Vol. I. Academic Press,
London

Green A H 1986 True and false allegations of sexual abuse in child custody
disputes. Journal of the American Academy of Child and Adolescent
Psychiatry, 25, 449–456

Haley J 1976 Conducting the first interview. In: Haley J (ed) Problem-Solving
Therapy. Jossey Bass, San Francisco.

Heller K 1968 Ambiguity in the interview interaction. In: Schlien J M (ed)
Research in Psychotherapy. III. American Psychological Association,
Washington D C

Hill P 1985 The diagnostic interview with the individual child. In: Rutter M,
Hersov L (eds) Child and Adolescent Psychiatry: Modern Approaches. 2nd
edn. Blackwell Scientific, Oxford

Royal College of Psychiatrists 1988 Child Psychiatry and the Law (In Press)

Shapiro M B 1979 Assessment interviewing in clinical psychology. British
Journal of Social and Clinical Psychology 18: 211–218

Steinberg D 1983 The Clinical Psychiatry of Adolescence. John Wiley,
Chichester

Steinberg D, Galhenage D, Robinson S 1981 Two years' referrals to a regional
adolescent unit: some implications for psychiatric services. Social Science
and Medicine 15: 113–12

Topper A B, Aldridge D J 1981 Incest: Intake and investigation. In: Mrazek
P B, Kempe C H (eds) Sexually Abused Children and their Families.
Pergamon, Oxford

Will D, Wrate R M 1985 Integrated Family Therapy. Tavistock, London

3

Developmental perspectives

Development in adolescence

The psychiatrist who treats adolescents must take into account the fact that they are going through a phase of rapid biological and psychosocial development. It is impossible to formulate and treat the adolescent's psychiatric disorder without reference to the state and manner of his or her maturational progress.

Adolescence is the developmental stage between childhood and maturity. Both anchor points are somewhat ill-defined. If the onset of puberty is taken as indicating the end of childhood proper, then most girls in the United Kingdom would no longer be children by the age of 11. Since other aspects of their development indicate a state of continuing dependency and immaturity, most people would regard them as children for a year or two more and suggest a marker such as menarche as indicating the abandonment of childhood at an average age of 13 for girls. Boys enter puberty some eighteen months later than girls but the fact that their first ejaculation is most likely to occur at the age of 13 enables a general consensus to be reached that the start of the teenage years can be taken as the onset of adolescence for many purposes. This is, of course, only a convention.

The definition of maturity poses more problems. There is no single age at which maturity is achieved. Table 3.1 lists various indices of responsibility; the fact that they are spread over a wide age-span suggests that there is an idea of relativity about legal maturity: it is defined according to the task or responsibility in question. For most purposes, the age of 18 is taken as indicating legal maturity as far as most basic adult social responsibilities are concerned. Entry into adult life in legal terms is, however, by no

Table 3.1 Legal ages of responsibility

Age	Entitlement or liability
7	Can operate post office savings account
10	Responsible for own criminal actions (if it can be shown that the child knew that what he was doing was wrong)
13	Entitled to hold a week-end job
14	Full responsibility for criminal actions
16	Can now: leave school and work full-time consent to sexual intercourse (girls) buy cigarettes and drink certain alcoholic drinks so long as they are taken with a meal consent to medical treatment hold a motorcycle licence join the armed forces (boys)
17	Can drive a car Girls can join the armed forces
18	Adult status for many legal purposes: voting jury service financial autonomy (cheques, credit cards, mortgage, hire purchase) buying and drinking alcohol in a pub betting in a betting shop can no longer be made a ward of court, adopted or taken into local authority care
21	Can: adopt a child stand in local and general elections engage in male homosexual activity hold HGV and PSV driving licences

means the end of personal maturation. What constitutes psychosocial maturity is a major question but may be answered in part by suggesting a list of indices (Table 3.2).

The conclusion must be that maturity in its fullest sense is not achieved until well into what is conventionally regarded as adult life; for many people it will not be realized until their fourth or fifth decade (if then). Once again, this goes beyond a consensus lay view as to when adolescence might end, whatever truth it might hold in developmental terms.

For clinical administrative purposes in the United Kingdom, most adolescent in-patient units admit boys and girls aged from 13 to 15 inclusive. The reason for an upper age limit of 16 is because this is the minimum age at which pupils are allowed to

Table 3.2 Indices of full maturity

Physical
  Cessation of physical growth
  Acquisition of reproductive capacity

Emotional
  Acceptance of ambivalence, frustration, and the ability to postpone gratification
  Minimal dependency needs
  Ability to give and receive affection without fear for own integrity; a capacity for selfless caring
  Capacity to control impulses and cravings without necessity for constant "patrolling" of one's own defences
  Ability to enjoy without guilt
  Even-temperedness and serenity; minimal resentment
  A gradation of intensity in relationships

Social
  Ability to be alone.
  Autonomy, self-determination, capacity for measured assertion
  Material independence
  A high priority for human relationships
  At ease with one's social identity and roles
  Accurate empathy and appreciation of the needs of others
  Freedom from pretence

Intellectual
  Capacity for abstract thought and hypothetical planning
  A sense of humour
  A depth of perspective which indicates "wisdom"
  Increasing generality and diminishing specificity in reasoning

Spiritual and moral
  Rational and consistent personal standards, not merely passively absorbed
  Consciousness of own mortality without panic
  Understanding of the point of view of others without having to adopt it
  Awareness of one's capacity for initiative and choice
  Capacity for continued adaptation

leave school. In-patients below this age will require schooling whilst in hospital and most units have schools attached. A split within a unit between those patients who are obliged to attend school and those for whom it is no longer obligatory is potentially destructive to a therapeutic milieu. Furthermore, most psychiatrists concerned with adolescents in the United Kingdom work within the framework of child psychiatry services which are organized and funded on the premise that they deal with school-age children. One result of this is that 16- to 18-year-olds fall uneasily between the child and adult psychiatric services, often to their own clinical detriment.

There is thus a disparity between socio-legal, developmental and administrative definitions of adolescence. For the sake of clarity, it seems reasonable to assume that adolescence occupies the years between the thirteenth and eighteenth birthdays.

In order to practise adequate psychiatry in the service of adolescent patients it is essential to understand normal physical and psychosocial development. For the sake of clarity, physical, cognitive, social and emotional aspects are here treated separately; yet it is important to recognize that these strands of development interact and that there is substantial difference between the sexes in both pace and content of maturation.

Physical growth

Some aspects of puberty appear to be triggered by the body's own growth. At a critical weight of about 48 kg (47.8 + 4.6 kg in Frisch & Revelle's 1970 study) menstrual cycles are established and menarche occurs in girls. If their weight subsequently falls back below this threshold, menstrual cycles are arrested. A related and probably more fundamental critical threshold for menarche is when body fat is 22% of total body weight (Frisch & McArthur 1974). It is well known that over the last 150 years menarche has occurred progressively earlier in the teens and it seems likely that this reflects improvement in the standards of nutrition which will affect both variables.

Menarche is preceded by two or more years of observable sexual development. The first sign of puberty in girls is the bud stage of breast development at about the age of 11. This is followed rapidly by the pubertal growth spurt and the appearance of pubic hair. Indeed, either of these developmental changes will sometimes precede breast development. The peak of the female pubertal growth spurt is at an average age of 12 so that at this age, girls are typically taller than boys.

In boys, the first sign of puberty is enlargement of the testes at an average age of $11\frac{1}{2}$, in other words six months later than girls. The pace of puberty is slower in boys, with pubic hair appearing about 6 months after initial testicular growth (i.e. age 12) and the growth spurt beginning at an average age of 13 and peaking at 14, two years later than in girls.

An absence of any signs of puberty by the age of 14 in either sex is abnormal and warrants investigation (Brook 1985).

Such changes are themselves the result of qualitative changes in endocrine activity. The negative feedback of oestrogens and testosterone on the hypothalamus which is evident during childhood is reduced, allowing hypothalamic releasing factors to increase the secretion of gonadotrophins by the anterior pituitary.

The rate of growth during the pubertal growth spurt is roughly double the rate during childhood and at the peak of this spurt (age 12 for girls, 14 for boys) an annual increase in height of 8 cm is to be expected. During the early phase, hands and feet grow rapidly in size and this may represent a source of embarrassment to the youngster. Linear growth slows to a virtual standstill by the age of 16 for girls, 18 for boys.

Differences exist between the sexes with respect to growth at puberty. Girls start earlier, and finish earlier than boys. Their peak velocity of growth is less than that in the male. They demonstrate a marked spurt in hip widening and do not lose fat as boys do. Boys show particular increases in shoulder width, muscle bulk and strength. Enlargement of the male larynx causes breaking of the voice. By the end of puberty, boys are, on average, taller, stronger and more able to sustain strenuous exercise than girls.

Such changes in the rate and pattern of growth are accompanied by the development of primary and secondary sexual characteristics. Although there is substantial variation between individuals as to the age at which such developments occur, the sequence of events is constant and can be staged according to Tanner's (1962) scheme illustrated in Table 3.3. In both sexes, pubic hair appears early but full reproductive competence is achieved comparatively late; the initial menstrual cycles of girls are anovulatory and the first ejaculations of boys do not contain viable sperm.

The increase in circulating androgens, oestrogens and progesterone of both gonadal and adrenal origin is associated with an increase in sexual behaviour. The evidence is less complete than one would like but suggests quite strongly that androgens make an important contribution to the generation of sexual drive in both sexes. It would be wrong to suppose that libido depends solely upon androgens; it does not, and the differences between individuals with respect to sexual drive cannot be reduced to a comparison of circulating testosterone levels. What can be asserted with confidence is that the rise in androgen production

21

Table 3.3 Stages of puberty (Tanner 1962)

Girls: breast development

B1	Prepubertal: elevation of papilla only
B2	Bud stage: slight elevation of breast and papilla
B3	Small pubescent breast, areola within breast contour
B4	Areola and papilla project above breast contour
B5	Mature breast: areola recedes leaving only papilla projecting

Both sexes: pubic hair

P1	None
P2	Sparse, slightly pigmented downy hair along labia or at base of penis
P3	Darker, coarser, curly hair spreading sparsely over pubic symphysis
P4	Hair adult in type but smaller in area, not spreading onto thighs
P5	Adult quantity with spread to medial side of thighs

Boys: genital development

G1	Prepubertal: genitals same size and general proportions as in childhood
G2	Enlargement of testes with reddening of scrotum
G3	Lengthening of penis, further growth of testes
G4	Penis thickens and glans enlarges, scrotum darkens
G5	Adult form and dimensions

at puberty accounts for the enormous increase in sexual awareness and interest which is such an obvious feature of adolescence.

Although animal studies demonstrate that androgens increase assertive behaviour in both sexes, there is rather little evidence to support such a conclusion for human adolescents. It seems highly likely that prenatal endocrine influences shape certain social behaviours (see Rutter 1979) but evidence for an effect on non-sexual social behaviour during adolescence is sparse. For instance, a study of male criminals by Kreuz & Rose (1972) suggested that violent crime in adolescence was associated with a higher testosterone level than was non-violent crime though the levels of testosterone among their total sample of young adult prisoners were not obviously abnormal compared with a rather ill-chosen control group (army volunteers). Certainly there appeared to be non-criminal individuals in the study with testosterone levels just as high as those of prisoners with convictions for violence in adolescence; any link between violence and testosterone cannot be straightforward.

High levels of circulating androgen promote sebaceous gland activity in the skin and acne is likely to ensue in the majority of both boys and girls during the mid-teens. As is generally appreciated, this can cause affected teenagers considerable apprehension about their own sexual attractiveness.

Social demands

Society has expectations of adolescents. They are expected to seek increasing independence from their families of origin in financial, instrumental and emotional terms. During their middle or late teens they are obliged to leave school, a process that may be synchronised with national examinations. It is generally anticipated that they will seek social recreation within their own peer group. In particular, they are expected to discover heterosexual friendships and experiences. Linked with this is a general anticipation that they will take an interest in their own appearance and dress.

Certain constraints apply. Thresholds for various activities are set by law (Table 3.1). Outrageousness in dress, speech or sexual behaviour is condemned, albeit in a somewhat ambivalent way as though society relishes a certain challenge to its own conformity.

Not all pressures are channelled through family, school and the law. The spending power of the employed teenager is courted by manufacturers of cosmetics, electrical toys and entertainments. In their advertisements they generate more than a desire to buy a particular product; by suggesting that its possession will result in instant popularity they imply that it is also desirable to be popular. A commercial for a cosmetic defines current tastes in facial beauty and makes the implication that having an attractive face is important for social success.

Some social expectations are likely to be in line with the aspirations of the teenagers themselves. Many adolescents find themselves in conflict with their families or wider society because they want greater independence for themselves. Their problem is not that their wish conflicts with the expectations of others, rather that they want it too soon or that they demand autonomy in one area whilst remaining dependent in another. The conflict is over rate and consistency, not the ultimate purpose. It is well known that acquiring independence is not a simple linear, incremental progression but includes a tidal process of ebb and flow with advances being followed by regression if new autonomy results in anticipatory anxiety or actual failure in some independent endeavour. Nor is autonomy a unitary entity: independence in one field of life (such as living away from family of origin) does not necessarily predict self-sufficiency in another (such as handling personal finances).

The moves away from family into peer group and from school into work increase the number of social roles occupied by the adolescent. Before puberty, a girl may be the eldest daughter, favoured niece, the pupil with the neatest writing in the class, and big sister to her brother. By her late teens, the same girl may have become someone's lover, someone else's ex-girlfriend, supervisor at work, apple of her boss's eye, the one who can't quite get her clothes looking right, a confidante for the new girl in accounts, life and soul of the office party and the one who always clears up afterwards. Roles are likely to have changed at home too. She may now be the authority on wine bars, mother's companion on shopping trips, the one who always blurts out the truth in family discussions and a better cook than her mother.

It may be difficult for the individual teenager to judge what the exact social expectation of any role or attribute is. Pressure (particularly commercial pressure) to make oneself heterosexually attractive is accompanied by a legal prohibition on sexual intercourse below the age of sixteen, and a measure of moral disapproval even after that threshold is crossed. Having spent the school years within a group of friends most of whom would have been the same age, a move to work or social activities wherein colleagues or associates may be the same age as parents or grandparents can expose the older adolescent to a wide range of attitudes, behaviour or beliefs, particularly those of earlier generations.

As well as a general view as to how personal development should proceed during adolescence, there are stereotypes of adolescents. They are commonly assumed to be rebellious, oppositional, hedonistic and difficult, superficial and fickle in their interests, and estranged from their parents' generation. Every now and then one sees an adolescent in clinical practice who is behaving abominably in a conscious effort to live up to such an image.

Cognitive development

The style of thinking in middle childhood is characteristically bound to the specific and particular; it is concrete. This is adequate for considering the world as it exists in the present but insufficient for making flexible plans for the future. For a child whose care is in the hands of adults, this is no problem, but the ability to weigh and compare alternative future solutions to a problem is of considerable survival value for an adolescent who is increasingly becoming independent of adult care.

In Piaget's terminology, this ability to sift options and speculate about possibilities is a feature of the stage of formal operations (Inhelder & Piaget 1958). This follows the stage of concrete operations which is generally held to occupy the years 7–11 and in which the relationships between things and the properties of objects are the crucial elements of thought. Formal operational thought, according to Piaget, is the crucial feature of cognitive development in adolescence. His theory is by far the most refined and penetrating description of adolescent thought though it is not beyond criticism.

Formal operational thought consists of several components:

1. Single abstractions

The capacity to form an idea about an intangible characteristic or a concept: justice, responsibility, socialism etc. A plurality of concrete instances can be simultaneously considered and an abstraction grasped. With this skill, political thought, reflections upon human relationships, and personal identity can be accommodated within thought. Before the age of about 12, the concept of law can only be considered by referring to specific offences and particular punishments. By 16 or so, the purpose of law can be discussed in terms of "freedom", "standards of conduct" and so on without reference to any concrete examples (Adelson et al 1969).

2. Hypothetico-deductive thinking

The power to set up competing hypotheses with which to explain events enables the solution of problems in imagination without recourse to the actual situation in which the problem was manifest. This facilitates thinking about reasons for events or phenomena by weighing alternative solutions. It uses logic to process ideas; the idea takes precedence over the concrete instance.

3. Reflective (recursive) thinking

The ability to think about one's own thought processes and

evaluate them. By such means, the strength and weakness of different viewpoints can be considered: the adolescent can strike mutually contradictory stances and examine each, he can speak in a debate on either side if forced to and propose an argument to support either side.

4. Interpropositional logic

Although the child can test the truth of a single proposition, the teenager becomes able to test the logic that links propositions. Statements prefaced by "if" can be manipulated irrespective of their content by a teenager whereas the child is sidetracked by whether a proposition is true in the first place: if it is unlikely, he cannot think about it further. Thus Osherson & Markman (1975) showed their experimental subjects a blue chip before hiding it and then asked them to consider whether a statement such as "Either the chip is green or it is not green" could be true. Children were not able to reason the logic of such a statement since they could not move beyond the evidence of their own eyes: the chip was blue and they could not say whether the statement was true or false. Adolescents and adults could make judgements on the truth of the statement irrespective of concrete evidence, they could detach logic from the specifics of the situation.

5. Systematic manipulation of interacting abstract variables

The ability to construct a complete political ideology or understand fully a complex theory such as neo-Darwinism involves comprehending the laws of interaction between abstractions and a mental facility which can examine their interplay. Few adolescents attain such an intellectual level.

These skills enable adolescents to argue with adults on their own terms, recognising the principles behind laws and rules, moving beyond child-like acceptance of fairness or authority as a justification for an action to an understanding of ethics, an appreciation of the motives and perceptions of others and a composite view of a self defined in relations with others. Formal operational thought enables idealism and philosophical thought; the more articulate and intelligent teenagers rehearse such abilities in writing or discussion. It allows reflection on ideas about the world, the self, the purpose of things. As a newly acquired skill it is rehearsed exploratively and can thus lead to fierce degrees of existential doubt, to political questioning, to moralising and to endless argument with parents and teachers.

From a clinical standpoint, it facilitates verbal interviewing since adolescent and adult now share a common mode of thinking to underpin their mutual discussion. Generalisations, concepts, hypotheses about the future, patterns of behaviour, styles of relating and so forth can be brought into a conversation without the dependence upon the concrete and specific which is characteristic of child-like thought.

What infuriates families is the way in which a young adolescent can use his new-found capacity for intellectual reasoning to question rules or standards of conduct by appealing to general ethical principles and by so doing generate a fierce argument. Characteristically, as soon as recriminations arise and the atmosphere sours, emotions are aroused and the adolescent regresses defensively into concrete operational thought and a return to specifics, just as the parents are warming to the argument in formal operational mode. This sequence can easily enter a cycle, with the adolescent returning to the attack having drawn breath whilst in the familiar mental territory of concrete operational thought, and feeling able to return to formal operational mode. Meanwhile the parents have stepped down their intellectual thought patterns to take into account the more child-like arguments now being put and find themselves flat-footed by their adolescent child's return to more abstract reasoning.

By no means all individuals attain formal operational thought. In laboratory experiments (which typically examine only one aspect of formal operations), only about half or fewer of those adolescents studied can solve problems that require it (Connell et al 1975, Dale 1970, Jackson 1965). In one large study Shayer et al (1976) demonstrated that less than one-third of mid-adolescents were at the level of early formal operational thought and only one-tenth were capable of advanced formal thinking. Nor is this only a matter of chronological age since only just over half of Towler & Wheatley's (1971) college students could demonstrate that they understood conservation of volume and only half of Tomlinson-Keasey's (1972) middle-aged women had reached the first stages of formal operational thought with less than one-fifth at an advanced level. Nevertheless, the capacity for advanced thought does increase with age with most people achieving their ultimate level of functioning at about 25 (Fischer et al 1983).

Neimark (1975) in a detailed review of intellectual development in adolescence points out the general poverty of knowledge in this area. What influences the acquisition of formal operational thought is largely unknown. Overall intelligence seems to have to reach a particular threshold level and may partially compensate for lack of experience. The extent to which formal education can stimulate intellectual development is speculative and findings on the impact of individual personality variables such as reflectiveness/impulsivity (Cloutier & Goldschmid 1976, Neimark 1975) appear to be contradictory. Nor is it known how adolescent thought might differ from the thought of adults. It seems at least possible that the obvious self-centredness of much adolescent behaviour and the familiar tendency to regard adult intervention as part of a conspiracy of constraint indicate that there is a disparity between what the adolescent might be capable of in terms of reasoning and what ordinarily happens in everyday thinking. Conceivably it is the effect of practice and experience that enables the adult to rise above such egocentric attitudes and, in similar vein, to temper idealism with pragmatism.

One attempt to deal with the phenomenon of adolescent egocentrism is the contribution of Elkind (1978). His argument is that formal operational thought allows the adolescent to think about how other people think but in its early stages this leads to the adolescent confusing his own thoughts and those of others; his own preoccupations are also attributed to others. Certainly, whilst capable of single abstractions or comparing competing alternative abstract hypotheses, even older adolescents have difficulty with constructing a full system of abstractions (Richards & Commons 1983) although this is what is required in order to place a concept of oneself in a social field. This limitation can lead to the adolescent imagining that others take him as seriously as he does, and his creation of an "imaginary audience" which observes him according to his own preoccupations (such as physical appearance), applauding or decrying him as he does himself. In a related discussion, Elkind suggests that adolescents are also prone to see themselves as extremely special, any uncertainty about their own developing identity or competence fuelling a self-preoccupation intensified by their capacity for reflective conceptual thought to the point where they create an explanatory "personal fable" for themselves. The introspective individual sees his feelings, ideas and perceptions as verging on the unique and may stray into fantasies of omnipotence. This interacts with the naïve idealism characteristic of mid-adolescence which may also result from over-simplified abstractions. Studies of political idealism in adolescence (Adelson 1975) give a clue as to how egocentrism is abandoned. It seems likely that peer contact and discussion moderates extreme positions (Youniss 1982) and increasing cognitive sophistication and self-confidence allows the capacity for compromise and reformulation of ideas without feeling threatened by loss of face.

Language development

The cognitive developments described above allow adolescents to use language more subtly. This is particularly obvious with respect to what psycholinguistics terms "pragmatics": the ability to use language in social contexts. By taking the entire situation into account, meaning can be conveyed by fewer words or different inflections. Hints can be dropped, oblique questions asked in order to camouflage the real purpose behind an enquiry, badinage distinguished from determined insult. *Double entendre*, irony, parody and sarcasm can be used and understood. Teenage humour relies heavily on such figures of speech and the way in which they can illustrate incongruity. Not that all this is accomplished overnight. In developmental terms, understanding precedes expression and it is easy to underestimate the sophistication of a teenager's language by relying only on his use of speech.

In parallel with speech, writing becomes more elegant and structured. The capacity to advance an argument in writing and to structure an essay is acquired by many and the perspective of a potential reader can be grasped. Obviously the extent to which such skills are developed is a function of the interaction between education, experience and native wit.

Aspects of development discussed elsewhere

Moral and sexual development during adolescence are described in Chapters 8 and 13 respectively. The impact of adolescence upon the family is discussed in Chapter 4 and the process of socialisation mentioned in Chapter 8. Interpersonal development is mentioned in Chapter 7.

The process of psychosocial development

Development is more than growth; the term carries an implication that there is an increase in complexity which can include qualitative changes that are more than quantitative accretion. In general terms, theories of development are better at describing developmental change than in explaining how it happens. With respect to adolescence, there are partial explanations for how changes occur but an equal number of unknowns, too.

Puberty as a physical process seems to be triggered by aspects of physical growth such as weight or fat mass (see above, p. 20). These factors are themselves influenced, within limits, by environmental elements such as available nutrition. The physical changes resulting include both quantitative aspects (such as linear growth) and qualitative innovations (sexual fertility), the latter representing a discontinuity in the train of development since features appear that were not previously present.

To what extent the psychosocial changes which are components of adolescence are a direct result of physical changes is unclear. It is unlikely that a direct causal mechanism operates since children with precocious puberty are not small adolescents in anything but physical terms; psychologically they are children. It seems more likely that the physical changes of puberty interact with the expectations held by the adolescent, his family, school, employer, friends and society generally about what is appropriate behaviour and standards for a teenager and ultimately an adult.

The outward physical changes of puberty can affect the adolescent by demanding that he or she adjust to them as well as to the differing attitudes of those around him or her. The girl becomes a young woman and elicits sexually-tinged responses from the men around her. Thus she has to adapt both to her own bodily changes (of which she may approve or feel disappointed, ashamed or awkward) which are happening outwith her own control, as well as to the way in which she is for the first time, for example, courted and pursued by teenage boys when on a family beach holiday and realises that she is sexually attractive to men.

Boys may be affected not just by the physical changes in terms of the form they take and the altered expectations of others which ensue but also by their timing. Once again, there is an interaction between physical changes and social responses. Early entry into puberty is associated with popularity in the peer group, late maturation with teasing and rejection (Clausen 1975). This may reflect other influences such as the overall association between low intelligence and delayed puberty but it seems likely that a major explanatory factor is that pubertal muscularity breeds success at sporting activities. Furthermore, pubertal boys are remarkably intolerant of difference from arbitrary group norms and will persecute the fat, the foreign and the feeble. To a certain extent this reflects their own anxieties at being acceptable or physically entire. Girls are apparently much less affected by the timing of pubertal changes though some nervousness about eventual adult height is not uncommon at the time of the growth spurt.

How far endocrine changes at puberty affect behaviour and emotions is obscure. The tenuous evidence suggesting that androgens support but do not completely account for libido and aggressive behaviour has been referred to above (p. 22). Whether oestrogen/progesterone cycles can be implicated in any explanation as to why depression becomes a more frequent clinical problem in adolescence than in childhood is still controversial, with an absence of unequivocal evidence either way.

Precisely how the cognitive stage of formal operations is entered is unknown. To a certain extent it depends upon general intelligence but whether physical changes in the brain such as the rapid spurts in brain growth which typically occur at ages 10–12 and 14–16 are relevant is unresolved. Earlier claims by Epstein (1974, 1980) that biological changes in the rate of brain growth and EEG wave pattern correlate with entry to the stage of formal operational thought have not been well substantiated.

For much psychosocial development in adolescence, a task-mastery model is useful. The changes which occur in the adolescent's body and thought are paralleled by the social demands mentioned above and represent challenges which have to be met by the adolescent who has to adjust, cope, learn and accommodate. In doing so, new patterns of adjustment, new behaviours and fresh attitudes appear. Mastery of such developmental hurdles may be creative, maladaptive or sterile. It may

31

have clinically relevant consequences in terms of emotions, self-image or behaviour.

Table 3.4 sets out a summary of the developmental challenges to be faced during adolescence. A few are timed by chronological age or physical development but otherwise there is rather little to determine in which order they arise or what a particular adolescent may be preoccupied with at any particular age. Coleman's (e.g. 1980) focal theory of adolescent development referred to below (p. 37) suggests that certain issues are likely to arise at particular ages but any one issue may not be a particularly crucial concern for a given individual of that age; other variables such as family support or previous experience combine to accentuate or defuse it.

Table 3.4 Maturational tasks of adolescence

Tasks set by biological maturation

Accommodating to linear growth which shapes the expectations of others (e.g. by being thought to be older or younger than actual chronological age)
Accommodating to changes in body shape
Coping with libido and fertility without precipitating pregnancy
Feeling comfortable with physical appearance and attractiveness (including acne)
Managing powerful emotions such as crushes and falling in love
Developing the capacity for abstract conceptual thought

Tasks set by the drive for independence (the origins of which are to be found in the adolescent, the family and social expectations generally)

Increasing independence from parents in terms of money, dress, self-care, and leisure activities
Increasingly individual moral standards
Self-sufficiency in dealing with practical and emotional difficulties
Retaining links with parents whilst becoming a more separate person: balancing the demands of peer group standards against parental constraints

Tasks set by general expectations

Taking (or not taking) examinations; making a career choice
Leaving school and starting work (or not being able to work if in an area of high unemployment); developing a work identity
Conforming to fashions established by friends or the mass media
Acquiring new skills or liberties related to age thresholds (driving, legal sex, legal drinking)
Having heterosexual relationships: boy- and girl-friends
Managing opportunities for intoxication and dangerous excitement without harm
Preserving satisfactory status in the peer group
Maintaining and developing a stable and secure personal identity
Balancing self-preoccupation and self-sacrifice

Personal identity

For those who espouse earlier developmental theories identity is the prime concern of adolescence. Given all the changes and demands cited above, it is easy to see why. In Erikson's scheme of psychological development (see Fig. 3.1) the developmental task of adolescence is to achieve and maintain a sense of inner sameness and continuity which is personal, unique and consistent. Failure in this task results in role diffusion (sometimes also termed role confusion). In Erikson's (1965) words, such adolescents "temporarily overidentify, to the point of apparent complete loss of identity, with the heroes of cliques and crowds." Otherwise put, a sense of being unique and worthwhile with a recognisable individuality and personality may be difficult to achieve or retain. For some adolescents, such a sense of self may only be obtainable by sacrificing their own individuality in adopting the characteristics of a charismatic other or by joining a group who share a mode of dress or style which enables its members to see themselves in each other, using each other as mirrors.

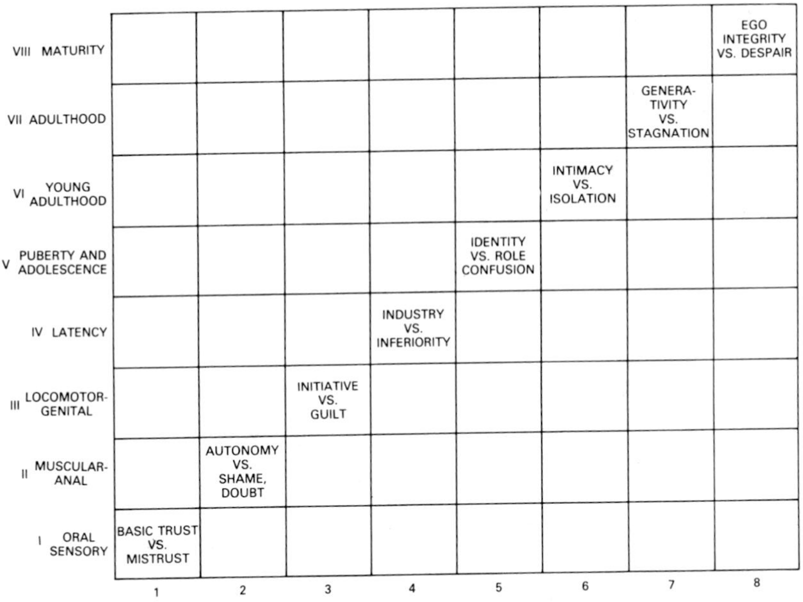

	1	2	3	4	5	6	7	8
VIII MATURITY								EGO INTEGRITY VS. DESPAIR
VII ADULTHOOD							GENERA-TIVITY VS. STAGNATION	
VI YOUNG ADULTHOOD						INTIMACY VS. ISOLATION		
V PUBERTY AND ADOLESCENCE					IDENTITY VS. ROLE CONFUSION			
IV LATENCY				INDUSTRY VS. INFERIORITY				
III LOCOMOTOR-GENITAL			INITIATIVE VS. GUILT					
II MUSCULAR-ANAL		AUTONOMY VS. SHAME, DOUBT						
I ORAL SENSORY	BASIC TRUST VS. MISTRUST							

Fig. 3.1 Erikson's model of human development: "Eight Ages of Man" (Erikson 1965)

Undoubtedly there are some adolescents who feel this putative crisis of identity acutely. Blos (1967) quotes a patient as saying:

> If you act in opposition to what is expected, you bump right and left into regulations and rules. Today when I ignored school — just didn't go — it made me feel very good. It gave me a sense of being a person, not just an automaton. If you continue to rebel and bump into the the world around you often enough, then an outline of yourself gets drawn in your mind. You need that. Maybe when you know who you are you don't have to be different from those who know or think they know who you should be.

The patient was a patient, of course. Various studies of normal teenagers indicate that it is not likely that such a way of going about things is universal among adolescents even if the notion of an "identity crisis" is part of the celebration of adolescence by the psychologically minded.

Engel (1959) carried out a Q-sort test to assess the self-concept of 13- to 15-year-old boys, followed up the sample and repeated the assessment two years later. The correlation between the two results was high, implying that most of the boys maintained a stable concept of themselves. A minority did alter their view of themselves and these were likely to have had a negative self-concept at the outset and a high score on indices of maladjustment. This finding is one of several which suggest that too many of the traditional assumptions about adolescent development derive from observations of patients rather than normal teenagers.

Coleman and his colleagues (1977) examined the relationship between two conceptions which an adolescent might hold about himself — what he is, and what he will become — and found that possession of a negative future self-image was increasingly common in late as opposed to early adolescence though a majority of boys possessed a positive present self-image, throughout the age range.

This kind of approach to self-concept, which assumes that it consists of several dimensions and exhibits various facets, has been best developed by Offer and his associates, particularly through the use of the Offer Self-Image Questionnaire which covers 11 areas to yield a picture of five different "selves" (see Table 3.5). A number of studies, conveniently summarized in Offer et al (1984), demonstrate that normal adolescents are not in the throes of a crisis of personal identity. Such a conclusion supports other studies using different instruments: the develop-

Table 3.5 The Offer Self-Image Questionnaire (Offer et al 1984)

Psychological self
  1. Impulse control
  2. Emotional tone
  3. Body and self-image

Social self
  4. Social relationships
  5. Morals
  9. Vocational and educational goals

Sexual self
  6. Sexual attitudes

Familial self
  7. Family relationships

Coping self
  8. Mastery of external world
10. Psychopathology
11. Superior adjustment

ment of personal identity does not reach crisis proportions in normal adolescence. Certainly adolescents do have doubts and curiosities as to what sort of individual they are or might become but it is not clear from empirical research how much they differ from young adults or those in mid-life in their preoccupation with personal identity. Coarse measures of single aspects of self-image suggest that adolescence itself should not be treated as if it were homogeneous in considerations of self-concept. There is a trend for studies to note that older adolescents (17–18-year-olds) are likely to admit to pessimistic views of their own future (e.g. Coleman et al 1977) whereas it is 12-year-olds who are most prone to low self-esteem and heightened self-consciousness (eg. Simmons et al 1973).

Although there is absolutely no evidence that most adolescents suffer from what Erikson (1968) termed a "normative crisis" in their development of personal identity, there is considerable usefulness in the idea when applied to disturbed adolescents. Young teenagers with low self-esteem or a negative evaluation of themselves are those who are likely to manifest an unstable self-concept in the next few years, and they are also the individuals who are most likely to show "maladjustment" on personality questionnaires (Rosenberg 1965). The personal circumstances most likely to support an adequate sense of self-worth are also those associated with healthy psychological development:

interested and supportive parents with adequate self-esteem who provide clear guidance on expectations of conduct and enforce limits upon unacceptable behaviour whilst tolerating a degree of free individual expression and unconventionality within those limits (Coopersmith 1967, Baumrind 1975).

It is reasonable, therefore to return to Erikson's ideas in order to inform clinical practice with disturbed adolescents so long as it is borne in mind that these ideas should not be taken as indicating that most adolescents suffer from turbulence in forging a concept of their own identity. In Erikson's framework, the establishment of a coherent identity is at the expense of a defeat for the process of identity diffusion. One aspect of this process has already been mentioned above — identification with heroes and groups. His later (1968) analysis of the topic identified four major concepts:

- **Intimacy**. The adolescent avoids commitment and closeness in personal relationships because of a fear of loss of identity. Isolation or reliance upon excessive formality in relationships results.

- **Diffusion of time perspective**. A partial denial of the challenge of growth is associated with an inability to plan ahead and a suspension of awareness of the passage of time.

- **Diffusion of industry**. A difficulty in committing effort to study or work. As a result there may be complaints of difficulty concentrating on a task, or conversely an excess of effort thrown into one activity to the exclusion of all else.

- **Negative identity**. The individual defines himself as the converse of expectations held by others. By sarcastically rejecting their standards and assumptions, the adolescent defines himself as someone different. A tone of hostile disdain is a usual accompaniment. Note that this differs from the idea of negative self-concept mentioned earlier (which means a self-depreciatory stance in self-evaluation).

Testing Erikson's assumptions is not easy as he nowhere defines what degree of identity crisis he considers to be usual. Marcia (1966, 1977) attempted to explore identity development in college students and identified four stages:

—**Identity diffusion**. This is the state of affairs which antedates any identity crisis. The adolescent has not yet committed himself to any system of beliefs or aspirations.

—**Identity foreclosure**. The individual commits himself to a set of values and beliefs but these are derived passively from others.

—**Moratorium**. A state of crisis within which the individual searches and selects alternatives in a quest for identity.

—**Identity achievement**. Following a crisis, resolution has resulted in an ideological and vocational commitment.

Criticism of this work is conveniently summarized by Coleman (1980) who points out that such stages do not necessarily follow in strict sequence and that it may be that adolescents undergo a series of "crises" with one area of life being comparatively stable whilst another is in a state of uncertainty. In this respect, Coleman finds himself in agreement with Matteson (1977): concerns about different issues reach a peak at various different

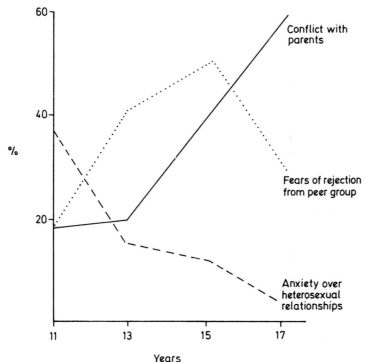

Fig. 3.2 Peak ages for the expression of different themes (from Coleman's 1974 data)

times during adolescence (Fig. 3.2). In Coleman's "focal" theory of adolescent development, particular sorts of relationship patterns and issues come into focus at different ages. Each may or may not be critical for a given individual, may overlap with another issue and need not follow or precede others in a rigid sequence. Most youngsters will find themselves dealing with only one issue at a time, and it is likely (but not inevitable) that others of similar age and sex will also be concerned with it to greater or lesser degree. The march toward maturity does not take place on a broad front with each area of development in step with every other. Empirical support for such a notion is available in Coleman's own work (1974, 1978) and Abramowitz et al (1984).

Coleman's focal theory provides a plausible solution to the puzzle posed by the observation that most teenagers do not seem to suffer from distress provoked by the necessity of maintaining a sense of stable identity whilst negotiating numerous developmental challenges. Rather than being obliged to face a mass onslaught of demands for maturational adaptation it seems that there is breathing space available. Single issues can be dealt with in isolation from others and may not have to be completely mastered before moving on to another challenge.

REFERENCES

Abramowitz R H, Petersen A C, Schulenberg J E 1984 Changes in self-image during early adolescence. In: Offer D, Ostrov E, Howard K I (eds) Patterns of Adolescent Self-image. Jossey-Bass, San Francisco
Adelson J 1975 The development of ideology in adolescence. In: Dragastin S E, Elder G H (eds.) Adolescence in the Life Cycle. Halsted Press, London
Adelson V, Green B, O'Neil R 1969 The growth of the idea of law in adolescence. Developmental Psychology 1: 327–332
Baumrind D 1975 Early socialisation and adolescent competence. In: Dragastin S E. Elder G H (eds.) Adolescence in the Life Cycle. Halsted Press, London
Blos P 1967 The second individuation process of adolescence. Psychoanalytic Study of the Child 22: 162–186
Brook C G D 1985 Management of delayed puberty. British Medical Journal 290: 657–658
Clausen J A 1975 The social meaning of differential physical and sexual maturation. In: Dragastin S E, Elder G H (eds) Adolescence in the Life Cycle: Psychological Change and Social Context. Halsted Press, London
Cloutier R, Goldschmid M 1976 Individual differences in the development of formal reasoning. Child Development 47: 1097–1102
Coleman J C 1974 Relationships in adolescence. Routledge and Kegan Paul, London
Coleman J C 1978 Current contradictions in adolescent theory. Journal of Youth and Adolescence 7: 1–12

Coleman J C 1980 The Nature of Adolescence. Methuen, London

Coleman J C, Herzberg J, Morris M 1977 Identity in adolescence: present and future self concepts. Journal of Youth and Adolescence 6: 63–75.

Connell W F, Stroobant R E, Sinclair K E 1975 Twelve to Twenty: Studies of City Youth. Hicks and Sons, Sydney

Coopersmith S 1967 The Antecedents of Self-Esteem. W H Freeman, San Francisco

Dale L G 1970 The growth of systematic thinking: replication and analysis of Piaget's first chemical experiment. Australian Journal of Psychology 22: 277–286

Elkind D 1978 The Child's Reality: Three Developmental Themes. Lawrence Erlbaum, Hillsdale

Engel M 1959 The stability of self-concept in adolescence. Journal of Abnormal and Social Psychology 58: 211–215

Epstein H T 1974 Phrenoblysis: special brain and mind growth periods. Developmental Psychobiology 7: 217–224

Epstein H T 1980 EEG developmental stages. Developmental Psychobiology 13: 629–631

Erikson E 1965 Childhood and Society. Hogarth Press, London

Erikson E 1968 Identity: Youth and Crisis. Norton, New York

Fischer K W, Hand H H, Russell S 1983 The development of abstractions in adolescence and adulthood. In: Commons M L, Richards F A, Armon C (eds) Beyond Formal Operations: Late Adolescent and Adult Cognitive Development. Praeger, New York

Frisch R E, McArthur J W 1974 Menstrual cycles: features as a determinant of minimum weight for height necessary for their maintenance or onset. Science 185: 949–951

Frisch R E, Revelle R 1970 Height and weight at menarche and a hypothesis of critical body weights and adolescent events. Science 169: 397–398

Inhelder B, Piaget J 1958 The Growth of Logical Thinking. Routledge and Kegan Paul, London

Jackson S 1965 The growth of logical thinking in normal and subnormal children. British Journal of Educational Psychology 35: 255–258

Kreuz L E, Rose R M 1972 Assessment of aggressive behavior and plasma testosterone in a young criminal population. Psychosomatic Medicine 34: 321–332

Marcia J E 1966 Development and validation of ego-identity status. Journal of Personality and Social Psychology 3: 551–558

Marcia J E 1967 Ego identity status: relationships to change in self-esteem, general adjustment and authoritarianism. Journal of Personality 35: 118–133

Matteson D R 1977 Exploration and commitment: sex differences and methodological problems in the use of identity status categories. Journal of Youth and Adolescence 6: 353–374

Neimark E D 1975 Intellectual development during adolescence. In: Horowitz, F. D. (Ed.) Review of Child Development Research, Vol. 4. University of Chicago Press, Chicago

Offer D, Ostrov E, Howard K I 1984 Patterns of Adolescent Self-Image (New Directions for Mental Health Services No. 22). Jossey-Bass, San Francisco

Osherson D N, Markman E 1975 Language and the ability to evaluate contradictions and tautologies. Cognition 3: 213–226

Richards F A, Commons M L 1983 Systematic and metasystematic reasoning: a case for stages of reasoning beyond formal operations. In: Commons M L, Richards F A, Armon C (eds) Beyond Formal Operations: Late Adolescent and Adult Cognitive Development. Praeger, New York

Rosenberg M 1965 Society and the Adolescent Self-Image. Princeton University Press, Princeton

Rutter M 1979 Changing Youth in a Changing Society. Nuffield Provincial Hospitals Trust, London

Shayer M, Kuchemann D E, Wylam H 1976 The distribution of Piagetian stages of thinking in British middle and secondary school children. British Journal of Educational Psychology 46: 164–173

Simmons R, Rosenberg F, Rosenberg M 1973 Disturbance in the self-image at adolescence. American Sociological Review 38: 553–568

Tanner J M 1962 Growth at Adolescence. Blackwell Scientific, Oxford

Tomlinson-Keasey C 1972 Formal operations in females from eleven to fifty-four years of age. Developmental Psychology 6: 364

Towler J O, Wheatley G 1971 Conservation concepts in college students: a replication and critique. Journal of Genetic Psychology 118: 265–270

Youniss J 1982 Parents and Peers in Social Development: A Sullivan-Piaget Perspective. University of Chicago Press, Chicago

4

The families of adolescents

Most adolescents live in families, generally those that they were born into. Nearly one half of all psychiatric disorder in adolescence is a continuation of childhood psychological difficulties (Rutter et al 1976) in the aetiology of which it is recognised that family influences play a large part. It follows that the role of the family in causing or maintaining adolescent psychiatric disorder is likely to be substantial though there is some evidence to suggest that its influence is rather less than with childhood disorder when conditions arising anew in adolescence are considered (Rutter et al 1976).

It pays to consider what type of family contemporary adolescents are likely to live in. Although most essays on the topic of family life and adolescents assume two parents and a single marriage, an increasing minority of teenagers live with single parents, "blended" (or "reconstituted") families resulting from remarriages, and foster families. Considering whether such variant family structures have specific influences upon adolescent development is hard to disentangle from the issue of the impact upon adolescents and children of relevant antecedents such as divorce and its aftermath. For the sake of simplicity it is proposed to assume a conventional two-parent structure (which is the family that most adolescents will grow up in) and take divorce or other causes of family disruption separately.

Family development

The task-mastering approach to individual psychosocial development outlined in Chapter 3 can be applied to family development. The usual model is to consider the tasks set by child-rearing and the maturation of children, particularly the eldest child (Solomon 1973). Thus, by the time the eldest enters puberty, parents, siblings and grandparents will have mastered subsidiary tasks: parents separating from their families of origin and establishing a shared lifestyle with role allocations between themselves, a mutually satisfactory sex life, early parenthood and the demands of dependent babies, dealing with attachment behaviour in the infant and toddler stages, encouraging separation of the child from home at school entry and so forth. There is an epigenetic notion within such a model: unless the tasks set by one stage are met satisfactorily, subsequent tasks cannot be mastered appropriately. For instance, unless separation from early attachment figures is promoted by parents, establishment of the young adolescent into the peer group cannot be accomplished since he will be unable to leave his parents without overwhelming anxiety. If sexual boundaries between the marriage system and the parenting system have not been soundly established and a father sexually abuses his daughter in childhood, then her own adolescent adjustment to sexual maturity will be compromised, with frigidity or promiscuity as likely consequences.

At first sight, the tasks set for the family by the first child entering and passing through adolescence include:

— providing a sense of continuity of identity for the adolescent in spite of imposed physical changes at puberty; maintaining a graded approach to responsibilities and autonomy by avoiding both infantilisation and premature release into adulthood

— reinforcing sexual boundaries within the family system to contain marital sex within the marriage, separate from the activities of sexually maturing adolescent offspring

— adjusting but not abandoning discipline and limit-setting, particularly with respect to aggression, sexual behaviour and risk-taking inside and outside the home; creating a balance between allowing privacy and preserving sufficient supervision.

— providing adequate information about the world outside the home, and what are acceptable standards of behaviour, safety and sex

— teaching social skills such as negotiation and self-presentation

— providing realistic feedback on styles and postures without damaging self-esteem; tolerating experimentation

— letting go and allowing the peer group to set certain (safe) standards and contain friendships beyond the direct scrutiny of parents

— being prepared to rescue disasters

— allowing the older teenager to leave home free of guilt or rancour.

To a large extent, these tasks are the obverse of those faced by the individual adolescent, and one way of summarising the responsibilities of parents in this area is to say that they should support the individual adolescent in his or her mastering of developmental tasks. The qualities required to carry this out do not differ fundamentally from those aspects of good-enough parenting which have been delineated in the rearing of younger children: a warm, child-centred approach which combines common sense and sensitivity to the teenager's viewpoint coupled with democratic (but not permissive) control, and consistency in discipline as well as personal example.

This is not to say that parents can retain their views and methods of child-rearing without attention to the fact that their child is becoming adult. Even when both parents agree about the needs of their adolescent, they may be out of tune with his or her developmental status; a situation commoner in families with a disturbed teenager (Fischer 1980). They may, for example, have difficulty separating their own needs from those of their adolescent child. For many families, adolescence in the children coincides with a mid-life crisis in one or both parents. Fathers are likely to question themselves about their own career since this will have established a particular trajectory and the fulfilment or otherwise of earlier dreams achieved. Mothers, who have probably sacrificed vocational ambition for child-rearing and sought alternative satisfactions in their relationships with their children, become aware that these are soon to leave the nest. With the departure of the youngest child from home, each parent will find themselves alone with the other; not always an encouraging prospect. Freed of child-care burdens, the mother may find herself in a vocational vacuum, yet her attempts to discover worthwhile occupation can produce conflict with her husband who has grown used to her provisions as a homemaker. Both parents will be aware that they are past their conventional physical prime, a realisation heightened by the presence of adolescent youth in the home. Such preoccupations can prejudice the degree with which middle-aged parents can separate their own emotional needs from those of their teenage children and will impair their ability to support them in mastering developmental hurdles.

Control and communication

The two issues of control and communication, often bracketed together, arise frequently in clinical practice with families containing adolescent children. Work on the qualities of parenting by Baumrind (1975) draws an important distinction between "authoritative" and "authoritarian" parenting. Whereas authoritarian parents impose control upon an adolescent by means of forceful measures intended to produce obedience to a set standard of conduct, authoritative parents use rational explanation and allow discussion to encourage autonomy as well as self-disciplined behaviour; however, unlike "permissive" parents who are permissive or even indulgent, they retain final responsibility for their child's activities and retain a veto. In some studies, such a style of parenting is also known as "democratic". In a number of studies of early human development, the combination of attributes which can be termed authoritative will, when combined with adequate parental affection, yield the character traits valued in Western society: independence, friendliness, creativity and assertiveness without hostility. In contrast, authoritarian households will encourage compliance, neatness, conformity and dependency when such a style of parenting is coupled with parental love, but should this be in limited supply, the result is classically the young person who internalises hostility and is excessively anxious or neurotic. Permissive households tend to yield uncontrolled adolescents who, in contrast to those from more controlling homes, often appear to lack purpose and self-direction and may well be drawn into drug and alcohol abuse (Jessor & Jessor 1974), their parents apparently fearful of assuming authority and losing an opportunity to instruct and model responsible behaviour. Such crude generalisations about parenting styles should be treated with some circumspection since they neglect the contribution of the temperament of the child or adolescent. Nevertheless, there is substantial confirmation of the broad thrust of the above associations (Baumrind 1975, Becker 1964).

In any case, given the greater freedom granted to adolescents as opposed to children and the acquisition of formal operational thought (see Ch. 3) with which adolescents can imagine competing alternatives to parental injunctions, their parents will increasingly need to justify themselves rationally to remain in effective control: a considerable communicative task. Parental authority comes to depend upon reason rather than domination, the latter being rejected by teenagers (Pikas 1961). Small wonder that many disturbed adolescents complain that they are not listened to, that people talk at them rather than to them and do not explain themselves, thus seeming unfair and providing a focus for resentment. Clearly communication must be quantitatively sufficient but it becomes difficult to separate out intimacy and empathy from such considerations. For instance, Elder (1963) showed that adolescents were more likely to model themselves on their parents when the latter used reasoned explanations to justify decisions, and extremes of permissiveness or autocracy were found by Middleton & Snell (1963) to equate with a lack of closeness between parent and adolescent with a greater risk of rebellious rejection of parental views.

Parents' memories of their own adolescence are more retrievable and more vivid than those of their childhood. The potential for rivalry ("when I was your age...") and envy of greater recreational opportunities than they enjoyed themselves is therefore that much greater, as is the temptation for parents to obtain satisfaction vicariously through the experiences and achievements of their offspring. Although usually benign, such mechanisms can prove pernicious, particularly when a muddled parent allows or even subtly encourages a teenage son or daughter to run dangerously wild in order to experience imaginatively both the pleasures denied to themselves and the satisfaction of seeing illicit excitements punished; a vicarious enactment of their own psychic struggle between conscience and impulse. In such circumstances it is easy to see how an adolescent can become thoroughly confused as to what it is that parents expect; communication is distorted, there is a lack of clarity.

This aspect of the quality of communication (as opposed to its

45

quantity) is examined in rather a different way by assessing the relative proportions of positive, supportive comments and negative, critical ones. In general, there is an excess of negative communications: harsh, critical, demeaning, in families where there is a disturbed adolescent (West 1981). Naturally, it would be wrong to conclude that this is necessarily causal since it may result from the strain of living with a difficult teenager but there is a little evidence that communication problems can precede the manifestation of disturbance (Goldstein et al 1978). Certainly adolescents themselves contribute actively to displays of negative affect and measures of this are as predictive of outcome as parental contributions are (Asarnow et al 1982). Rather than a linear model of causality, a systems model with continuing interaction and reciprocal modification becomes more useful in understanding the perpetuation or origin of disturbance.

Alienation

Contrary to popular supposition, serious arguments between adolescents and their parents are by no means common. For instance, two-thirds of the adolescents on the Isle of Wight studied by Rutter et al (1976) said that they never disagreed with their parents, and about the same number denied any altercations with them. The parents' accounts parallel these findings: only 18% of parents reported arguments with their adolescent offspring. This does not mean that there were no disagreements between the two generations but the sources of such differences were usually fairly trivial and concerned with such matters as dress or what time young people had to be in by. Communication difficulties as seen from the parents' side were similarly reported only by a minority (24% for boys and 9% for girls) and physical withdrawal by the young teenager (going off to his room, staying out, not doing things with the family) was still more uncommon, being shown by 12% of boys and 9% of girls. Disagreements between sons and mothers tend to precede those between sons and fathers by a few years in adolescence (Steinberg 1981) and the higher rates for boys in this study of 14–15-year-olds probably reflects some of this.

Altercations with parents, communication difficulties with them and physical withdrawal from family life were all commoner among disturbed adolescents in the same study but none of the three variables was present in a majority of such young people.

Ghodsian & Lambert's (1978) report from the National Child Development Study offers general confirmation of such findings with British 16-year-olds, 88% of whom described themselves as getting on well with their mothers and 77% with their fathers. From the viewpoint of their parents, the generally positive view of family relationships is reciprocated and most parents in the study held favourable attitudes to their adolescent children's behaviour and friends (Fogelman 1976).

Such findings are generally in line with American studies (Coleman 1961, Douven & Adelson 1966, Epperson 1964, Meissner 1965, Offer & Offer 1975) which each asked slightly different questions of adolescents but, taken together, suggest that:

— most adolescents trust and admire their parents

— parental disapproval is harder for adolescents to take than disapproval expressed by friends

— about half of all teenagers feel that their parents understand them adequately or well

— minor disagreements with parents about clothes and going out are common and many, perhaps most, teenagers consider their parents old-fashioned or over-restrictive.

Alienation is something of an over-used term with a broad meaning. If it is used to extend to feelings of being unwanted by parents, then it is interesting to note that, although uncommon overall according to such studies, it was experienced by over half of the adolescents reared by "permissive" parents and nearly half of those with autocratic parents in Elder's (1962) study, rates many times greater than for democratic households with authoritative parents.

Psychiatrists and other mental health professionals make their greatest errors of judgement about adolescent normality and abnormality when they are asked to indicate the quality of intra-familial relationships. When asked to predict the responses of normal, healthy adolescents on the Offer Self-image Questionnaire, the professionals in one study seriously overestimated the degree of alienation of adolescent from parents, so that a majority of them thought that items indicating the perception of parents as unfair, incomprehensible and intolerant were typical of normal teenagers, whereas only a minority of normal adolescents did, in fact, respond to these items (Offer et al 1981). A replication of this finding demonstrated with remarkable irony that it was in just this area of family relationships that depressed and conduct-disordered adolescents differed most from normal adolescents on the questionnaire used (Hartlage et al 1984).

In parallel with such a professional tendency to romanticise about psychopathology in normal adolescents, the notion of a "generation gap" between adolescents and their parents in terms of basic values has been well-rehearsed in the clinical literature. The above findings suggest that differences over minor disciplinary matters are certainly common enough though not obviously universal. Nevertheless, there is no support for statements such as that of Miller (1975):

> Adolescents seek out extreme positions with parental figures in periodic confrontations which form a necessary part of the normal developmental process

or Coleman (1961):

> [The adolescent] is cut off from the rest of society, forced inwards toward his own age-group, made to carry out his whole social life with others his own age. With his fellows he comes to constitute a small society, one that has most of its important connections within itself, and maintains only a few threads of connection with the outside adult society.

Indeed, Meissner's (1965) study emphasised that the vast majority of teenage boys were proud of their parents, enjoyed having their friends meet them and were content to spend most of their leisure time at home, certainly until their late teens. Disengagement from home life was gradual and not marked by serious confrontation. Nor was there serious disagreement about social values between the adolescents in Gustafson's (1972) Swedish study and their parents: most accepted the conventional values of the community in which they had grown up. Noting broad agreement between various studies which have examined the consensus between parents and adolescents on basic social values, Rutter (1979) stated:

> Taken together, the findings from all studies seem to indicate that adolescents still turn to their parents for guidance on principles and on major values but look more to their peers in terms of interests and fashions in clothes, in leisure activities and other youth-orientated pursuits.

This echoes the statement made nearly thirty years ago by Bandura and Walters (1959) who observed:

> The view that adolescence is a period of rebellion is often supported by references to superficial and external signs of nonconformity, such as the adolescent fondness for unorthodox clothing, mannerisms and language. Too often his fundamental deep-seated acceptance of fundamental values is overlooked.

Divorce

At current rates, some 80 000 British adolescents each year will have parents who divorce (Central Statistical Office 1982). Their reactions to this disruption of family life will be various, according to the extent of family discord before the divorce itself, to their own personality development, and to the kind of relationship they continue to have with each parent subsequently. Wallerstein & Kelly (1980) point out how important it is to relate adolescent responses to normal psychosocial development: the normal oscillatory progress towards independence from the family of origin can be disrupted by the loss of the earlier two-parent home as a sufficiently secure base. Normally, one can expect adolescents to show episodic assertions of independence interspersed by temporary regressions to more child-like behaviour but with an overall progression towards personal autonomy. This requires a stable family structure, tolerant of such variations in stance and granting a background of consistency and continuity which allows experimentation with style and identity. Disruption of the family unit by divorce prejudices this and is experienced by some adolescents as a foreshortening of the amount of time in which they have to grow up. It is as if the parent who leaves has forestalled their own future departure from the family. Feelings of being exposed and made vulnerable were found to be quite frequent among Californian adolescents in divorcing families, as were feelings of sorrow at the loss of the intact family of their childhood, though both tended to be masked by anger, the young people scolding their parents for their selfishness and insensitivity for divorcing at such a time and apparently finding some release from their sense of powerlessness in so doing (Wallerstein & Kelly 1980).

For some of the teenagers in Walczak & Burns' (1984) study, divorce came as a relief from previous family disturbance and it is clear that the experience of parental divorce can accelerate personal development by catapulting the adolescent into a position where he or she has to cooperate with the full-time parent in maintaining the household, is obliged to take a moral view of the rights and wrongs of parental behaviour, and is likely to have to face a life with fewer material resources. A greater degree of closeness with either parent is achieved by some teenagers following the divorce, provided that sensible custodial and access arrangements are made.

However, there are many adolescents who are affected adversely by the divorce process, particularly by the behaviour of their parents after the divorce itself. Release from their marriage precipitates a crisis of identity for some parents, who may adopt an inappropriately youthful style which embarrasses the adolescent, especially as it may parallel their own concerns about personal identity. Rather similarly, details of their parents' sex life may be revealed during the divorce procedure (particularly by a parent seeking sympathy) or the newly-divorced parent may celebrate their new freedom with a series of new sexual partners whose visits to the home emphasise to the adolescent that parents are sexually active, a fact many adolescents would apparently prefer not to notice. Some adolescent girls react to such experiences by a burst of sexual behaviour outside the home and may voice anxieties about their own future competence as sexual partners in marriage. The youthfulness of their parents' lovers may produce considerable discomfort for the teenager and a resulting hostility towards them.

A new view of parents as vulnerable and dependent, to be seen as individuals rather than a combined presence, can variously provoke reactions of cooperation or rage at the inability of adults to behave maturely and responsibly. The temptation to dichotomise and polarise is perhaps not as marked as in a younger age group (Wallerstein & Kelly 1980) but the pressure from a parent to take sides in the dispute may be overwhelming.

Under such pressures, four types of response may be seen:

1. accelerated maturity with a healthy maturity and poise, associated with helpfulness and cooperation in the home
2. regression to childhood pursuits and companions and clinging to the full-time parent and home life
3. a "strategic withdrawal" with a distancing and aloofness

from home life, a turning to activities outside the home but without serious risk-taking or "acting out"

4. an escape into chaotic social and sexual activity, beyond parental control.

Such a categorisation is crude but helps to underline the distinction between a good outcome for Groups 1 and 3 and a poorer prognosis for Group 2 and 4. Nevertheless, the general outlook for the adolescents involved in parental divorce is reasonably good in the longer term though a continuing concern for such young people is the risk that their parents' unhappy experiences may find an echo in their own married lives.

In helping adolescents survive the process of divorce, most authorities suggest that counselling coupled with sensitive arrangements concerning custody and access are the important components (Fine 1987) but these will depend upon a suitable legislative and social framework, the nature of which is still under consideration in the UK.

Single-parent families

For most adolescents living in single-parent families, their situation will have followed parental separation or divorce, though in some instances parental death or the decision by a parent to have a child without marriage will have produced the present family structure. To generalise economically about the effects of living with a lone parent it is necessary to gloss over such antecedents, although it is evident that they will have considerable influence on parental behaviour and mental state as well as on the adolescent's development in childhood. For instance, the adverse impact on children of the discordant family relationships which commonly precede divorce is well documented and is usually contrasted with the less pernicious effects of parental loss by death. Bearing such caveats in mind, it is possible to make some comment on the effects of father absence, the commonest situation in one-parent families.

Boys from homes without a father are more likely to resemble girls on formal measures of intellectual and academic functioning. They tend to score higher on scores of verbal ability than on mathematics, the reverse of the usual male profile (Carlsmith 1964) and to show a field-dependent conceptual style more typically found in girls (Barclay & Cusumano 1967). The longer

51

the duration of father absence, the more typically feminine such profiles become, a finding which applies to psychological absence of the father as well as physical absence (Biller 1974), and can be reversed by the presence of a supportive stepfather (Chapman 1977). Adolescent boys from homes which lack a father are, across the board, more likely to be impulsive and irresponsible, have less satisfactory peer relationships, possess lower self-esteem and to be at risk for delinquency (Biller 1974), but it is hard to distinguish the effects of absence of father from those secondary to parental discord leading to the father leaving home in the first place. It has been argued that it is more essential for boys to have an adequate example of adult masculinity and that they suffer more from the divorce process than girls (Hetherington 1979). It is important to note that the qualities of the boy's mother can probably balance any deficit secondary to the absence of his father: a positive attitude to typically masculine assertiveness, for instance can result in more positive masculine behaviour in the boy (Biller 1974).

The effects of father absence on girls are less striking. A study by Hetherington (1972) showed that adolescent girls from homes where the father had died were less confident with boys and men than girls from homes with a father present. Those from homes where the father had left following divorce, though, were heterosexually active at an earlier age than usual in spite of being apparently anxious in male company. There is some suggestion that these differences may even out in early adult life (Hainline & Feig 1978).

How much such results follow from mere absence of a father is unclear. The mother's attitudes to the father and to men generally will obviously have an effect, and a demeaning attitude to him coupled with the increased conflict between parents in the year which follows their divorce can produce psychological harm which is not directly related simply to his absence. The presence of another adult in the home may mitigate the effects of disciplinary inconsistency or maternal overinvolvement without that person having to be in a paternal role. Also, it is important to remember that, following divorce, the common consequences for the mother and her children include a reduction of income, a move of house and school and the attenuation of social support for the mother, all of which can have deleterious effects upon an adolescent.

Step-families

Remarriage by the surviving parent of a divorce or bereavement may be difficult for adolescent children of either parent. The common issues that arise include:

— divided loyalties provoked by having three parental figures; feeling unable to be fond of a step-parent because that betrays old affections to the absent parent

— feeling displaced from a parent's affections by their new spouse or by his or her children

— refusing to accept that the step-parent has a disciplinary role

— distaste for open affection or sexuality between parent and step-parent

— accommodating to a new set of (step-)grandparents

— demands for instant love from the new step-parent, followed by a refusal to have anything to do with them

— hatred of the new arrangement because it signifies the death of a previous two-parent family and abolishes the fantasy that it can be re-created

— sexual attraction between step-parent and adolescent step-child or between step-siblings

— a failure to distinguish between dislike and hatred in step-relationships.

Sensible advice for step-parents about the above complications is available from The National Stepfamily Association (Maris House, Maris Lane, Cambridge) and particularly in a booklet published by them (De'Ath 1985).

Fostering

Adolescents may be cared for by parents not their own according to short, intermediate or long-term fostering arrangements. About half of the children in Local Authority Care in the UK are fostered, an arrangement which includes a number of adolescents. The closeness of links with the family of origin will depend upon the anticipated duration of care though, as Hersov (1985) points out, social work aims in this aspect do not always correspond to actual practice and many adolescents in long-term fostering have lost contact with their biological parents. Partly because of this, the uncertainties about returning to original parents especially when these are not in contact, and because foster parents have no formal commitment to their foster children beyond the age of 18, various authorities have recommended that many children and adolescents in long-term fostering would be better off in terms of emotional security and adjustment to the foster family by being adopted by the foster parents though Hersov (1985) sounds an appropriately cautious note when pointing out that this would not necessarily benefit all such foster children and should not be seen as a rigid principle.

The experience of Kent Social Services in establishing a fostering service for adolescents with serious behaviour problems (Hazel 1980) has spawned many imitators though commonly with less success than the original scheme, probably because the provision of support services for foster parents, extensive in the original project, has been less assiduously adhered to by other social service departments. Nevertheless, the Kent project deserves imitation: two-thirds of foster placements survived and, overall, three-quarters of the adolescents placed were thought to show significant improvement.

Adoption

Current good practice in adoption advocates telling the child about his or her adoptive status early in life and certainly well before puberty. Adopted adolescents who had not been told until late were found to be angry at this in a study by Triseliotis (1973). The issue of biological parents, their nature and whereabouts, sometimes surfaces in adolescence in association with concerns about identity but this is not particularly common and contemporary findings do not support the idea of "genealogical bewilderment" proposed by Sants (1964) who suggested that not knowing one's heredity would prejudice the development of a secure self-image. The re-appraisal of the concept by Humphrey & Humphrey (1986) contains an apposite comment:

The adopted or foster child's search for a firm sense of identity has to be seen in the context of family relationships, both past and present. Where these are open and loving there may still be a demand for ancestral knowledge. . .but there need be no untoward implications for mental health. It is primarily where family relationships are disturbed, or in some other way unsatisfactory, that the syndrome of genealogical bewilderment is likely to arise.

It appears from studies such as that by Triseliotis (1973) that only a minority of adopted people take advantage of the right to inspect their birth certificate and those who follow this by a search for their biological parents are more likely to have a history of disturbed family relationships or personality problems, especially when they betray a sense of fervent intensity of purpose in doing so. They are also likely to have been told late: about two-thirds of the searchers in Triseliotis's study had not learned of their adoptive status until after the age of 11.

Leaving home

At the end of adolescence, the prospect looms of leaving the family home to live separately. It seems likely that this is achieved gradually and without drama by most late adolescents, though some will fight their way out abusively on the basis that attacking or denigrating something to which one has previously been attached is a way of diminishing its importance and thus minimise the pain of losing it. For others, leaving home may be postponed by external factors such as a high rate of local unemployment, by elements within the individual adolescent such as mental handicap, or by dynamics within the family such as the reluctance by parents to face the "empty nest" and each other should the adolescent in question be the youngest and thus the last to depart. Stierlin & Ravenscroft (1972) describe various ways in which parents may bind adolescents, locking them into the family by exploiting their dependency, making them feel guilt at leaving, or disqualifying any statements they make suggesting a bid for autonomy. They further suggest that some teenagers may be allowed a partial freedom to leave in order to perform vicarious duties for parents who wish their own conflicts resolved at second hand; others may be expelled prematurely by neglectful or rejecting parents with the result that the outcast's resentment is displaced onto figures outside the family in aggressive or delinquent behaviour. Such ideas are untested scientifically but are useful in generating hypotheses in the treatment of families with adolescents who are apparently in conflict about leaving home. The seminal book by Haley (1980) performs the same purpose with respect to family therapy in an area neglected by scientific study.

Mundane truculence at home

The ill-tempered adolescent who is grumpy and rebarbative at home is a common enough figure. Psychiatric advice may be sought though the problem, if conceptualised as medical, is more likely to come to the notice of the general practitioner. It may be possible to understand the problem in terms of chronic difficulties in family functioning: long-standing disharmony in family relationships, a cold unfeeling style of parenting and so forth. When the issue arises in an ordinary family the parents' irritation and puzzlement as to why their erstwhile compliant child has become argumentative, rude and uncooperative frequently leads to suspicions that he or she is troubled by some private concern. This may be so but it should not lead to an abandonment of an interactive perspective which takes into account how other family members live and deal with the difficult adolescent. Commonly both arenas — private preoccupations and family relationships — combine to exacerbate each other in a vicious cycle.

One instance of this is what might be called the "strop cycle" (Fig. 4.1). An adolescent who is particularly concerned with his personal identity, individual autonomy, and the possible ways in which he might be and become different from his parents may also lack the self-confidence to assert positively his own tastes and beliefs. Instead he forges a negative identity, defining himself as different from everything suggested; self-definition by opposition — not like this, not like that. His parents' and siblings' characteristics, dress, attitudes, beliefs and possessions are decried as "stupid", "fascist", "boring" or some such adjective. At the same time he is reluctant to nail his own colours to the mast and stand up for his own ideas; the attributes of others are criticised but nothing of his own is suggested in turn because he lacks the self-esteem to risk the danger of humiliation.

In return, parents and older siblings react with withering scorn since they feel attacked and respond aggressively by returning the

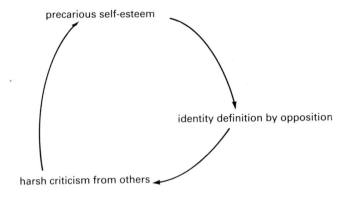

Fig. 4.1 The "strop cycle"

flak. In consequence, the teenager's self-esteem is further damaged and the defensive stance of choosing to criticise others rather than make a declaration about oneself in a positive way becomes more entrenched. At the same time, mutual resentment between the adolescent and the rest of the family causes tempers to flare and helpfulness or generosity to disappear because of the risk that they will be hurtfully rejected.

Simultaneously there are developmental concerns affecting parents, siblings and the adolescent himself. The newly-found capacity for formal operational thought can be rehearsed in endless arguments. These can be protracted if there is a lack of negotiating skills on either side and may escalate to aggressive outbursts (see p. 117). Irritability secondary to mood swings or even depression will foster argumentativeness which obscures the underlying affect. The same can be said about anxious preoccupations which are unvoiced and may be difficult for an adolescent to mention to family members, particularly if loss of face through an admission of weakness is feared.

Such preoccupations may be realistic, e.g.

— trouble at home: divorce, secrets, too much responsibility, sexual abuse

— trouble at school: unpopularity, bullying, academic failure, exams

— trouble with others: police, friends, differing peer-group standards, pregnancy, racism.

Others will be morbid: dysmorphophobic fears; obsessions; anorexia nervosa; drugs; hypochondriasis.

The psychiatric contribution is firstly to determine whether family issues such as chronic discord, communication failure, trust, abuse, infantilisation, or vicarious satisfactions are the pivotal factor or whether the individual has his own concerns, whether these are realistic or morbid, or whether an underlying factor such as fatigue or depression is exaggerating them. Secondly, there is the need to examine how family and individual issues might interact; thirdly, the need to intervene in order to alleviate the situation. To a large extent the latter will obviously follow accurate formulation of the problem. If this understanding is communicated to the family it can often lead to a re-framing of the original complaint against the adolescent so that his motivations can be seen as more than vindictive or malevolent. The trap for the psychiatrist is the danger of being unwittingly drawn into taking sides or colluding with the pressures and habits which are maintaining the situation (being "drawn into the system").

In those instances where explanation proves insufficient, recourse to managing the problem in terms of mainstream treatment as dictated by formulation is logical. In a number of the milder instances, particularly those wherein a variant of the strop cycle operates, reciprocal contracting (Ch. 22, p. 334) enables family members to place positive demands upon each other and to communicate more clearly what their mutual expectations of each other are. It is often sensible to combine such an approach with attempts to change communicative style so that the adolescent's (and parents') self-esteem can be heightened by, for instance, the trading of positive comments and praise.

REFERENCES

Asarnow J R, Lewis J M, Doane J A, Goldstein M J, Rodnick E H 1982
    Family interaction and the course of adolescent psychopathology: an analysis
    of adolescent and parent effects. Journal of Abnormal Child Psychology
    10: 427–442
Bandura A, Walters R 1959 Adolescent Aggression. Ronald, New York
Barclay A G, Cusumano D 1967 Father absence, cross-sex identity, and field
    dependent behaviour in male adolescents. Child Development 38: 243–250
Baumrind D 1975 Early socialisation and adolescent competence. In: Dragastin
    S, Elder G (eds) Adolescence in the Life Cycle. Halsted Press, London
Becker W C 1964 Consequences of different kinds of parental discipline. In:
    Hoffman M L, Hoffman L W (eds) Review of Child Development Research.
    Vol. I. Russell Sage Foundation, New York

Biller H B 1974 Paternal Deprivation. Lexington Books, Lexington Ky.

Carlsmith L 1964 Effect of early father absence on scholastic aptitude. Harvard Educational Review 34: 3–21

Central Statistical Office 1982 Social Trends. HMSO, London

Chapman M 1977 Father absence, stepfathers and the cognitive performance of college students. Child Development 48: 1155–1158

Coleman J S 1961 The Adolescent Society. Collier-Macmillan, London

De'Ath E 1985 Teenagers Growing Up in a Stepfamily. National Stepfamily Association, Cambridge

Douvan E, Adelson J 1966 The Adolescent Experience. Wiley, London

Elder G 1962 Structural variables in the child rearing relationship. Sociometry 25: 241–262

Elder G 1963 Parental power legitimation and its effect on the adolescent. Sociometry 26: 50–65

Epperson D C 1964 A re-assessment of indices of parental influence in "The Adolescent Society". American Sociology Review 29: 93–96

Fine S 1987 Children in divorce, custody and access situations: an update. Journal of Child Psychology and Psychiatry 28: 361–364

Fischer J L 1980 Reciprocity, agreement and family style in family systems with a disturbed and non-disturbed adolescent. Journal of Youth and Adolescence 9: 391–406

Fogelman K (ed) 1976 Britain's Sixteen-Year-Olds. National Children's Bureau, London

Ghodsian M, Lambert L 1978 Mum and Dad are not so bad: the views of sixteen-year-olds on how they get on with their parents. Journal of the Association of Educational Psychologists 4: 27–33

Goldstein M, Rodnick E, Jones J, McPherson S, West K 1978 Familial precursors of schizophrenia spectrum disorders. In: Wynne L, Cromwell R, Matthyse S (eds) The Nature of Schizophrenia. Wiley, New York

Gustafson B 1972 Life Values of High School Youth in Sweden. Institute of Sociology of Religion, Stockholm

Hainline L, Feig E 1978. The correlates of childhood father absence in college-aged women. Child Development 49: 37–42

Haley J 1980 Leaving Home. McGraw-Hill, New York

Hartlage S, Howard K I, Ostrov E 1984 The mental health professional and the normal adolescent. In: Offer D, Ostrov E, Howard K I (eds) Patterns of Adolescent Self-Image. Jossey-Bass, San Francisco

Hazel N 1980 Normalisation or segregation in the care of adolescents. In: Triseliotis J (ed) New Developments in Foster Care and Adoption. Routledge and Kegan Paul, London

Hersov L A 1985 Adoption and Fostering. In: Rutter M L, Hersov L A (eds) Child and Adolescent Psychiatry: Modern Approaches. Blackwell Scientific, Oxford

Hetherington E M 1972 Effects of father absence on personality development in adolescent daughters. Developmental Psychology 7: 313–326

Hetherington E M 1979 Divorce: A child's perspective. American Psychologist 34: 851–858

Humphrey M, Humphrey H 1986 A fresh look at genealogical bewilderment. British Journal of Medical Psychology 59: 133–140

Jessor S L, Jessor R 1974 Maternal ideology and adolescent problem behaviour. Developmental Psychology 10: 246–254

Meissner W W 1965 Parental interaction of the adolescent boy. Journal of Genetic Psychology 107: 225–233

Middleton R, Snell P 1963 Political expression of adolescent rebellion. American Journal of Sociology 68: 527–535

Miller M 1975 Adolescence and authority. In: Meyerson S (ed) Adolescence:

The Crises of Adjustment. Allen and Unwin, London

Offer D, Offer J 1975 From Teenage to Young Manhood. Basic Books, New York

Offer D, Ostrov E, Howard K I 1981 The mental health professional's concept of the normal adolescent. Archives of General Psychiatry 38: 149–152

Pikas A 1961 Children's attitudes toward rational versus inhibiting parental authority. Journal of Abnormal and Social Psychology 62: 315–321

Rutter M 1979 Changing Youth in a Changing Society. Nuffield Provincial Hospitals Trust, London

Rutter M, Graham P, Chadwick O F D, Yule W 1976 Adolescent turmoil: fact or fiction? Journal of Child Psychology and Psychiatry 17: 35–56

Sants H J 1964 Genealogical bewilderment in children with substitute parents. British Journal of Medical Psychology 37: 133–141

Solomon M A 1973 A developmental, conceptual premise for family therapy. Family Process 12: 179–188

Steinberg L D 1981 Transformation in family relations at puberty. Developmental Psychology 17: 833–840

Stierlin H, Ravenscroft K 1972 Varieties of adolescent "separation conflicts". British Journal of Medical Psychology 45: 299–313

Triseliotis J 1973 In Search of Origins: The Experiences of Adopted People. Routledge and Kegan Paul, London

Walczak, Y, Burns S 1984 Divorce: The Child's Point of View. Harper and Row, London

Wallerstein J S, Kelly J B 1980 Surviving the Breakup. Grant McIntyre, London

West K L 1981 Assessment and treatment of disturbed adolescents and their families: a clinical research perspective. In: Lansky M (ed) Major Psychopathology and the Family. Grune and Stratton, New York

5

Adolescent turmoil: myth and substance

The phrase "adolescent turmoil" is imprecise and over-used. It is employed in association with a number of assumptions about the developmental psychology of adolescence which need examination.

Assumption: adolescence is a time of psychic turbulence. The traditional view of adolescence is that it is a time of emotional turmoil. This may be seen as resulting from the developmental tasks discussed in Chapter 3 or from the surge of endocrine activity at puberty which activates sexual drives so that "the unresolved Oedipal situation froths to the surface again" (Hyatt Williams 1975). Adolescence is said to be "by its nature an interruption of peaceful growth" (A Freud 1958) and the associated turbulence is held to be characteristic and normal:

> Without doldrums, pain, hurt, experiment, stimulation, aggression, tenderness, flatness, excitement, defiance, exaltation, responsibility, concern, love, hate, mood swings, rebellion etc., it would not be adolescence. (Hyatt Williams 1975).

Such a view — that adolescence is a curious developmental phase characterised by a special type of psychic simmering — is seductive. It also appears to refer to a contagious condition: Meyerson (1975) says "Everybody's head is set spinning when confronted by adolescence". But should it be? The evidence clearly needs to be drawn from the general population rather than those adolescents who attend psychiatric clinics. There is a strong suspicion that the authors of statements such as the above have been seeing too many patients and not enough ordinary teenagers. It is easy to sympathise with Offer et al's (1984) barely masked irritation when they note that mental health professionals "are not very familiar with the extensive empirical literature on normal adolescent development". They could have said with justification that such unfamiliarity is irresponsible.

Douvan & Adelson (1966), in a study of over 3 000 American teenagers, found little evidence of emotional turmoil or rebelliousness. Offer (1969), Grinker et al (1962), Silber et al (1961), and Westley & Elkin (1957) have all published studies which lead to the same conclusion: most adolescents rise to the developmental challenges of the teenage years without emotional turmoil. Offer & Offer (1975) in a prospective study categorised the development of boys aged 14–22 as continuous (smooth and adaptive), surgent (adaptive but irregular progress) or tumultuous. Less than one-quarter of their sample fell into the tumultuous category which involved anxiety, depressed mood, lack of self-confidence, mood swings and distrust.

On the other hand, there is no point in denying that adolescence is a period of considerable difficulty in terms of *potential* stress and that a proportion of teenagers will react with the development of emotional symptoms. Thus nearly half (45%) of the 14–15-year-olds on the Isle of Wight interviewed by Rutter et al (1976) admitted to misery or unhappiness to the extent that caused tears or a wish to get away from it all. About one-fifth (22%) stated that they didn't, as themselves, matter very much and were self-depreciatory. Suicidal thoughts were admitted by nearly 8% and occasional sensitive ideas of self-reference by 29%. On a self-administered questionnaire just over one-fifth rated themselves as "often miserable or depressed", a considerably higher proportion than among their mothers. There was little difference between boys and girls. These emotions were not handicapping and usually not evident to parents or teachers. The prevalence rate for misery and upset among the same population four years earlier when aged 10 was 12%, indicating that a higher rate for such feelings is found during adolescence when compared with both middle childhood and adult middle life as indicated by the self-report of the mothers of the adolescents studied.

General confirmation that a fair-sized minority of teenagers experience mild emotional distress is provided by D'Arcy & Siddique (1984) who found that 41% of a general population sample of Canadian 14–18-year-olds reported between 2 and 13 symptoms on the 30-item General Health Questionnaire (11% admitted to more than 13 symptoms and 48% reported none). In case such cross-sectional studies should overlook the possibility of different youngsters experiencing minor private turmoil at different stages of adolescence, reference needs to be made to retrospective questioning about emotional symptomatology as in Mechanic & Greenley's (1976) study of university students. In this sample about one-third of 18–24-year-old students had never experienced nervous symptoms and two-thirds had never had spells when they couldn't cope very well. Bearing in mind that university students as a group are pre-selected by criteria such as intelligence which correlate positively with mental health, it is curious to note that 18–24-year-olds in the general population provided even lower rates of positive reports to the same questions (National Center for Health Statistics survey, cited in Mechanic & Greenley 1976): half had never been bothered by nervousness, three-quarters had never been unable to "take care of things because (they) couldn't get going".

A reasonable summary of the above findings would be that emotional turmoil is not an essential or normal feature of adolescence. Up to half of all adolescents at any one time will have recently experienced subjective symptoms of private emotional distress which are not evident to others and are not handicapping. It is probable that the frequency of such private turmoil is higher than at other stages of life but it is by no means universal and may, indeed, not affect most adolescents.

Assumption: adolescent turmoil is polymorphous, may mimic serious pathology, yet has a good outcome.

Adolescence resembles in appearance a variety of other emotional upsets and upheavals. The adolescent manifestations come close to symptom formation of neurotic, psychotic or dissocial order and merge almost imperceptibly into almost all the mental illnesses (A Freud 1958).

Such a view implies that psychopathology in adolescents is to be expected yet does not really constitute disorder: "At times one can hardly differentiate between psychopathology and normal growth crises" (Ekstein 1968).

There have been a number of prospective studies, all of which demonstrate the opposite. Masterson (1967) demonstrated that adolescents who were psychiatric patients possessed more (and different) symptoms than a control group and that such symptoms were likely to have been persistent. Indeed they were likely to have persisted since childhood. A number of other authorities make the same point about persistence: much adolescent psychopathology has arisen before puberty and shows strong continuity of type with its childhood form (see e.g. Rutter 1979).

Serious psychiatric pathology in adolescence is not very difficult to distinguish from normality. Koenig et al (1984) illustrate how even a self-administered questionnaire can show not just differences between a clinic population and the general population but differences between diagnostic groups. The difficulty that some mental health professionals have in distinguishing between normal adolescence and pathology is a function of their ignorance of normal adolescent development (Hartlage et al 1984) and is abolished by the provision of guidelines (Gallemore & Wilson 1972). A variety of studies (Capes et al 1971, Ford et al 1978, Gossett et al 1977, Masterson 1967, 1968, Pichel 1974, Shea et al 1978, Weiner & Del Gaudio 1976, Welner et al 1979) all emphasise that psychiatric disorder in adolescence breeds true to type on follow-up and does not change or vary over the medium term in the form of its presentation, is not polymorphous in the manner suggested by Anna Freud in the quotation above, and has prognostic characteristics governed by the type of the disorder rather than by the stage of development; these prognostic indices being comparable to those applicable to the same disorders when manifest at other times of life (see below).

The point is more than just academic:

> Greta, the 16-year-old daughter of a wealthy American couple temporarily resident in London, developed auditory hallucinations in the third person and felt her personality "taken over" by Satan. She was admitted to an adolescent unit and a provisional diagnosis of schizophrenia was made. Her parents were alarmed and requested a second opinion from a visiting Californian psychologist who stated that she was experiencing "a normal adolescent adjustment reaction" Much relieved, her parents discharged her. Two days later she committed suicide by leaping in front of a train.

Psychiatric pathology should be considered just as seriously as during adult life or childhood. It has the same degree of associated suffering and the same destructive consequences. Disturbed teenagers require equally full assessment and treatment as any other person. There is no evidence that they will "grow out of it" any more than anyone else will or will not.

The prognostic status of private emotional turmoil characterised by feelings of anxiety, misery, self-depreciation and sensitivity, not handicapping and unrecognised by parents or teachers, is unknown when it is separated off from handicapping psychiatric disorder and treated in its own right. As discussed above, turmoil so defined is not uncommon among adolescents yet is clearly not what earlier writers had in mind when they described "adolescent turmoil". Its outcome has not been studied. A large number of epidemiological studies of adults in the general population (e.g. Binder et al 1981; Srole et al 1962) report high prevalence figures for rather similar emotional symptoms but continuities or otherwise with adolescence have not been explored.

Assumption: adolescent turmoil is necessary for healthy development Does it matter if many adolescents show no sign of disturbance and experience no emotional turmoil? The traditional view is that "many crises are normal in adolescence, and in fact necessary . . . . adolescence without normative crises is not adolescence" (Hyatt Williams 1975). The corollary of this is that the absence of psychic disturbance is, paradoxically, a cause for concern. Lindemann (1964) states:

> We have learned to become equally concerned about those adolescents who show no evidence of disturbance and retain the patterns of allegiance, obedience to common family goals, and unmarred achievement throughout the puberty period. We know that such persons are likely to become profoundly disturbed at a later time when adult behaviour is unquestionably demanded.

Fortunately this is nonsense, as common sense would decree. In fact the reverse is true. Psychological functioning shows remarkable continuity across the teenage years as far as disturbance or its absence are concerned. Much early adolescent psychiatric disorder has already been evident in childhood (Capes et al 1971), and this seems particulary true for severe disorder (Warren 1965). As far as personality functioning is concerned, Vaillant (1978) was able to show a close relationship between the social functioning of undergraduates and their social adjustment 35 years later. Bachman et al (1979) followed 16-year-olds for 8 years and similarly found considerable consistency in ratings of attitudes and self-concepts. Weiner (1982) (p 30), reviewing the issue concluded:

> Adolescents who manifest obvious signs of behaviour disorder rarely outgrow them. Those who appear disturbed are likely to be disturbed and to remain disturbed unless they receive adequate treatment.

Conversely, psychiatric health is more likely among adolescents who have harmonious relationships with their parents (Rutter et al 1976), evidence good academic progress (Gossett et al 1977), and show little antisocial behaviour (Masterson 1967), in direct contradiction to Lindemann's assertion above.

Conclusion

Adolescent turmoil exists but needs to be redefined. It is private, consists of subjective emotional symptoms and social doubts which are not evident to parents or teachers. It is not associated with impaired functioning in social or educational areas though the feelings are distressing to those teenagers who experience them. Many, possibly most, teenagers will not be subject to it. By all accounts it is composed of feelings which can be experienced at other stages of life and may well be related to the difficulties encountered in psychosocial development though there is no conclusive evidence for this. By no stretch of the imagination can it be confused with major psychiatric disorder though it may be hard to differentiate from mild affective disorder. It is not a necessary experience for future mental health.

REFERENCES

Bachman J G, O'Malley P M, Johnston J 1979 Adolescence to Adulthood: Change and Stability in the Lives of Young Men. Institute for Social Research, Ann Arbor

Binder J, Dobler-Mikola A, Angst J 1981 An epidemiological study of minor psychiatric disturbances. Social Psychiatry 16: 31–41

Capes M, Gould E, Townsend M 1971 Stress in Youth. Oxford University Press, London

D'Arcy C, Siddique C M 1984 Psychological distress among Canadian adolescents. Psychological Medicine 14: 615–628

Douvan E, Adelson J 1966 The Adolescent Experience. Wiley, London

Ekstein R 1968 Impulse-acting out-purpose: psychotic adolescents and their quest for goals. International Journal of Psycho-Analysis 49: 347–352

Ford K, Hudgens R W, Welner A 1978 Undiagnosed psychiatric illness in adolescents: a prospective study and 7-year follow-up. Archives of General Psychiatry 35: 279–282

Freud A 1958 Adolescence. Psychoanalytic Study of the Child 13: 255–278

Gallemore J L, Wilson W P 1972 Adolescent maladjustment or affective disorder? American Journal of Psychiatry 129: 608–612

Gossett J T, Barnhart D, Lewis J M, Phillips V A 1977 Follow-up of adolescents treated in a psychiatric hospital. Archives of General Psychiatry 34: 1037–1042

Grinker R R, Sr, Grinker R R, Jr, Timberlake J 1962 A study of mentally healthy young males (homoclites). Archives of General Psychiatry 6: 405–453

Hartlage S, Howard K I, Ostrov E 1984 The mental health professional and the normal adolescent. In: Offer D, Ostrov E, Howard K I (eds) Patterns of Adolescent Self-Image. Jossey-Bass, San Francisco

Hyatt Williams A 1975 Puberty and phases of adolescence. In: Meyerson S (ed.) Adolescence: The Crises of Adjustment. George Allen and Unwin, London

Koenig L, Howard K I, Offer D, Cremerius M 1984 Psychopathology and adolescent self-image. In: Offer D, Ostrov E, Howard K I (eds) Patterns of Adolescent Self-Image. Jossey Bass, San Francisco

Lindemann E 1964 Adolescent behavior as a community concern. American Journal of Psychotherapy 18: 405–417

Masterson J F 1967 The Psychiatric Dilemma of Adolescence. Churchill, London

Masterson J F 1968 The psychiatric significance of adolescent turmoil. American Journal of Psychiatry 124: 1549–1554

Mechanic D, Greenley J R 1976 The prevalence of psychological distress and help-seeking in a college student population. Social Psychiatry 11: 1–14

Meyerson S 1975 Adolescence: The Crises of Adjustment. George Allen and Unwin, London

Offer D 1969 The Psychological World of the Teenager. Basic Books, New York

Offer D, Offer J B 1975 From Teenage to Young Manhood: A Psychological Study. Basic Books, New York

Offer D, Ostrov E, Howard K I (eds) 1984 Patterns of Adolescent Self-Image. Jossey Bass, San Francisco

Pichel J I 1974 A long-term follow-up study of 60 adolescent psychiatric outpatients. American Journal of Psychiatry 131: 140–144

Rutter M 1979 Changing Youth in a Changing Society. Nuffield Provincial Hospitals Trust, London

Rutter M, Graham P, Chadwick O F D, Yule W 1976. Adolescent turmoil: fact or fiction? Journal of Child Psychology and Psychiatry 17: 35–56

Shea M J, Hafner J, Quast W, Hetler J H 1978 Outcome of adolescent psychiatric disorder: a long term follow-up study. In: Anthony E J, Koupernik A C, Chiland C (eds) The Child in his Family: Vulnerable Children. Wiley, New York

Silber E, Hamburg D A, Coelho G V, Murphey E B, Rosenberg M, Pearlin L I 1961. Adaptive behavior in competent adolescents. Archives of General Psychiatry 5: 354–365

Srole L, Langner T S, Michael S T, Opler M K, Rennie T A C 1962 Mental Health in the Metropolis. McGraw Hill, New York

Vaillant G E 1978 Natural history of male psychological health. VI. Correlates of successful marriage and fatherhood. American Journal of Psychiatry 135: 653–659

Warren W 1965 A study of adolescent psychiatric in-patients and the outcome six or more years later. I. Clinical histories and hospital findings. Journal of Child Psychology and Psychiatry 6: 1–17

Weiner I B 1982 Child and Adolescent Psychopathology. Wiley, New York

Weiner I B, Del Gaudio A C 1976 Psychopathology in adolescence: an epidemiological study. Archives of General Psychiatry 33: 187–193

Welner A, Welner Z, Fishman R 1979 Psychiatric adolescent inpatients: eight to ten-year follow-up. Archives of General Psychiatry 36: 698–700

Westley W A, Elkin F 1957 The protective environment and adolescent socialization. Social Forces 35: 243–249

6
Epidemiology

Prevalence of psychiatric disorder

A number of issues bedevil any attempt to make a simple statement as to how many adolescents are psychiatrically ill. There
are differing thresholds used to determine pathology in various
studies. The relative prevalence of different types of disorder
changes with each year of age within the teenage years. It is
likely that higher prevalence rates obtain in inner urban areas
than in rural ones and that this represents one aspect of a correlation between social disadvantage and the likelihood of psychiatric disorder. Uncertainty exists as to how much weight to give
to subjective accounts of symptoms by youngsters whose general
demeanour gives their caretakers and teachers no cause for
concern and who suffer from little or no social impairment.

The range of disorders which is seen among young adolescents
is generally similar to that found in older children. By the age
of 18 this has changed to resemble more closely the spectrum
seen in a young adult population. This shift, which is clearly
developmental, is paralleled by a change in the conceptual
approach of clinicians from the formulative emphasis of child
psychiatry to the diagnostic style of adult psychiatry. There is a
tendency for adult psychiatrists to recognize psychiatric disorder
only when its presentation conforms to specified diagnoses; the
informing model is that of mental illness even when this is not
explicitly espoused. Conversely the concept of disorder
commonly adopted by child psychiatrists is that of extreme
deviation in behaviour or emotions accompanied by social
impairment or substantial suffering; the model is that of distorted
psychosocial development. In child psychiatry the reports of

others such as parents and teachers are crucial in diagnosis and tend to overwhelm information derived from direct interview with the child, the converse of the usual state of affairs in adult psychiatry. All of this leads to some uncertainty as to whether the prevalence rates found at the onset of adolescence are comparable to those obtained for the late teenage years.

Thus Banks (1983) found a case rate of 3.5% in a sample of 200 17-year-olds as a result of individual interviews using the Present State Examination, an instrument designed from the standpoint of adult general psychiatry and solely dependent upon the mental state as determined at interview alone. On the other hand, Rutter, Graham and their colleagues (1976) from the standpoint of child psychiatry found a rate of 21% among Isle of Wight 14–15-year-olds for psychiatric disorders when the adolescents' own account of symptoms was taken into account, a figure which seems to have given rise to some unease among the authors since Graham and Rutter elsewhere (1985) suggest that a rate of 10–15% would be more reasonable. If just the information provided by teachers and parents in the Isle of Wight study was used, this showed but a moderate increase (35%) in rate of disorder over that found among 10-year-olds in an earlier study on the same island. However, a considerable number of teenagers gave good accounts of subjective affective symptoms in spite of their parents and teachers reporting no observable abnormality. Such interviews appeared valid but the practice of inferring psychiatric disorder from the patient's subjective report alone is not one with which child psychiatrists feel comfortable; corroboration is usually sought.

Nevertheless, there is support for a prevalence figure approaching Rutter et al's (1976) estimate of 21%. Leslie (1974) interviewed 141 teenagers aged 13–14 living in Blackburn, a 94% sample of 105 individuals selected on the grounds of a high score on a questionnaire issued to the parents of 1198 schoolchildren of that age attending ordinary schools in that town and 45 randomly selected from the remainder as a check. Forty-four adolescents attending special schools (and thus a high risk group for the detection of disorder) as well as 130 who were pupils at direct-grant schools (probably a low risk group on the grounds of high intelligence) were omitted from the survey. It was judged that the failure to include such groups would not alter the final prevalence rates substantially.

Combining data derived from interviews with both teenagers

and parents, and from teacher questionnaires, a judgement as to the presence, type and severity of psychiatric disorder was made in each case. Moderately severe disorder was "sufficient disturbance to be in no way distinguishable from [that] normally and appropriately referred to a child psychiatrist", severe disorder indicated definite suicidal risk, psychosis or was "seriously disabling". Case vignettes were published to illustrate this distinction.

The minimum total prevalence rate for severe disorders among boys was 6.2% and for moderate and severe cases combined was 20.8%. Among girls, 2.6% were rated severely disordered and the combined figure for both severe and moderate cases was 13.6%. The rate for moderate and severe disorder in boys and girls combined was 17.4%.

Among boys, the commonest diagnoses were conduct and mixed (i.e. combined conduct and emotional) disorder. Taking these together accounted for 65% of male cases. On the other hand, emotional disorders affected just over half of disturbed girls. Given the fact that boys outnumbered girls by three to two in the disturbed group, the overall figures indicate that conduct and mixed disorders accounted for just over half of all cases in this age group. Only a single case of psychosis was detected.

It is of interest to note that only 65% of the parents of moderately and severely disordered youngsters thought their child was abnormal. This compares with Rutter et al's (1976) finding that in 28% of their cases the diagnosis of psychiatric disorder was made solely on the teenager's account of their symptoms, there being no indication of abnormality in the descriptions given by parents and teachers.

Leslie's study gives a reasonable picture of psychiatric morbidity in a young adolescent population in an industrial town with a higher rate of socio-economic adversity and a lower level of psychiatric services than the Isle of Wight. It is thus a little surprising that her figures are generally comparable to Rutter et al (1976).

Krupinski and his colleagues (1967) found rates for psychiatric disorder of 16.4% for boys and 19.3% for girls aged 15–19 living in Heyfield, a rural Australian town. Similar rates (14.8% and 13.8% respectively) were obtained by a comparable process of door-to-door interviews in metropolitan Melbourne (Krupinski & Stoller 1971). These studies do not show the increase in rate associated with urban living demonstrated by Lavik (1977) who found a prevalence rate of 19.6% in Oslo compared with 7.9%

in a rural Norwegian valley, presumably because the contrast between Melbourne and Heyfield is less great.

To this general picture may be added the prevalence rates for psychiatric disorder obtained by the following American studies: 23% of 12–19-year-old non-psychiatric hospital patients (Hudgens 1974), 22% of first-year college students (Kysar et al 1969), 20% of a randomly selected group of 12–18-year-olds (Masterson 1967), 21% of 73 typical male high school students (Offer & Offer 1975), 15% of first-year college students (Rimmer et al 1978). Most such studies have been carried out on urban populations, though not necessarily deprived ones.

Such rates, of around 15–25%, are not seriously different from the rates for psychiatric disorder among adults (see e.g. Dohrenwend et al 1980), but could mask smaller differences in prevalence between the two epochs. In addition there is the problem of variation within adolescence and within adulthood when each is taken as a whole. D'Arcy's studies (D'Arcy 1982, D'Arcy & Siddique 1984) on a Canadian population using the General Health Questionnaire provide a clue but the conclusions can only be partial in view of poor response rates. Whereas 20.5% of boys and 34.4% of 14–17-year-old girls reported a score of 6 or more on the GHQ–30, 17% of young adult (age 20–29) males and 26% of young adult females reported a similar score; a slight fall in rate when young adulthood is compared with adolescence. With progression through adult life, rates fell to a plateau of around 13% for males and 18% for females in subsequent age decades until an increase in old age (70+).

It is difficult to know how prevalence rates might change year by year with passage through adolescence. In the same Canadian studies, there was a trend towards more frequent reporting of symptoms with advancing age from 14 to 19. This needs to be set against the fact that the GHQ does not tap antisocial behaviour which is pre-eminent among younger, rather than older, adolescents (West 1982). On the other hand, various studies suggest an increase in the prevalence of emotional and psychotic disorder with advancing age during adolescence (discussed in Graham & Rutter 1985) leaving the overall picture somewhat confused.

The relationship between psychiatric disorder in adolescence and social disadvantage or urban living is not as clear as is the case with children (described in Wolkind & Rutter 1985). Although there is probably a relative excess of disorder among urban adolescents compared to their rural counterparts (Lavik 1977), this is largely due to the persistence of conditions previously evident in childhood and likely to be mediated through effects upon family life (Rutter 1979). Disorder arising anew in adolescence is rather less likely to be caused by family disturbance than is the case with childhood disorder (Rutter et 1976). No convincing evidence exists to indicate any relationship between the overall rate of disorder in adolescence and parental social class.

As a general conclusion it is suggested that a range of 15–20% is a suitable approximation for a single prevalence figure for psychiatric disorder among teenagers. Within this range it needs to be recognised that boys will be affected more than girls in early adolescence, when antisocial behaviour is a common accompaniment or manifestation of disorder. In later adolescence, girls will outnumber boys and the relative predominance of affective disorder in this age group is associated with this. It is generally believed that social disadvantage is associated with a higher prevalence of disorder and this may underpin the urban–rural differences in rate that some studies show.

The pattern of disorders

In early adolescence there is an evident continuity with childhood. A number of children with conduct, emotional or developmental disorders will continue to be affected during their teenage years; their conditions persist. This is particularly true for conduct disorder: of the Isle of Wight 10-year-olds with conduct disorder, three-quarters would still receive the same diagnosis four years later (Graham & Rutter 1973), which corresponds to the findings by Farrington (1978) and Lefkowitz et al (1977) on the remarkable persistence of aggressive behaviour. The coexistence of pervasive hyperactivity with conduct disorder in childhood worsens the prognosis as far as behaviour in adolescence is concerned (Schachar et al 1981).

Antisocial behaviour outside the home peaks in the mid-teens though the prevalence of different types of offence changes with age, shoplifting being more typical of young offenders, and crimes of violence rising proportionally with age (West 1982). Theft and vandalism are remarkably common among urban teenage boys (Clarke 1978, Belson 1975), though conduct disorder was not appreciably more prevalent among Isle of Wight 14–15-year-olds than it had been when they were 10 years old. Antisocial behaviour, delinquency and conduct disorder are, of course different entities (see Ch. 8).

For conditions in which a selective developmental delay is important, the general picture is of diminishing prevalence rates with progression through the teens. Most instances of encopresis and enuresis abate during early adolescence as do most simple tics. Severe developmental problems do not share such a benign prognosis. For instance, profound developmental disorders of language such as the dysphasias present a persisting handicap, as do those cases of specific reading retardation which are derived from a language (rather than e.g. a "perceptual") difficulty though in such instances it is the associated spelling disability which comes to the fore clinically.

The continuity from childhood to adolescence for emotional disorders is rather low. Just under half of the children diagnosed as having an emotional disorder at 10 proved to have an emotional disorder on follow-up four years later (Rutter 1979). The corollary of this is that most emotional disorder in Isle of Wight 14–15-year-olds had arisen in adolescence. With increasing age, the somewhat amorphous emotional disorders of childhood become more discrete and differentiated so that the spectrum of emotional pathology resembles increasingly the pattern of adult neuroses. Agoraphobia and social phobia, neither of which are seen pre-pubertally, become increasingly prevalent. Anxiety states, hysteria, hypochondriasis and obsessional disorder may all be seen before puberty but become more frequently recognised during adolescence.

The prevalence of depression and depressive symptomatology increases markedly after puberty and may rise further during the teens. Parasuicide rates also show a dramatic surge, peaking in the late teens. Suicide rates rise even more rapidly throughout the teens. Mania, exceptionally rare before puberty, may now present and enable the diagnosis of bipolar affective disorder to be made. Most depression in adolescence is not, however, bipolar. The rise in the prevalence of neurotic and affective disorder during the teens is the factor largely responsible for the change from a male excess among psychiatrically disordered young teenagers to a female excess in the late teens.

Anorexia nervosa is most likely to appear at around the age of 17 (Crisp 1980) and is, perhaps, the only disorder which can be said to have a specific relationship to the adolescent developmental process (although a case could be made out for social phobia also being so regarded).

Schizophrenia is very rarely diagnosed before puberty but the condition is recognised increasingly throughout the teens.

Abuse of a variety of psycho-active substances becomes widespread during adolescence though there is a suspicion that the patterns of substance choice vary with age: solvent abuse in the early teens, alcohol and opiates later on.

Severe developmental deficits such as mental handicap and autism are lifelong disabilities and will persist throughout the teenage years.

REFERENCES

Banks M H 1983 Validation of the general health questionnaire in a young community sample. Psychological Medicine 13: 349–353

Belson W A 1975 Juvenile Theft: The Causal Factors. Harper and Row, London

Clarke R (ed,) 1978 Tackling Vandalism. (Home Office Research Study No. 47) HMSO, London

Crisp A H 1980 Anorexia Nervosa: Let Me Be. Academic Press, London

D'Arcy C 1982 Prevalence and correlates of nonpsychotic psychiatric symptoms in the general population. Canadian Journal of Psychiatry 27: 316–324

D'Arcy C, Siddique C M 1984 Psychological distress among Canadian adolescents. Psychological Medicine 14: 615–628

Dohrenwend B P, Dohrenwend B S, Gould M S, Link B, Neugebauer R, Wunsch-hitzig R 1980 Mental Illness in the United States: Epidemiological Estimates. Praeger, New York

Farrington D 1978. The family backgrounds of aggressive youths. In: Hersov L A, Berger M, Shaffer D (eds) Aggression and Antisocial Behaviour in Childhood and Adolescence. Pergamon, Oxford

Graham P, Rutter M 1973 Psychiatric disorder in the young adolescent: a follow-up study. Proceedings of the Royal Society of Medicine 66: 58–61

Graham P, Rutter M 1985 Adolescent disorders In: Rutter M, Hersov L (eds) Child and Adolescent Psychiatry: Modern Approaches. 2nd edn. Blackwell Scientific, Oxford

Hudgens R W 1974 Psychiatric Disorders in Adolescents. Williams and Wilkins, Baltimore

Krupinski J, Stoller A 1971 The Health of a Metropolis. Heinemann Educational, Melbourne

Krupinski J, Baikie A G, Stoller A, Graves J, O'Day D M, Polke P 1967 A community health survey of Heyfield, Victoria. Medical Journal of Australia 1: 1204–1211

Kysar J E, Zaks M S, Schuchman H P, Schon G L, Rogers J 1969 Range of psychological functioning in 'normal' late adolescents. Archives of General Psychiatry 21: 515–528

Lavik N J 1977 Urban-rural differences in rates of disorder. A comparative psychiatric population study of Norwegian adolescents. In: Graham P J (ed) Epidemiological Approaches in Child Psychiatry. Academic Press, London

Lefkowitz M M, Eron L D, Walder L O, Rowell Huesmann L 1977 Growing Up to be Violent. Pergamon, New York

Leslie S A 1974 Psychiatric disorder in the young adolescents of an industrial town. British Journal of Psychiatry 125: 113–124

Masterson J F 1967 The Psychiatric Dilemma of Adolescence. Churchill, London

Offer D, Offer J B 1975 From Teenage to Young Manhood: A Psychological Study. Basic Books, New York

Rimmer J D, Halikas J A, Schuckit M A, McClure J N 1978 A systematic study of psychiatric illness in freshman college students. Comprehensive Psychiatry 19: 249–251

Rutter M 1979 Changing Youth in a Changing Society. Nuffield Provincial Hospitals Trust, London

Rutter M, Graham P, Chadwick O F D, Yule W 1976. Adolescent turmoil: fact or fiction. Journal of Child Psychology and Psychiatry 17: 35–56

Schachar R, Rutter M, Smith A 1981. The characteristics of situationally and pervasively hyperactive children: implications for syndrome definition. Journal of Child Psychology and Psychiatry 22: 375–392

West D J 1982 Delinquency. Heinemann, London

Wolkind S, Rutter M 1985 Separation, loss and family relationships In: Rutter M, Hersov L (eds) Child and Adolescent Psychiatry: Modern Approaches. 2nd edn. Blackwell Scientific, Oxford

7

Personality and personality disorder

In child psychiatry and child development the term "temperament" is used to describe differences between children which are essentially aspects of the style of their behaviour (see Berger (1985) for a review of the concept). There is a thriving research industry involved in the examination of this concept (see Plomin & Dunn 1986, Porter & Collins 1982). Emerging from this seems to be a consensus that qualities such as activity level, emotional reactivity, sociability, behavioural inhibition, impulsivity and aggressivity are important individual differences in the style of behaviour which are measurable and relatively stable over the medium term. What is more, they are important in determining the experiences a child has and in particular the way in which other people react to the child and influence his or her psychosocial development. It has to be said that there remains appreciable disagreement as to the number of such characteristics which can be reliably identified.

Different patterns of temperamental characteristics have attracted specific labels: "slow to warm-up", or "difficult", for instance (Thomas & Chess 1977). It appears likely that various combinations of characteristics represent a vulnerability or resistance to psychiatric disorder in childhood (Graham et al 1973, Rutter et al 1964, Garmezy 1984). Most children, though, have temperaments which do not fall cleanly into such categories and must therefore be described according to a number of dimensions, usually including the qualities mentioned above. There is no generally accepted scheme of categorising the temperaments of all pre-adolescent children into different groups but it is possible to describe the temperamental profile of an individual according to the extent to which he or she exhibits particular qualities or styles of behaviour.

76

The study of temperament began with very young children as subjects. This probably explains the way in which the variables chosen to describe the style of behaviour have been those readily inferred from observations of small children's activities in everyday situations, commonly using parental reports as a source of information. Other sources of individual differences such as physical characteristics or intelligence are generally set aside and those such as styles of private thought are not explored. Thus temperament comes to comprise "a relatively small number of simple, non-motivational, non-cognitive, stylistic features" (Rutter 1987).

"Personality" is a term which encompasses much more than temperament. It has many definitions but at core refers to the individuality of the organisation of attitudes and behaviour. It includes motivational elements and cognitive components, indeed it is these derivatives of mental activity which play a major part in organising a coherent pattern of understanding experience and responding to the world. Concepts of the self-system and social relationships are central so that both intrapsychic and interpersonal processes influence and are influenced by personality in a dynamic and developing system.

In adolescence, the move away from the family into a wider range of social roles and experiences requires an expansion of coping strategies, a reappraisal of childhood attitudes and assumptions together with new expectations and understandings of social relationships. If coupled with the development of formal operational thought, this allows an exploration of ideas about the self which underpin ideas about identity. A notion of coherence must buttress any stable sense of identity and also any system of understanding others so that they are seen as people rather than as sources of unconnected behaviours. This coherence probably relies upon cognitive evaluation at one level but upon assumptions about relationships and self-esteem at another. A number of metaphorical systems attempt to illustrate how such evaluations and assumptions arise; in clinical use, psychoanalytic theories and attachment theory have probably been used most frequently. In such a way, an organisational approach to personality has developed which lays stress upon general personal functioning.

In parallel with this sort of thinking about personality is the idea of personality traits which may, when exaggerated or present to an extreme degree, indicate categories of personality or even

personality disorder. Any approach which leads towards a classification of personality according to categories and groupings will
have an intuitive appeal to the medical mind. Accordingly the
trait approach has been enshrined in much clinical teaching and
in the categorisation of personality disorder according to the
International Classification of Diseases though there are grounds
for thinking this could be simplified (Tyrer & Alexander 1979).

Which general approach to personality — the organisational
approach or the trait system — should be adopted cannot be
determined unless reference is made to how reliable and how
useful each is clinically. There is very little evidence available on
either score, and what there is appears unhelpful or contradictory
(Rutter 1987).

Obviously personality develops throughout childhood and most
people would argue that it continues to evolve during
adolescence. A sense of an emerging coherence to behaviour
with advancing age throughout the teens is a common observation. In part this may be spurious for two reasons. Firstly, it
is common for adolescents to experiment somewhat with
different styles of dress, attitudes and behaviour in order to
explore how such variations feel subjectively and function
socially. Such experimentation will diminish with time as experience is gained. Secondly, the individual adolescent can explain
himself or herself in a way which a child cannot. The behavioural
style and apparent motivation of a child are necessarily obtained
from the reports of others: caregivers and teachers in particular.
These adults see the child in different situations (home and
school) which elicit different aspects of psychosocial functioning.
In the late teens, the individual becomes the chief source of
information about his or her self and can present it plausibly in
a coherent, congruent, single frame.

Nevertheless, there is a genuine developmental aspect to
personality development which hinges upon the accumulation of
experience and the cognitive integration of meanings and attitudes associated with it. Thus an adolescent with personality
difficulties may be understood in terms of either delayed or
deviant personality development. Clinical reality frequently
involves an interaction between the two since maladaptive
responses may be learned because an appropriately mature level
of personality organisation has not yet been achieved but, for the
sake of simplicity, the two can be considered separately.

Personality development

The term "immature" when applied to adolescents generally means relatively immature, since all adolescents are technically immature. In colloquial use it is most likely to be used of young people who are child-like in their interests and sense of humour, seek help and reassurance too readily, show little initiative, are emotionally labile, anxious to please, and are lacking in independence particularly by remaining reliant upon the presence of attachment figures in order to manage anxiety. It is possible to move beyond the simple view that immaturity is revealed by behaviour that is child-like by considering the way in which attitudes and expectations alter with maturation.

A number of models exist for illustrating these aspects of psychosocial maturation during adolescence. The commonest type is a stage model, typically epigenetic in conception so that each stage needs to be resolved before the next is tackled. If one stage in such a model is not resolved satisfactorily, this will have adverse repercussions on attempts to master subsequent stages. Individuals may function predominantly at one level and if this is judged to be below the norm for their age they are said to be fixated at that stage. In such a vein Erikson's eight ages of man and Kohlberg's scheme for moral development are mentioned elsewhere (see Chs. 3 and 8) and are familiar to most clinicians working with adolescents. Less well known but strikingly similar are the schemes suggested by Sullivan et al (1957) and Selman (1976). Both concern social perspective-taking and the under-

Table 7.1 Stages of interpersonal maturity (Sullivan et al 1957): seven stages, each defined by a crucial interpersonal problem.

1. Discrimination between self and not-self

If fixated: individual behaves as if he were the whole world
expects partners to be so close that there is a unison of wishes, needs etc.
magical thinking typical
cannot postpone gratification, little distinction between having a wish and fulfilling it
non-striving but feels buffeted by society without knowing why or apportioning blame
unintegrated into society: drifters or in institutions

2 Differentiation of environment into persons and things

If fixated: sees others in terms of own needs; blames them if satisfaction not forthcoming

Table 7.1

people seen as instrumental, treated as unfeeling tools in very crude manipulations

roles allocated to people are very simple: givers, takers

expects world to be composed of providers, essentially a trusting stance

if thwarted, walks out avoiding a major showdown

typically feels misunderstood and resentful

outward ineffectual demeanour, docile, compliant without long-term goals

3. Perception of rules governing relationships between people and things

If fixated: premise that society regulated by rigid rules

seeks rules which define what is expected and what is due in order for needs to be met

external controls of reward and punishment only, no internalised guilt

believes that if conforms to rules, needs will be met

tests limits to discover "house rules"

trusts no-one; acquaintances but no long-term friends

may manipulate defensively in the belief that each person in a relationship is trying to make a sucker out of the other

if delinquent, typically confidence tricksters, swindlers, self-justifying

chameleon: adapts easily to new settings and institutions, appears to recognise codes of prosocial conduct but is also fearful of authority and power (may be in conflict)

friendly, unemotional, superficially co-operative

4. Perception of influence and demands of others (Can have a sense of self as seen by others. Use of identification by internalisation of attributes of others)

If fixated: assumes qualities of powerful figures in own experiance but then cannot live up to them

inner sense of inadequacy and guilt at not attaining standards he has set himself, can lead to splitting and projection onto outside world with others seen as all bad in order to preserve own sense of goodness, tendency to dichotomise

may become petty tyrant: tense, suspicious, hostile

prone to spells of boredom and feeling useless; may seek compensatory excitement

may offend in order to assuage internal guilt

5. Perception of stable action patterns in self and others (can deal with others without being overwhelmed by them, can empathise and enjoy others as individuals)

If fixated: concern about core identity among various roles

6. Perception of distinction between core identity and roles (Can establish long-term relationships of depth and consistency. Can set long-term goals)

If fixated: generally recognised as mature

7. Perception of integrating processes in self and others (Obtains a perspective on previous modes of experiencing, capacity for empathy with less mature)

"It is probable that no one completes this stage in the society of today"

Table 7.2 Stages of social perspective-taking (Selman 1976): six stages considered to be prerequisites for moral development

1. Egocentric point of view
Cannot recognise that the interests of others differ; no capacity to relate two points of view. Actions of others perceived just as actions with no understanding of the psychology behind them.

2. Concrete individualistic perspective
Awareness that others also have psychological interests to pursue and that these might conflict.

3. Placing self in interpersonal relationships with others
Recognition that shared feelings or expectations might take primacy over individual interests. Now has the capacity to put self in other's shoes; this becomes a golden rule.

4. Differentiation societal point of view from interpersonal agreement
Able to take the point of view of the system which has expectations and defines roles. Interpersonal relations can be located within the system.

5. Prior-to-society perspective
Perspective of a rational individual who is aware of rights and values which are prior to agreements and attachments. Understands that moral and legal processes may conflict. Integrates different perspectives by formal processes of contract and objective impartiality.

6. Moral perspective
Brings rationality to bear on an assumption that individual people are ends in themselves and should be treated as such. Social arrangements seen to derive from the perspective of a moral point of view.

standing of interpersonal transactions. Both are illustrated in Tables 7.1 and 7.2 from which their essential similarity can be seen. In each case it is arguable whether a pure stage theory is required or whether what is described is a continuum with well-described anchor points. As neither has a very substantial under-pinning from independent scientific evidence, this need not be taken as a crucial issue; the value is in providing a framework for clinical thought: the creative use of "soft" developmental theories in providing a stimulus to clinical practice mentioned by Berger (1985).

The reasons why an individual adolescent should demonstrate delayed psychosocial maturation according to any of these schemes are not well explored in the scientific literature. The work of Baumrind (1975), previously referred to on page 44, is a notable exception. Although concerned more with the relations between parental styles of child-rearing and the ways in which their children develop their own personalities than with rate of personality development, her findings are helpful in under-standing developmental delay in this area. Those she terms "authoritative" parents are those most likely to have adolescent children who would generally be thought of as being mature for their age: self-reliant, ambitious, individualistic and socially responsible. Such parents are interested in their children, use warmth and praise to encourage approved activities but do not hesitate to criticise undesirable ones, have high self-esteem and are generally warm and supportive whilst setting firm limits on behaviour. They are very similar in such respects to the parents of children with high self-esteem studied by Coopersmith (1967).

In contrast, parents who are more controlling and restrictive and who are inflexible in their edicts and attitudes ("authoritarian-restrictive") tend to have extremely conformist adolescent offspring, generally classified as less mature. Less easy to fit into a single developmental parameter are those adolescents who come from homes which are more laissez-faire or indulgent ("permissive"). They are likely to produce adolescents who are aimless and uninterested in conventional career achievements though they may be very creative, paticularly if their families are "harmonious", with parents who use discussion and principles rather than rules when resolving differences with their children.

This is broadly in line with the conventional clinical view that the socially and emotionally immature adolescent is likely to have parents who are overprotective and display a quality of restrictive infantilisation. The combination of low parental expectations in terms of social maturation and the general constriction of life experiences which is often associated means that there is little press or drive to solve developmental tasks and mature. A degree of indulgence or a conflict of attitudes between an overprotective, indulgent mother and a cold, harsh, authoritarian father is classically associated with antisocial behaviour coupled with moral and interpersonal immaturity, but the notion is over-simplified to the point of cliché and tends to breed therapeutic pessimism.

Such thinking tends to minimise the effects of inheritance upon personality, seeing variations in terms of the consequences of parental caretaking behaviour rather than considering how parents might produce an adolescent with a similar personality to their own through genetic effects. Thus a constitutionally nervous teenager with a tendency to withdraw in the face of novelty might elicit overprotective behaviour from a parent who is likewise anxious. This would not necessarily mean that a treatment approach which sought to change parental behaviour would be misplaced, however, since virtually every study which has attempted to unravel the genetic and environmental contributions to personality development confirms an interactive effect between the two sources of influence.

Personality disorder

Most general psychiatrists find the concept of personality disorder useful but the definition and study of such a condition remains rather unsatisfactory (Lewis 1974, Widiger & Frances 1985). In virtually all definitions there is a requirement that a basic fault in personal functioning, present since childhood or adolescence, gives rise to ingrained and maladaptive behaviours, attitudes and emotional responses which cause suffering to the self or others and are associated with social impairment.

It is generally assumed that the personalities of adolescents are immature by definition, so that the diagnosis of personality disorder is not one which many child and adolescent psychiatrists feel easy about making (Wolff 1984), particularly because it implies a fixity of reaction patterns and personality which can lead to prognostic pessimism and therapeutic inertia. Indeed, one of the criteria for antisocial personality disorder in DSM-IIIR (the American Psychiatric classification system) is age 18 or over.

In addition, there is an unresolved tension between the two major systems used to conceptualise personality disorder. One approach, exemplified by many of the ICD diagnoses (the WHO classification system), is to label according to the presence of exaggerated personality traits which have been thought to distort personality functioning. Thus there are types of personality disorder such as paranoid, affective, schizoid, anankastic and so forth. The difficulty with such an approach is that the specificity, reliability and stability over time of such labels is rather poor (see e.g. Mann et al 1981, Tyrer et al 1983).

The second general approach is exemplified by an emphasis on patterns of behaviour with special reference to personal relationships and some assumptions about underlying psychopathology. This pervades much of DSM-III which groups personality disorder into three major groups: odd or eccentric behaviour (paranoid, schizoid, schizotypal), dramatic behaviour (histrionic, borderline, narcissistic, antisocial), and fearful behaviour (avoidant, dependent, compulsive, passive-aggressive).

An important review by Rutter (1987) suggests that the classification scheme based on extreme traits should be abandoned since the traits can more profitably be defined in dimensional terms. He further recommends locating some apparent disorders of personality in other sections of a classification system for psychiatric disorder. For instance, schizotypal personality disorder would be grouped with schizophrenia rather than with personality disorder and Asperger's syndrome with autism. Another suggestion is that the group of personality disorders termed "dramatic" by DSM-III could be lumped together since all reflect a persistent and serious abnormality in maintaining social relationships.

There are two disorders of personality which seem to be worthy of special mention with respect to adolescence: borderline disorder and what is often identified as schizoid personality disorder (interestingly, Steinberg's (1983) text comes to a similar conclusion in selecting borderline state, schizoid personality and Asperger's syndrome for specific discussion).

Borderline personality disorder

Originally a psychoanalytic concept, borderline personality disorder was operationally defined in DSM-III-R and it is this definition (see Table 7.3) which has been most widely used in recent years. The status of the condition is controversial and it is not listed in ICD-9. Tarnopolsky & Berelowitz (1987) argue that "the scale has now tipped in favour of [its] diagnostic status" but at the same time they point out that patients with borderline personality disorder may well also fulfil the criteria for other personality disorders. The gibe recorded by Kaplan & Sadock (1981) that borderline personality disorder is the personality disorder which decided not to specialise, deserves repetition. The same authors also point out that the condition is rarely made in patients aged over 40 which suggests that it might reflect immaturity of some sort.

The diagnostic criteria seem as though they might well describe a number of psychologically troubled adolescents, particularly those with a decreased tolerance for stress and a relative inability to regulate strong emotions. Such a parallel is reinforced by the developmental views of writers like Kernberg (1975); borderline patients continue to use primitive defences such as splitting which ordinary people grow out of. Similarly, they are prone to the use

Table 7.3 Diagnostic criteria for borderline personality disorder (DSM-III-R)

A pervasive pattern of instability of mood, interpersonal relationships, and self-image, beginning by early adulthood and present in a variety of contexts, as indicated by at least *five* of the following:

1. a pattern of unstable and intense interpersonal relationships, characterised by alternating between extremes of overidealisation and devaluation

2. impulsiveness in at least two areas that are potentially self-damaging, e.g. spending, sex, substance use, shoplifting, reckless driving, binge eating (do not include suicidal or self-mutilating behaviour)

3. affective instability: marked shifts from base-line mood to depression, irritability, or anxiety usually lasting a few hours and only rarely more than a few days

4. inappropriate, intense anger or lack of control of anger, e.g. frequent displays of temper, constant anger, recurrent physical fights

5. recurrent suicidal threats, gestures or behaviour or self-mutilating behaviour

6. marked and persistent identity disturbance manifested by uncertainty about at least two of the following: self-image, sexual orientation, long-term goals or career choice, type of friends desired, preferred values

7. chronic feelings of emptiness or boredom

8. frantic efforts to avoid real or imagined abandonment (do not include suicidal or self-mutilating behaviour).

of dichotomous categorisation such as dividing people into all-good and all-bad. Once again, this is common amongst disturbed teenagers.

The emphasis within the DSM-III-R criteria upon impulsivity and poor control of risk-taking behaviour, upon identity disturbance, and upon the chronic sense of emptiness and boredom with a fear of being left alone, similarly evoke ideas of disturbed adolescents. The more clinical accounts of borderline personality (see e.g. Hartocollis 1977) stress the argumentative, demanding, dismissive attitude that so-called borderline patients often exhibit. Once again, the parallels with disturbed adolescents are striking. These are not echoes of adolescence itself since emotional turmoil is not a universal adolescent phenomenon but the general description of the borderline state will do well for a crude generalisation as to how the non-specifically disturbed adolescent is likely to behave under stress or in crisis.

Since a number of adolescents with psychiatric disorders or adjustment reactions viewed as "turmoil" will develop healthy personalities there would appear to be good reasons for avoiding the use of the term "borderline personality disorder" when an adolescent is being considered. Just as with a number of other personality disorder categories which stress interpersonal problems, particularly dependence–independence issues and socialisation, what constitutes pathological disturbance in adulthood does so by virtue of its persistence over time since adolescence. The fact that adolescents are, of necessity, immature in terms of interpersonal relationships, the development of a robust self-system, and affective control means that they will, when upset or struggling socially, adopt immature coping strategies, manifest immature defences, suffer instabilities of mood and identity, and irritate their associates or doctors. Their personality functioning may be inadequate or maladaptive but to label it as personality disorder (in the conventional sense which implies chronicity) may be premature and is best avoided in order to prevent self-fulfilling prophecy. Such a conservative approach may also spare a number of adolescents the consequences of psychopharmacological enthusiasm bred by reports such as that of Goldberg et al (1986) claiming that adults with borderline personality disorder benefit from low-dose neuroleptics. The developing personality of the adolescent requires education and counselling rather than medication. Although it is admittedly not beyond possibility that the latter might facilitate the former and make maturation easier for some troubled teenagers there seem to be no grounds for advocating this in the absence of specific studies.

Schizoid personality disorder and Asperger's syndrome

Wolff & Chick (1980) demonstrated the stability from childhood through to adult life of a personality pattern which they described as schizoid. There is little doubt about the reliability of such a finding but there has been some debate about the terms used. Elsewhere, Wolff makes it clear that she used the term because it was in wide use in adult psychiatry but that the children and adolescents she described were "identical in all respects to those described by Asperger" (Wolff & Barlow 1979) and would thus be described by many as having Asperger's syndrome (Tantam 1988, Wing 1981). The trouble with the former label is that, to many clinicians, it hints at a predisposition to schizophrenia which is unproven. Difficulties arise with the latter term since, although most clinicians would use Asperger's syndrome to refer to mild autistic impairment, the children originally described by

Asperger (1944) were to all intents and purpose identical to those described by Kanner (1943), even though Asperger has subsequently protested that they were different.

As generally used, the term "Asperger's syndrome" refers to people who:

— are unable to empathise with others and lack emotional warmth

— are didactic and inflexible in their social encounters, lacking much capacity for give-and-take or turn-taking in conversation and being unable to grasp intuitively the unspoken rules of social interaction

— use stilted, pompous, grammatically correct speech which lacks inflection and metaphor

— lack much capacity for abstract conceptual thought and sophisticated humour

— are wooden and gauche in body posture and gait

— have hypertrophied and dominating special interests of a categorical or mechanical kind which cannot easily be shared

— lack friends.

Individuals who possess such characteristics may sometimes have a past history of autism and the prevailing mainstream view is that the condition is linked to autism, conceivably on a continuum (Wing 1988). Some have a developmental history of early speech acquisition, attachment behaviour and imaginative play which would rule out typical autism, yet close enquiry often reveals that the nature of childhood speech and play were constrained and stereotypic whilst the attachments were mainly directed to objects rather than people. Perhaps the most sensible strategy is to assume that the overall syndrome can be seen as a particular sub-group within schizoid personality, which may arise out of a childhood picture of autism which has attenuated with maturation or as a mild form of autism in which individuals are licked rather than bitten by the fundamental impairments of that handicap.

Such adolescents need to have their shortcomings treated with respect. Too commonly they are pressurised into a level of social participation which is beyond them and which is alarming. Wolff

& Chick (1980) draw attention to a high rate of suicide attempts and I know of one successful suicidal bid by a teenager with Asperger's syndrome who left a note saying "I know I'm weird and I guess I always will be" after his school had, with the best of intentions, made him a monitor for his class. The least that psychiatrists can do for such unfortunate teenagers is advise their parents that what is manifest in behaviour is the result of a handicap and to refrain from trying to treat with medication or intrusive psychotherapy. It may be important to stress that the condition is not schizophrenia though, of course, there is no reason why affected individuals might not develop schizophrenia and a very few do (see Wolff & Chick, 1980).

REFERENCES

Asperger H 1944 Die autistischen Psychopathen im Kindesalter. Archiv für Psychiatrie 117: 76–137
Baumrind D 1975 Early socialization and adolescent competence. In: Dragastin S E, Elder G H (eds) Adolescence in the Life Cycle. Halsted Press, London
Berger M 1985 Temperament and individual differences. In: Rutter M, Hersov L (eds) Child and Adolescent Psychiatry: Modern Approaches. Blackwell Scientific, Oxford
Coopersmith S 1967 The Antecedents of Self-Esteem. W H Freeman, San Francisco
Garmezy N 1984 Stress-resistant children: the search for protective factors. In: Stevenson J (ed) Recent Research in Developmental Psychopathology (Journal of Child Psychology and Psychiatry Monograph No. 4) Pergamon, Oxford
Goldberg S C, Schulz S C, Schultz P M, Resnick R J, Hamer R M, Friedel R O 1986 Borderline and schizotypal personality disorders treated with low dose thiothixene vs placebo. Archives of General Psychiatry 43: 680–686
Graham P, Rutter M, George S 1973 Temperamental traits as predictors of behavior disorders in children. American Journal of Orthopsychiatry 43: 328–339
Hartocollis P (ed) 1977 Borderline Personality Disorders. International Universities Press, New York
Kanner L 1943 Autistic disturbances of affective contact. Nervous Child 2: 217–250
Kaplan H I, Sadock B J 1981 Modern Synopsis of Comprehensive Textbook of Psychiatry. III. Williams and Wilkins, Baltimore
Kernberg O F 1975 Borderline Conditions and Pathological Narcissism. Jason Aronson, New York
Lewis A 1974 Psychopathic personality: a most elusive category. Psychological Medicine 4: 133–140
Mann A H, Jenkins R, Cutting J C, Cowen P J 1981 The development and use of a standardised assessment of abnormal personality. Psychological Medicine 11: 839–847
Plomin R, Dunn J (eds) 1986 The Study of Temperament: Changes, Continuities and Challenges. Lawrence Erlbaum, Hillsdale N J

Porter R, Collins G M (Eds) 1982 Temperamental Differences in Infants and Young Children. Pitman, London

Rutter M 1987 Temperament, personality and personality disorder. British Journal of Psychiatry 150: 443–458

Rutter M, Birch H, Thomas A, Chess S 1964 Temperamental characteristics in infancy and later development of behavioural disorders. British Journal of Psychiatry 110: 651–661

Selman R L 1976 Social-cognitive understanding: a guide to educational and clinical practice. In: Lickona T (ed) Moral Development and Behavior. Holt, Rinehart and Winston, New York

Steinberg D 1983 The Clinical Psychiatry of Adolescence. Wiley, Chichester

Sullivan C, Grant M Q, Grant J D 1957 The development of interpersonal maturity: applications to delinquency. Psychiatry 20: 373–385

Tantam D 1988 Asperger's syndrome. Journal of Child Psychology and Psychiatry (in press).

Tarnopolsky A, Berelowitz M 1987 Borderline personality: a review of recent research. British Journal of Psychiatry 151: 724–734

Thomas A, Chess S 1977 Temperament and Development. Brunner/Mazel, New York

Tyrer P, Alexander J 1979 Classification of personality disorder. British Journal of Psychiatry 135: 163–167

Tyrer P, Strauss J, Cichetti D 1983 Temporal reliability of personality in psychiatric patients. Psychological Medicine 13: 393–398

Widiger T A, Frances A 1985 The DSM-III personality disorders. Archives of General Psychiatry 42: 615–623

Wing L 1981 Asperger's syndrome: a clinical account. Psychological Medicine 11: 115–129

Wing L 1988 The continuum of autistic characteristics. In: Schopler E, Mesibov G B (eds) Diagnosis and Assessment in Autism. Plenum, New York (in Press).

Wolff S 1984 The concept of personality disorder in childhood. Journal of Child Psychology and Psychiatry 25: 5–13

Wolff S, Barlow A 1979 Schizoid personality in childhood. Journal of Child Psychology and Psychiatry 20: 29–46

Wolff S, Chick J 1980 Schizoid personality in childhood: a controlled follow-up study. Psychological Medicine 10: 85–100

8

Antisocial behaviour

The teenager who is troubling to others by virtue of his anti-social behaviour is likely to be insufficiently socialised. This is not always true in its simplest sense since antisocial behaviour can reflect socialisation to inappropriate standards or arise from emotional conflict and distress, but it is a useful rule of thumb to assume that an antisocial teenager is effectively suffering from a deficit state: insufficient or inappropriate knowledge or practice in how to respond to boredom, challenge, impulse, temptation, or an invitation to offend.

Acquiring socially approved behaviours, attitudes and standards is essentially a process of learning which is therefore based upon the experience of the individual person. It is ultimately dependent upon environmental factors yet these do not exert blanket effects to which everyone reacts similarly. Individuals differ, one from another, and the ways in which they do so will interact with elements in their environment to yield different personal experiences. They may elicit different reactions from those around them, may interpret these reactions differently and may learn different responses. Some individual differences are largely constitutional in origin, others are themselves the product of experiences, but in most instances it is hard to draw a clear distinction between the two: each modifies the impact and expression of the other.

A simple rebuke from a female teacher addressed to an adolescent boy will, for example, impinge according to such variables as:

— the expectations the boy has of the adult, whether he likes and respects her and whether he desires her approval

— the context within which the rebuke is delivered: a generally warm and supportive relationship or a cold, hostile one

— the stage of development of the boy: his dependency, his understanding of social roles

— previous experience: whether there has been a long history of such remonstrances or whether this is the first

— how the boy copes with the criticism and preserves his self-esteem.

Some individual differences will make certain experiences more likely. Teenagers with "difficult" temperamental profiles are more likely to elicit negative reactions from parents; those adolescents with specific learning disabilities are likely to be exposed to more experiences of failure. Experience is also compounded by the effects of previous experience through such mechanisms as conditioning and internalisation, or by way of indirect pathways such as the manner in which repeated failure and criticism can damage self-esteem and lead to a reluctance to expose oneself to the risk of further disappointment. The establishment of vicious spirals wherein individual vulnerability and social environment mutually exacerbate each other's deficits is familiar clinically. It means that it is pointless to espouse simple models which select either nature or nurture, rearing or genetics even though these will always have a ready appeal to the inexperienced or the intellectually slothful. The process of social maturation is one of complex and subtle interaction. It is lifelong: the business of becoming a contributing member of society does not begin or end during the teenage years. Nevertheless the pace accelerates dramatically during adolescence after the comparative lull of middle childhood as the teenager emancipates himself from the family controls previously established and maintained since toddlerhood. Many antisocial adolescents have been somewhat troublesome children but the impact of adolescence is to dilute parental supervision, increase exposure to alternative standards and attitudes, and magnify the effect of aggressive behaviour. This may be contained by continuing socialisation or it may not.

There is a confusing overlap between the terms used to describe the end-result of failed socialisation. "Juvenile delinquency" refers to law-breaking behaviour, usually recognised by detection rather than self-report so that delinquents are those who have been found guilty in a court of law. "Conduct disorder" is a psychiatric disorder characterised by an excess of behaviours which give rise to social disapproval and which is associated with significant suffering or with impairment of personal functioning. For practical purposes, the suffering should be located within the adolescent since antisocial behaviour is likely to give rise to suffering in others in any case. Conduct disorder in adolescence is frequently an extension of childhood antisocial behaviour. It is a common psychiatric diagnosis but only affects a minority of teenagers and a minority of delinquents. Since not all antisocial behaviour is illegal, it is possible to be diagnosed as having a conduct disorder without being delinquent. As a criterion for the diagnosis is the presence of excessive antisocial behaviour, this would not include most delinquents since the defining characteristic of that group is offending, not in itself necessarily excessively antisocial. To be termed an "aggressive psychopath", an individual has to possess a handicapping disorder of personality. Some recidivist delinquents and some cases of conduct disorder may fall into such a category but most will not.

Juvenile delinquency

Juvenile delinquency — law-breaking behaviour by young people — is common though typically undetected. All of the 1425 London boys interviewed confidentially by Belson (1968, 1975) admitted to stealing at some point in their past. Information obtained by confidential self-report is difficult to validate and many self-report schedules include a number of rather minor offences such as travelling on public transport without a ticket and vandalism. Nevertheless, in Belson's study, those boys who privately claimed most offences were also those who were most likely to be convicted and West & Farrington (1973, 1977) noted that boys with the highest criminal involvement according to self-report were also those who were nominated by their peers as most criminal. These findings provide indirect validation that delinquent acts are widespread among urban teenage boys yet do not usually result in conviction (see Hindelang et al 1979 for a review).

If law-breaking behaviour is widespread, how is it that a number of studies demonstrate a difference between delinquents and so-called normals? The answer is in two parts. Firstly, those delinquents that have been studied are official delinquents; they have been convicted. Consider the steps involved in becoming an official delinquent. An offence is committed but the perpetrator may not be caught. If caught, he may not be taken to the police. The police may take no further action in any case, or they may hand the boy over to his parents or the social services. Similarly, a formal caution may mean that the boy never reaches court. Even if the case does go to court, only a conviction will result in the boy entering the statistics as an official delinquent. In spite of such attrition, some 20–30% of urban male teenagers will be convicted during their teens (see West 1982). In general, these will be the most criminally active but other forms of selection operate at each stage of the process. Offences such as breaking and entering or assault are more likely to result in conviction than others such as vandalism. Factors such as the area the offence was committed in, behaviour when caught, dress, race, previous contact with the police and so on all affect the chances of being charged and convicted.

This does not mean that official delinquents are no different from their counterparts in the general population. They are more likely to exhibit non-criminal antisocial behaviours such as lying, more likely to smoke, drink excessively, take drugs, gamble heavily, and get into more fights or behave aggressively to others (West 1982, West & Farrington 1977). Their family and social circumstances, detailed below, are also different from those of a non-convicted group. Bias in the processing of offenders is real enough but does not overwhelm the fact that various important individual, family and social factors are associated with official delinquency as causes and correlates. The term delinquency is henceforth used here as shorthand for official (convicted) delinquency.

The second part of the answer as to why delinquents are different from unconvicted teenagers hinges upon the phenomenon of recidivism. One-half of all convicted delinquents are never convicted again and, of those that are, half will only be convicted once more. Only a minority will re-offend repeatedly and receive several convictions; they are recidivists. The correlates of delinquency apply most strongly to this group and they are likely to manifest signs of psychological disturbance and psychiatric disorder (Stott & Wilson 1977). Almost certainly, it is the presence within any sample of delinquents of a recidivist minority which has the greatest effect upon the mean of any measured characteristic of the group. As far as can be demonstrated, once-only offenders occupy a half-way position between normals and recidivists on any measure. They differ rather little from normality and are not usually of great interest to psychiatrists. Recidivists, however, are quite commonly deviant in a number of characteristics and merit psychiatric interest, even though delinquency is a socio-legal category and in no way a psychiatric disorder.

Juvenile delinquency, across the board, is nevertheless a considerable social problem. One-half of all indictable (serious) crime is committed by individuals aged between 10 and 21, and in large cities about one boy in four will be convicted during those years, usually between the ages of 14 and 18. Although about one-quarter of offenders will go on to more than two convictions, most criminal careers peter out by about age 25 (see West 1982).

The contribution of psychiatry to the management of the problem is largely in the area of research and in providing consultation to the social agencies which process delinquents. In order to assist with the latter, some understanding of aetiology is required and is dealt with here under three main headings: social, family, and individual factors.

Social factors

There are two principal disciplines, sociology and criminology, involved in the study of how social elements might create delinquency. Sociology has primarily considered social processes, three of which have been well articulated in association with delinquency.

a) Identification with a subculture or group.

Local or peer-group attitudes and standards of behaviour might be at variance with national legal standards and sanction behaviour which is technically illegal but does not infringe local mores. According to Mays (1954), the characteristic life-style of those living in Liverpool dockland sanctions shoplifting, theft from shipping consignments, fare-dodging on public transport, and fighting in the street as normal teenage activities wherein local adolescents might discover excitement and prestige in the eyes of their mates.

Such a notion is plausible but there remains the difficulty of demonstrating that identification with so-called subcultural standards is a cause rather than an effect of delinquency. It is not clear that all dockland inhabitants in Mays' study would sanction such delinquent activities; within a community there might be various subcultures, including a delinquent one. The latter might be formed by delinquents rather than forming them. Given the phenomenon of delinquency areas (see below), individual delinquents are likely to live near each other. Male adolescents characteristically form small friendship groups and delinquents, it is well known, are also likely to commit crime in small groups. In a review of the evidence, Hirschi (1969) concluded that delinquent activities affected a young person's choice of friends rather than vice versa, a view consonant with the conclusion of Duck (1973): close friends serve to validate one's own point of view. It becomes possible to see how a local delinquent subculture might perpetuate delinquency by allowing certain illegal activities but it is not quite so clear how it might provoke them in the first place. General experience of delinquents suggests that it is peer-group activities rather than standards which can precipitate antisocial behaviour in vulnerable individuals: those who cannot control their impulsiveness, who crave excitement or esteem, or who lack the social skills needed to oppose the group's choice of delinquent activity. The aetiological mechanism becomes imitation of behaviour rather than identification with standards. This is consonant with the developmental observation that in early adolescence a friendship group is formed by individuals who share the same activities and precedes by several years the formation of a group by seeking out like-minded individuals as friends: the phenomenon of associating with people who like doing the same things together comes a few years before the search for like-minded friends with whom one can identify.

Irrespective of how delinquency might be initiated, there are grounds for thinking that preferential association with delinquents can perpetuate antisocial behaviour, since West & Farrington (1977) found that breaking off relationships with delinquent friends appeared to be a factor in terminating a delinquent career. The isolated power of group influences in determining delinquency does not appear to be great in that Jensen (1972) found that parental discipline had an association with delinquency independent of relationships within the peer group. This may reflect the difficulty which many recidivists have in establishing and maintaining the close relationships with others which would support identification with them. Typically the delinquent's peer group is a shifting collection of acquaintances with immature social development: not the most conducive setting for the learning of internalised standards.

b) Alienation of the individual from the wider social group

Bitterness, envy or protest may cause an individual adolescent to repudiate official values. Such a mechanism is less prone to the criticism of identification offered above since it hinges less upon personal relationships, hardly the strongest area of personal development as far as delinquents are concerned. If an adolescent feels prohibited from involvement in a successful materialistic culture on account of unemployment, class or racial discrimination, or poverty, he may set himself against the culture which allows such discrimination and oppose its restrictive legislation. Alternatively he may feel it appropriate to turn to crime in order to gain the things which society encourages him to desire without providing the means for him to obtain them.

However, Rutter & Giller (1983) provide a brief, damning critique of such a theory, pointing out (1) that high aspirations in working-class youths do not lead to delinquency, (2) that most delinquent boys become law-abiding adults, (3) the lack of a sufficiently strong association between social class and delinquency. To this might be added the fact that some racial groups may be discriminated against yet yield remarkably few delinquents: the Jews are an obvious example. Furthermore, alienation theories which might apply readily to minor antisocial acts such as scrumping or writing graffiti on walls cannot explain why most victims of serious crime in high delinquency areas are the poor and the elderly.

c) Labelling

Labelling theory assumes that attributing a "delinquent" label to an individual defines an identity and fosters future antisocial behaviour by a process of encouraging self-confirmation in that role. Some support for the relevance of this comes from Farrington's work (Farrington 1977, Farrington et al 1978). Boys with high and low levels of delinquent activity revealed by self-report at the age of 14 were re-examined at age 18 on self-report scores. Those who had, in the meantime, been found guilty in court increased their scores. Not appearing in court was associated with a fall in self-reported crime. Other variables such as family background could not be found to explain this difference.

Once again, the power of an explanatory sociological hypothesis lies in explaining the maintenance or escalation of antisocial behaviour rather than original causation. It may also, in this instance, reflect a paucity of alternative, more positive, roles available to the more advantaged (socially and personally) adolescent, a situation which may change for the better through employment (if available) and the development of closer personal ties (West & Farrington 1977); labelling can operate beneficially too. One problem is in ascertaining the magnitude of the effect: studies which yield empirical support for the labelling hypothesis in other areas of social development are extremely sparse. Rutter & Giller (1983), having examined such studies, concluded that the effects of labelling are substantially weaker and less widely applicable than often assumed.

Delinquency areas

The second major discipline involved in the study of social and economic factors associated with delinquency is criminology which has historically made a particular contribution by the study of the way in which ecological variables, measured in objective terms, covary with crime rates. Prominent among such work is the concept of delinquency areas (see Baldwin 1975).

Studies in North America and the UK have repeatedly confirmed that certain geographical areas consistently have higher rates of crime than others, whatever kind of delinqency is sampled. The prevalence of delinquent activity is highest in overcrowded, urban industrial areas with inferior housing, over-crowding, and poor facilities for recreation. High unemployment, poor educational achievement, and indices of poor health are also typical of such areas. Delinquency rates differ between city boroughs, between electoral wards within boroughs (Power et al 1972) and between streets (Jephcott & Carter 1954). Such differences are remarkably stable over time. Wallis & Maliphant (1967) found a significant correlation between their findings on delinquency rates in different areas of London and the figures reported by Burt (1925), forty years earlier.

Why all this should be so cannot be answered simply. Clearly there are potential artefacts: most of the differences between Nottingham streets in Jephcott & Carter's (1954) study could be accounted for by the activities of members of a few families. But area rates which are stable over decades are unlikely only to reflect the criminal habits of certain families, especially since discontinuities between generations in a family outweigh continuities (Rutter & Madge 1976). Nor are the variations in practice which bias police activity according to where the crime was committed (Landau 1981) sufficient to account for such enduring area differences. Physical dilapidation in its own right is an inadequate explanation (Rutter & Madge 1976) though the plausible suggestion has been made that in high delinquency areas there are opportunities for crime presented by untended business premises and unsupervised warehouses, the fabric of which allows for undetected entry with minimal force (Mayhew et al 1976). Similarly, a lack of alternative local recreational facilities may facilitate antisocial activities as an alternative source of excitement; certainly their absence correlates with a high rate of delinquency (Central Policy Review Staff 1978).

Family factors clearly interact with the material circumstances within which families live. Poverty does not appear to exert a direct influence upon delinquency but compromises adequate family functioning through factors such as overcrowding which can affect family relationships, disciplinary practices, supervision of children, and parental health, all of which link with delinquency and psychiatric problems among adolescents. High delinquency rates in an area correlate with high rates of parental depression and psychiatric disorder in children and adolescents (Gath et al 1975). The association between delinquency and psychiatric disorder in an individual adolescent applies principally to recidivists. Curiously enough there is no focussed work on the prevalence of recidivists in particular within delinquency areas. Selective migration of families into or out of such areas does not seem to be a substantial element (Rutter & Madge 1976).

It has been shown that schools have an independent effect upon the social development of their pupils and that particular schools can have a high or low rate of delinquency among their pupils, independent of which area they are drawn from (Power et al 1967) or how they are selected at entry (Rutter et al 1979).

The effects exerted upon pupils' behaviour seem to be mediated by the way in which the school operates as a social institution rather than as a function of its physical characteristics (Hargreaves 1967, Rutter et al 1979). Relationships between staff and pupils are highly significant in this and such relationships would, on common-sense grounds, appear to be dependent upon the qualities of the staff. Since it is well known that inner-city schools have chronic problems in recruiting and keeping staff and that schools with high delinquency rates suffer from high staff turnover (Rutter et al 1979), it is at least possible that a lack of relevant staff expertise may play a part in fostering delinquency among school-age adolescents.

The effect of the local peer group and prevailing subculture has been discussed above. It seems to be evident that ecological factors are not direct causal influences in their own right. They are elements which facilitate or impede socialisation processes, orthodox or deviant, which are themselves dependent upon personal interaction and individual vulnerabilities. Not all adolescents within a high-delinquency area or in a high-delinquency school are delinquents; other influences within the family and the individual are significant.

Family factors

Delinquency runs in families. For instance, young offenders are at least twice as likely to have a criminal father as non-offenders. If both parents have criminal records, about 60% of their sons will be delinquent (West & Farrington 1973). The strongest association is with delinquency in brothers (Ferguson 1952).

What mechanism might be involved? A genetic contribution is speculative. Parents with criminal records appear usually to have abandoned their criminal careers before bringing their sons up (West & Farrington 1973) so that setting a bad example seems unlikely. Nor do such parents hold unorthodox moral views: they appear to deplore delinquency in their offspring and indeed may punish it vigorously. They are not the culture carriers for illegal sub-cultural standards.

It is possible that criminal parents transmit attitudes to property or violence by more subtle means than direct instructions or sanction. Most clinicians have met families wherein parental anti-authoritarian views have been handed down to the children. This may be direct ("Don't let them put you down, son") or covert, as when parents experience vicarious satisfaction from a son's abusive attack upon his teachers.

> Gary, 14, was in perpetual trouble for attacking his teachers at school and had been suspended several times. On each occasion he was punished, his father marched up to the school and, in his own words, "sorted things out" with the teachers involved. More than once this resulted in an exchange of blows. Father, who appeared to have a reading disability, felt very bitter about his own childhood experience of schooling. Whilst mildly censorious towards Gary — "You really shouldn't do that sort of thing" — his own behaviour towards the school on each occasion conveyed a different message. When describing how Gary had vigorously abused a particular teacher both parents became quite excited "She really asked for that . . . . . . and he gave it to her, good and proper. She won't do that again in a hurry . . . . . ."

The teenager's conscience may be patchy as a result of parents giving mixed messages about the desirability or otherwise of an activity, probably reflecting their own confusion about it.

> Mrs K., a single parent, was at a loss to know how to control her 15-year-old son's stealing. He did not steal from home but was repeatedly caught breaking into offices and pilfering from neighbours. She punished him on each occasion and nagged him about it continually but it made no difference, he seemed to have no compunction about helping himself to other people's property. She had two past convictions for shoplifting and a current habit of stealing plants from the rock garden in her local park, though she was convinced her son knew nothing of these misdemeanours. She defended her activities stoutly to the clinic staff: "The Council can afford it; I'm a ratepayer; nobody gets to know anyway . . . ."

An excellent description of such a phenomenon in terms of "super-ego lacunae" was offered by Adelaide Johnson (1949). Rather similarly, a parent's energy in proscribing an activity may stimulate curiosity in the youngster.

> Karen, the 16-year-old illegitimate only daughter of young Miss N, had been subjected to several years of warnings and exhortations not to "mess around with boys". Her mother was concerned that Karen should not fall pregnant in her turn as she had done herself. The strength and vehemence of Miss N's warnings excited Karen's interest in matters sexual yet her mother's prohibitive attitude made it impossible for her to discuss sex with her daughter. At the same time, sex provided a way for Karen of getting back at her mother for what seemed like unreasonable restrictions on party-going and the like. Karen was pregnant by a casual encounter before she left school.

The extent of such mechanisms is unstudied. They appear common to the clinician, though this may result from a non-psychiatric agency judging that such interactions are amenable to family therapy and referring accordingly. Almost certainly they overlap with what might be termed poor parenting. This pejorative term is intended to encompass a number of shortcomings or stresses well documented in the classic studies of Glueck & Glueck (1950) and McCord & McCord (1959):

— inconsistent discipline, either between parents or by one parent from one time to another

— over-harsh punishment, particularly in a context of a cold or aloof relationship between child and parent

— poor supervision of the teenager's activities by parents.

Quite clearly these overlap with each other, combining to compromise effective social training. Poor supervision results in fewer opportunities for parents to teach clear rules or coping strategies whether by instruction, example, or reward and punishment. Inconsistency in parental responses is confusing to the child and its very inefficacy breeds increasingly coercive behaviours on both the parents' and the adolescent's part. These yield acrimony and resentment, a climate in which identification with parental moral standards becomes strained and self-esteem threatened. In consequence the development of the ability to resist temptation and postpone gratification is retarded. Given suitable opportunities, delinquency is likely.

A number of studies have demonstrated a link between family size (more than four children) and delinquency. The possible significance of this is complex. Children from large families are also likely to have poor educational achievement and low IQ scores (Douglas et al 1968). This may reflect the association between large family size and social disadvantage: poor families are larger and delinquency increases with poverty. It also compounds any effect of overcrowding, the two going hand in hand. Clearly a large number of children will exacerbate either effect. Parents whose abilities to socialise their children are already undermined by preoccupations about money, unemployment or physical child care are at risk of being overwhelmed by having to cope with the demands of a large family. The usual parental response of delegating child care to the older children means that the calibre of parenting is further diminished whilst imposing extra demands on the older siblings. For any single child within the family, parental time and attention is curtailed. There are few opportunities for parents to involve themselves in promoting moral development by reasoning and induction (Kohlberg 1976) or teaching negotiating skills (Kifer et al 1974) or generally instructing their offspring in "sober strategies in coping with frustration" (Davitz 1952).

The association between broken homes, or prolonged separation from parents, and delinquency has been known for years. Behind the clarity of these findings, the mechanisms are less straightforward. Protracted separation from parents from an early age can impair attachment and the formation of affectional bonds with parental figures. This impairs socialisation for a variety of reasons: personal identification with the standards and behaviour of an adult is less likely; multiple caretakers in a children's home are more likely to be inconsistent one with another, supervision may be attenuated within an institution and so forth. A teenager from a home riven with acrimonious dispute may be removed from home at a late age because the family falls apart. In such circumstances it is likely that it is the discord preceding the broken home which is culpable.

A number of studies and reviews have made this latter view the reigning orthodoxy: that it is openly discordant relationships within the family rather than "broken homes" *per se* which breed antisocial behaviour (Rutter & Madge 1976). They may do this by creating inconsistencies in parental handling, by providing unsatisfactory models for conflict and resolution, by creating fear and resentment in the child, by encouraging triangulation or scapegoating of children, by souring relations between parent and child leading to harshness, rejection or resentment; and by generally preventing the conditions for the teenager to acquire appropriate self-esteem and social training.

Thus it has been shown that intra-familial discord without parental separation is also associated with antisocial behaviour (McCord & McCord 1959) and that separation from a parent by death is not nearly so strongly linked with it (Rutter 1966). It is important for the psychiatrist involved with adolescents to have a thorough understanding of attachment formation, though this is not considered further here since it is a topic central to child psychiatry (see Heard 1987, Hill 1986) and discussed at length by Bowlby (1969, 1973, 1980) and Rutter (1981).

Moving from a simple statement that broken homes cause delinquency to a more refined position which examines the effects of impaired attachment formation and of discordant family relationships is a clear advance. It seems likely though that other variables will still need to be evaluated, complicating the picture further. Substitute parental care varies widely: some children's homes appear effective at inculcating empathy, altruism and restraint in their charges, others less so. The experience of divorce itself has an emotional impact upon the children involved (Wallerstein & Kelly 1980) which can express itself in antisocial activity. Even bereavement, although not strongly implicated in the aetiology of delinquency in general can, in the individual child, precipitate delinquent behaviour.

> At the age of 16, Daniel lost his father through an unexpected brain haemorrhage. Over the next three days he became increasingly unstable with outbursts of tempestuous anger. Finally he took a 15lb hammer from his father's garage and, without explanation, wandered into town. On his way he demolished a sundial in a public ornamental garden, smashed a shop window and was heading for the hospital where his father had been taken to when he was picked up by the police. When seen later he was clearly extremely distressed but unable to put anything into words, literally speechless with grief.

Nevertheless such reactions are rare. More commonly a view may be taken which represents the family of the delinquent as failing in his socialisation rather than directly provoking antisocial behaviour. Such families lack resources and compound their own shortcomings by attempts to compensate which are themselves maladaptive: an escalation from verbal reprimand to harsh physical punishment is an instance. For the family as well as the individual, a notion of criminal behaviour (in the parental generation) as an expression of social incompetence also expressed in poor parenting is intrinsic. Criminal parents are also likely to drink excessively, have poor work records and high reliance on social welfare (Knight & West 1977), factors which associate with delinquency in the children even in the absence of parental criminality (Robins & Lewis 1966). Inadequacy in one social area is paralleled by inadequacy in another. Even the effects of discord may be seen as a consequence of failure to establish adequate boundaries between, for example, the marriage and the parent/child subsystems. Or harsh recrimination between parent and child may represent a shortcoming in parental empathy for a more immature personality.

Nor are there social shortcomings only within the family. Wahler (1976) has pointed out that the families of antisocial teenagers are also likely to be isolated within their own communities, so cutting themselves off further from community resources. That they may also frustrate the efforts of welfare agencies to assist them is also well recognised, the reasons for doing so similarly resting more on immaturity and incompetence than on malice.

Individual factors

No theory of delinquency can rely wholly on social factors. An idea of interaction between individual predisposition and social variables is necessary to account for the fact that not all young persons in a high delinquency area are delinquents.

Furthermore, longitudinal studies (e.g. Conger & Miller 1966, West & Farrington 1973) have demonstrated that many boys who became delinquent in adolescence could be identified during primary school by their teachers. At that stage they were more disobedient, aggressive, quarrelsome and likely to truant — different behaviours from those which later resulted in their conviction. It is important to note the discontinuities: most children with such behavioural abnormalities do not become delinquent and a little less than half of all delinquents exhibited such behavioural deviance when younger. Somewhat similarly, hyperactive children in Weiss et al's (1985) follow-up study were substantially at risk for becoming delinquent though most did not officially offend and most delinquents have not been hyperactive children.

Examining the differences between delinquents and non-delinquents yields but little useful information. Most delinquents are male. As a group their intelligence and academic achivements tend to be a little lower (West & Farrington 1973) and their impulsiveness higher (Riddle & Roberts 1977) than their non-delinquent counterparts. Such differences are small — e.g. IQ 90–95 as an average for delinquents as a whole — and there is substantial overlap with a non-delinquent population.

It is likely that such unpromising findings reflect the fact that delinquency is common and that half of all delinquents are single offenders. In all probability these once-only offenders are rather ordinary youngsters from a psychiatric point of view. Certainly that clinical impression is borne out by findings such as that of

Stott & Wilson (1977): that the number of repeated convictions for delinquency correlates proportionally with "personal maladjustment". Douglas et al. (1968) found lower levels of measured intelligence among recidivists than among single offenders. Similarly, Riddle & Roberts (1977) found increased impulsiveness among recidivists. The suggestion is that it is recidivists within a delinquent population which affect the group average scores on such variables.

Genetic factors

In comparable vein, although studies have shown little genetic effect for juvenile delinquency as a whole (McGuffin & Gottesman 1985), there is evidence that a genetic predisposition to adult crime can operate (Crowe 1974, Hutchings & Mednick 1974). The rate of recidivism in adult crime is self-evidently higher than among the young: adults have been at it for for longer and are well past the peak age for offending which is 15–16. It is quite likely that much of the crime committed by individuals in both adult studies cited was perpetrated when they were teenagers, since it was indictable crimes which were studied and these are more prevalent among a teenage population. If so, such studies would suggest that a significant genetic element might operate for recidivist juvenile delinquency but not for once-only offenders. Since the latter are by far and away the most numerous the general statement that there is no important genetic basis underlying juvenile delinquency as a whole still stands.

Studies of X and Y chromosome abnormalities among juvenile offenders have generally shown little of significance. A few delinquents will show such abnormalities (Kahn et al 1969) but the numbers are far too few to draw any conclusions for delinquency as a whole. Conversely, prospective studies of XXY and XYY children show the vast majority to be law abiding during adolescence (Gath 1985).

To start to understand what the quality is which might be genetically transmitted and predispose to recidivist delinquency, it is necessary to focus matters closer, even though the evidence is far from complete. One possibility is that inherited autonomic variables might be important. There has been considerable interest in how neurophysiological variation between individuals might impair social learning and thus produce socialisation deficits (Hare 1978). For instance, it has been recognised for some time that recidivist delinquents are likely to show impaired avoidance learning in an experimental situation (Davies & Maliphant 1974) and to exhibit generally lowered autonomic arousal as evidenced by such indicators as pulse rate (Davies & Maliphant 1971, Wadsworth 1976). Earlier attempts to explain such findings in terms of Eysenck's (1964) theory of personality — that delinquents are neurotic extroverts who score highly on "psychoticism" — have not been supported by findings (Hoghughi & Forrest 1970, West & Farrington 1973).

It can be argued (Mednick 1981) that a failure of autonomic arousal to decline rapidly will reflect a similar delay in fear subsidence. This would confuse any learned association between fear of punishment and a given punishable action; a defect in avoidance learning which will prejudice socialisation in childhood, particularly with respect to impulse control. Ordinarily, previous experience of a situation in which the child has been punished will result in anticipatory fear being experienced in the same situation. If the child decides not to do the action for which he has been previously punished, the fear will dissipate. The rapid reduction of fear provides reinforcement for the decision not to offend. Juvenile delinquents are more likely to show a slow decay of electrodermal excitation which may be taken to be an indirect indicator of fear (Hare 1978). Mednick (1981) reports a study in which the sons of criminal fathers who did not become delinquent themselves were shown to have higher intelligence and quicker electrodermal recovery than the criminal sons of criminal fathers. Similarly, the criminal sons of non-criminal fathers had remarkably slow electrodermal recovery rates, both findings being consonant with the hypothesis. Such autonomic variability is, however, not held to be the sole variable in producing delinquency, but interacts with intelligence (ability to learn) as well as family discipline: what form of censure is applied to which actions.

Studies of recidivist and incarcerated delinquents typically demonstrate a high rate of minor neurological abnormalities ("soft signs"), past head injury, specific learning disabilities and abnormal EEGs (see e.g. Lewis et al 1981). None of these individual characteristics are specific to delinquency and probably represent general vulnerabilities to psychological disorder. They are less prevalent among non-incarcerated delinquents and most medical authorities who have studied the topic have come to the conclusion that a continuum of neurological damage from normal to seriously compromised parallels a spectrum of antisocial behaviour from well-socialised to violent recidivism. Serious neurological abnormality can certainly be found in a number of delinquents but cannot account for the generality of delinquency (West 1982). There is no evidence that any specific form of neurological damage is associated with delinquency.

The general conclusion which can be drawn from studies of individual vulnerability to delinquency is that the predispositions which have been identified tend to be shortcomings and weaknesses; it is apparently not the case that delinquents possess an excess of anything which makes them offend. Rather, they seem to have an insufficiency of those attributes which would cause them to be easily socialised and resist the temptation to act carelessly, impulsively or greedily.

Moral development

The finding that delinquents as a group are morally immature (Hudgins & Prentice 1973) does not necessarily provide an explanation of delinquency in itself since it must be asked why they should be so.

There is the possibility that morality is merely one aspect of socialisation and subject to the same influences as, for instance, learning self-control. For example, Hoffman (1970) describes how parental discipline affects the development of conscience. The use by parents of power-assertive disciplinary techniques, didactic edicts and physical punishment yields, if anything, a fear of punishment following transgression without an anticipatory inhibition. Withdrawal of love is superior in producing a sense of guilt and tends to be associated conventional moral attitudes, with anxieties about the future consequences of transgression. The induction of guilt by explanation and reasoning about the consequences of actions is also powerful but the moral position so developed is more concerned with empathy and anxiety about the effects on others of the transgression.

So far, the argument suggests that the child-rearing conditions for promoting conscience and inhibiting antisocial behaviour are remarkably similar: moral development might simply be a reflection of behavioural socialisation. Moral development is not, however, merely the acquisition of attitudes as a result of

Table 8.1 Kohlberg's stages of moral development

Post-conventional
Stage 1 Avoidance of punishment, obedience to higher authority as a
consequence of its greater power.
Stage 2 Following rules only when in one's own interest; right is what is fair or
agreed.

Conventional
Stage 3 Living up to the expectations of significant others. Doing as you would
be done by. Notions of loyalty and trust.
Stage 4 Laws are to be upheld for the sake of the smooth running of society
and only to be broken in extreme instances.

Preconventional
Stage 5 Distinction between certain absolute values (life, individual liberty
etc.) and obligations entered into for the greatest good of the greatest
number according to a rational social contract.
Stage 6 Following self-chosen ethical principles, particularly those that are
seen as universally valid even when these conflict with local laws.

identification or learned contingencies. Piaget (1932) and Kohlberg (e.g. 1976) have demonstrated the importance of a cognitive
dimension, certainly as far as developing a sense of justice is
concerned. Kohlberg's scheme is illustrated in Table 8.1. Such a
model is not without its critics, though, general support for the
conceptualisation of the early stages has resulted from a number
of studies. The status of post-conventional morality is less well
supported. Gibbs (1977) has suggested that the final three stages
are parallel alternative forms of abstract moral reasoning and not
necessarily sequential stages. Weinreich-Haste (1979) has pointed
out that it is possible to divide the categories into two sets of
three stages each. Each stage progresses through authoritarian,
expedient, and compassionate levels, first on a concrete, then on
an abstract basis.

Kohlberg has essentially restricted himself to the study of
justice. Such a practice ultimately follows the demonstration by
Hartshorne & May (1928) that moral traits such as honesty
correlated poorly with each other and with themselves when
examined across different situations. In consequence, the notion
that moral virtue is a homogeneous entity has largely been abandoned by research psychologists, particularly since the experiments by Milgram (1963, 1965) showed how situational factors
can lead to outrageous acts being performed by apparently
virtuous individuals. Nevertheless, there is considerable con-
sonance between Kohlberg's model (which is essentially a model
of ego functioning, rather than super-ego derived) and those

schemes which illustrate "interpersonal" or "social perspectives" development discussed in Chapter 7.

The psychiatrist and the delinquent

Historically, antisocial behaviour in childhood has been seen to be a legitimate area of medical interest whereas similar behaviour in adulthood is understood to be a matter for the penal services. Antisocial activities in adolescence apparently occupy an intermediate position. Psychiatrists are quite commonly called upon to write reports on adolescents who seem to the courts before which they appear to be remarkable in their incorrigibility or the curious nature of their offence. In terms of quantity, the psychiatric contribution to the management of delinquency is mainly concerned with formulation, consultation and advice rather than direct treatment.

Providing advice to criminal courts in the form of reports has its own conventions; a guide to which is provided by Bebbington & Hill (1985). Some knowledge of the powers of criminal courts is required and these are summarised in Table 8.2

A most significant area of social work with young offenders in England and Wales, which has excited the interest of a number of psychiatrists, is intermediate treatment (IT). This was originally conceived as a method of dealing with delinquents without removing them fully into custody but going beyond the rather ineffectual supervision order. An intermediate treatment order can be made by a court as an addition to a supervision order and empowers a local authority social services department to remove the adolescent from home in order to take part in activity programmes for a period of up to 90 days in a three-year period. It was intended that such facilities would also be available to adolescents who were not offenders.

In practice, different local authorities have interpreted their obligations with considerable variation; a situation verging on the confused. In part this reflects a lack of a unified theoretical base (Cawson 1985), but there have also been local developments of practice towards specialised branches of IT such as intensive groupwork and vocational training. The adolescent psychiatrist needs to know what is available in terms of IT provision on his local patch and may well feel it appropriate that he be drawn into offering a consultative service to specific IT projects.

Table 8.2 The principal powers of criminal courts relevant to adolescent offenders

Discharge (all ages)
Absolute or conditional (further action to be taken if another offence committed during specified period)

Binding over (age 14 and over, or parents if under 14)
To keep the peace. Further action if breached.

Fines (all ages)
The court can also order compensation and costs.

Supervision order (up to and including 16)
A social worker or probation officer is given responsibility to "advise, assist and befriend" ordinarily by visiting and counselling for up to 3 years. Various requirements can be added:
— residence with a named individual
— treatment for a mental condition
— INTERMEDIATE TREATMENT (intermediate between supervision at home and committal to care): a range of constructive opportunities for social training, widening experience, skills development etc. provided by social service departments. Can include short spells away from home for residential courses, adventure programmes etc.

Probation order (age 17 and over)
Adult equivalent of supervision order. A probation officer offers supervision and can bring the offender back to court for non-compliance. Conditions can be added:
— residence in a probation hostel
— treatment for a mental condition

Care order (up to and including age 16)
Places a child in the care of a local authority social service department which assumes parental rights and powers. The court must be satisfied that the child is in need of care and control which would not result without the order being made, AND that one of the following applies:
— his health or development is being avoidably prevented or neglected, or he is being ill-treated
— another child in the same household is the subject of a care order for the above reason
— he is exposed to moral danger
— he is beyond parental control
— he is truanting from school
— he is guilty of a criminal offence
Once a care order is made, the decision to place the adolescent in a foster home, children's home, or CHE rests with the local authority. Care orders run until 18 unless made when the adolescent is 16, in which case they run until 19.

Community Service Order (age 16 and over)
A specified number of hours to be spent carrying out activities beneficial to the community under the supervision of the probation service. Only if local facilities exist, if the offender has not previously received a custodial sentence, and if the offence would be punishable by imprisonment.

Attendance Centre Order (age 14–20 inclusive)
For offences which merit imprisonment in adulthood. Boys spend a specified number of hours at a centre doing activities under a police supervision. Requires local facilities.

Detention Centre order (age 14–20 inclusive)

For serious offences otherwise punishable by imprisonment. A social enquiry report is required first and the boy must not have received a previous custodial sentence. Boys are sent to a residential centre with a militaristic ethos for a period of weeks for a 'short, sharp shock'.

Detention (age 14–16 inclusive)

For very serious offences. The Home Secretary decides the place of detention.

Youth custody (age 15–20 inclusive)

Replaces the old sentence of Borstal training with a fixed sentence, maximum 1 year for 15 and 16-year-olds. A social enquiry report is required.

Hospital or guardianship order (under section 37 of the Mental Health Act 1983)

Such psychiatric contributions should be separated off from the issue of psychological treatment of delinquents: an unfashionable area but one which deserves examination.

Treatment

Most delinquents will not be treated psychiatrically. For a number of years it has been the received wisdom that psychological and psychiatric approaches to delinquency are ineffective, a pendulum swing from previous optimism that psychodynamic interventions in particular would abolish the disease of crime. The pendulum appears to be about to swing back with the realisation that the process of becoming (or remaining) an official delinquent produces, and is itself subject to, psychological effects.

These are quite likely to be specific for the individual rather than true for all delinquents, so that large studies may show little effect because factors cancel each other out when the group as a whole is examined. For instance, although Farrington (1977) showed that a teenager's first appearance in court increased the likelihood of subsequent antisocial behaviour, his study paid insufficient attention to sentencing or other provisions made by the court, and these certainly can influence subsequent behaviour to such an extent that an opposite effect can be found. For instance, Berg et al (1978) demonstrated that adolescents before the court for truancy were more likely to return to school if the

111

court adjourned for a few weeks and then recalled the offender in order to test for attendance at school in the meantime than if, when first seen, the offender were made subject to a supervision order implemented by a social worker. This does not mean the latter was ineffective, merely less effective: the optimum management of truancy appears to be a combination of adjournment to test attendance coupled with counselling (see Berg 1985). The suggestion is that appearance in court may be counterproductive for some individuals but effective for others; at present there is no way of identifying which delinquents will be affected in which way.

Within the coarse provisions that may be implemented by (or as a consequence of) court action, some differential effects can be shown which depend upon variables in the staff of an institution. Reconviction rates following a spell in a residential establishment such as a CHE (community home with education on the premises) or a probation hostel can be related to staff characteristics. Good staff–pupil relationships, consistent kind firmness associated with emotional warmth, and high expectations seem significant in reducing antisocial attitudes and behaviour (Davies & Sinclair 1971, Sinclair & Clarke 1982).

A number of small-scale projects have shown that various interventions can reduce the likelihood of subsequent reconviction compared to untreated controls. For example, the Cascadia Project demonstrated the impact of cognitively-based social skills training (Sarason 1978), Persons (1967) did the same with a combination of individual and group psychotherapy, and Massimo and Shore (1963, Shore & Massimo 1973) showed an effect for a programme of vocational counselling, supportive psychotherapy and remedial education. Yet a number of studies of superficially similar interventions applied to larger samples show no effect for psychotherapy, counselling, educational provision and the like. The Provo (Empey & Erickson 1972) and Silverlake (Empey & Lubeck 1971) experiments, and the Borstal milieu study by Bottoms and McClintock (1973) are among those which showed no difference between groups given experimental and control interventions (usually traditional paternalistic residential care) as far as reconviction rates were concerned.

These negative results may in part reflect advantages in old-fashioned paternalism for some delinquents. Craft and his colleagues (1964) were able to show by a randomised study at Balderton Hospital that immature antisocial teenagers and youths of somewhat limited intelligence actually reoffended less after exposure to a paternalistic, traditional regime than those admitted to a therapeutic community. In addition, failure to show a positive result may be a consequence of poor matching between delinquent, type of intervention and type of staff. The Grants (1959), for example, demonstrated a trend for psychologically mature offenders to respond to groupwork by mature but not by immature staff, yet immature offenders could not be influenced, by groupwork, even when carried out by mature staff.

Differences between delinquents obviously matter in responses to particular treatments. For instance, it was the black rather than the white delinquent youths who responded to guided group interaction in the Highfields Project and showed lower reconviction rates on follow-up (Weeks 1958). Considering individual differences of a finer grain, the PICO Project offered incarcerated delinquents individual counselling/psychotherapy once or twice weekly for nine months. Candidates considered suitable for this treatment were verbal, intelligent, anxious and motivated to change, whereas those judged unsuitable were the converse. Although suitable candidates subsequently offended less than untreated controls, unsuitable candidates given psychotherapy actually did worse and offended more than controls on follow-up (Adams 1961).

The large study carried out for the California Youth Authority by Warren and her colleagues (Warren 1969, 1977, Palmer 1973, 1974) has only been partially reported, a regrettable fact since the key concept was the matching of delinquent and professional worker. The Jesness inventory (Jesness 1962, 1963) was used to assign to each delinquent a 'I-level' of interpersonal maturity derived from a scheme of seven levels of maturity described by Sullivan et al (1957) (Table 7.1). An experimental group of delinquents were treated in a community programme and results compared with a traditional institutional regime. So-called "power oriented" teenagers (Level 3) did better in the traditional regime, and "neurotics" (Level 4) showed lower reconviction rates in the community programme. The term "neurotic" here means a capacity for internalisation of standards and some understanding of motivation, whereas "power oriented" indicates that the boy understands interpersonal behaviour only in terms of authority and its manipulation. Attempts were made to match community parole officers with delinquents in terms of I-level scores, officers with an interest in intrapsychic mechanisms and emotions being allocated to "neurotic" delinquents, those with a direct approach emphasising external controls being paired with "power-oriented" offenders. There is some evidence that the general community strategy was more effective than an institutional approach for just over one-third of the boys but that some boys still did better in traditional institutions. Unfortunately, the results available are insufficient to allow more detailed comment but they serve to emphasise the heterogeneity of the delinquent population.

Most studies in the 1950s and 1960s used counselling techniques as psychological interventions and it is not possible to be very enthusiastic about the results overall; studies which do show an effect often have minor methodological problems and are generally outnumbered by those which do not (as discussed by Lipton et al 1975, and Rutter and Giller 1983). With the 1970s, behaviour modification came to be used and assessed with delinquents. Alexander & Parsons (1973; Alexander et al 1976), working with what is sometimes called "soft" delinquency on an out-patient basis using whole-family treatments, were able to obtain results which suggest the superiority of behaviourally-based family therapy (which also made use of cognitive and communicative training) over insight-directed psychodynamic and non-directive counselling family therapies. The Achievement Place studies have been the most influential in terms of planning interventions for young offenders in residential care. In the original Achievement Place, a residential unit run on family lines used a token economy which progressed to a merit system free of detailed contingency management, included social skills training and collaboration with parents. Various papers describe the project and its results (see e.g. Hoefler & Bornstein 1975, Phillips et al 1971). Clearly the boys change whilst in the unit but follow-up data are sparse and thus the ultimate efficacy of the project is still in question. Nevertheless, preliminary response to the concept has been enthusiastic, with imitators springing up in the United States and elsewhere (e.g. Liberman et al 1975) and attempts have been made to extend the basic principles to young people living at home and attending a special centre as in the Kentfields projects (Davidson & Robinson 1975).

Whether the short-term improvements that such studies usually demonstrate are due to the behavioural intervention itself is not always clear. Jesness (1975) was not able to show a significant overall advantage for a token economy regime over transactional analysis in a comparison of two residential establishments (though his figures show a trend towards a differential effect according to I-level for each regime), yet Seidman et al (1980) were able to demonstrate a separate and positive effect for the contingency contracting aspect of a community programme for delinquents on reconviction rates over a two-year follow-up, a finding comparable to that of Alexander's group (see above) in suggesting that in community work the behavioural component does seem to have an independent effect.

Taken as a whole, the effects of a number of psychological programmes are not sizeable and there appear to be interventions that can make some delinquents more likely to re-offend. Given this, it would seem wise to do as little as possible in terms of correctional work until there emerge clearer indications for particular methods to be carried out by certain types of staff with identified types of delinquents which can be shown to yield reliable and persisting results. This is caution and not nihilism; there is enough in the published studies to indicate some optimism. Nor does it mean that the psychiatrist should have no truck with delinquent youth. This account does not cover the entire field of psychological interventions with delinquents, merely the published scientific studies of planned interventions intended to reduce offending. In day-to-day clinical work, numerous other opportunities for psychiatric input arise since delinquents may also become depressed, be dependent upon drugs, exhibit relationship difficulties, have complex partial seizures and so forth. Lewis (1981) argues vigorously that the specifically medical needs of delinquents are frequently neglected by psychiatrists; a point of view with which it is hard to disagree. There is also the important field of psychiatric consultative work, particularly with social service departments and most specifically with intermediate treatment programmes. It would be a serious error to imagine that the responsibility of psychiatrists is to design or participate in projects intended to halt offending (even if that is what the courts often wish); their primary role is to alleviate suffering and treat psychiatric disorder. Delinquency is not a medical condition, but those who are delinquent may experience psychological suffering, may have a psychiatric or physical disorder, and their advisors and parents may need psychiatric and psychological advice and support in dealing with them.

Aggressive behaviour

The topic of aggression is dealt with in most books on child development to which reference should be made for a full account (see, e.g. Shaffer et al 1980). This section is only intended to provide a clinical perspective on a complex and imperfectly understood topic.

The existence of the noun "aggression" leads to an assumption that aggressive behaviour is motivated by a unitary drive. Thinking of aggression as an entity can lead to unreliable conclusions (see below) and it is probably better to use an adjectival approach and talk of aggressive behaviour: aggression is thus the quality of actions intended to harm or frighten another person and may have various causes. The use of the idea of aggression as a drive led to ideas of catharsis, yet these have proved to be ill-founded; catharsis is not an effective reducer of aggressive behaviour (see e.g. Berkowitz 1973, Mallick & McCandless 1966). Although aggression is not the same as hostility, there is an obvious, incomplete, mutual overlap with the emotional states of irritability, resentment, hatred, anger, and fear.

Aggressive behaviour is common in adolescence, particularly among boys. Commonly but not constantly it will be a continuity of an aggressive style of childhood behaviour. Aggressive reaction patterns are remarkably consistent over time (Olweus 1979), so much so that they are comparable to IQ in terms of their stability over the first two decades of individual development. Both individual and family characteristics interact to promote an aggressive behavioural style. Earlier formulations of the aetiology of aggression such as the frustration–aggression hypothesis tended to deal with single aggressive acts rather than a persistent (but not absolutely pervasive) quality of behaviour. In order to explain this remarkable stability of the trait, it is necessary to go beyond simple models of drive or precipitant.

It can readily be demonstrated that aggression as a quality of behaviour can be learned, particularly in terms of operant conditioning and modelling (see Eron et al (1974) for a typical study, or Hill (1983) for a brief review). Given that aggressive responses and initiatives exist within the repertoire of all individuals, it is possible to see how the likelihood of their occurrence may be increased or diminished over developmental time according to experience. It is particularly important to recognise the impact of vicarious as well as direct experience. The contribution of witnessed violence within the family and peer group is easy to understand but it is less well realised that there is good evidence that television is also aetiologically significant. Aggressive adolescents watch more television than those who are less aggressive, a finding most clearly described in Belson's (1978) large study but generally evident in a number of studies summarised in Eysenck & Nias (1978) and which, taken together, indicate strongly that watching television fosters aggressive behaviour rather than vice versa.

If a general tendency to behave aggressively, particularly when goal-directed behaviour is thwarted or the actions of others are perceived as hostile, can be encouraged by observational and direct learning, what other processes might influence this tendency? In the face of frustration, provocation or temptation, a number of responses are possible. Aggressive behaviour is primitive, often impulsive, sometimes the last resort. Other options necessitate a measure of self-restraint and the employment of more sophisticated skills such as negotiation, objectivity or the postponement of gratification. Such skills are also learned, hinge upon constitutional variables such as gender and temperament, and will therefore vary between individuals. For any individual, the final outcome in terms of a tendency to aggressive responses comes to be seen as the product of an interaction between experience and individual differences. This allows aggression to be manifest as the result of a deficiency of socialisation in terms of acquired alternative responses as well as deviant socialisation as far as learned aggressive responses are concerned. Faced with an aggressive teenager, one avoids simply asking the lay question "what's got into him?", and asks additionally what has not got into him. An aggressive tendency can be conceptualised as a deficiency state as well as the result of maladaptive learning.

A crude, clinical rule of thumb divides aggressive behaviour into three groups. Type 1 adolescents have a long history of habitual aggression, and a developmental formulation along the above lines will be appropriate. There are two particularly common themes. In the first (1a), there has been a family background of quarrelling parents who are emotionally cold, use harsh physical punishment (Farrington 1978) and engage in coercive interactive processes (Patterson 1982). Family relationships are soured and distant so that there has been little opportunity to learn more constructive coping skills and ample opportunity to learn aggressive and violent behaviours. Where the balance tilts towards excessive and repressive punishment, the adolescent may act compliantly at home but aggressively at school because punishment there is understandably less severe; the parents' response to this is to express incredulity and to blame the school. In the second sub-group (1b), emotional coolness or even frank rejection is the relatively dominant component, the child enters adolescence with low self-esteem and poor self-confidence, likely to behave grumpily (fearing failure, the preferred response is to sneer, denigrate and refuse to participate) and react explosively to perceived threat especially when status or "face" is at risk. In such circumstances, a general lack of social and interpersonal skills is usually evident following from a lack of basic nurturance. Not unsurprisingly, there is an association between Type 1 habitually aggressive behaviour and delinquency: many adolescents who have been exposed to deficiencies in one area of parenting have also suffered from shortcomings in another.

The other type (2) includes the habitually undercontrolled, sometimes overindulged child who has become a tyrannical adolescent: a spoilt brat now larger than his parents and taking control within the family by tantrums, abuse and bullying. Like a younger child, the discovery that one can outpower one's erstwhile protectors is tinged with anxiety; where is safety now? In an attempt at self-reassurance, the adolescent may behave increasingly omnipotently at home in order to demonstrate to himself that he is indeed powerful, yet this underlines the point that only he can protect himself now. Family life becomes punctuated with tantrums and wilful, bullying behaviour on the part of the adolescent. The impact of all this is often accentuated by a lack of social life outside the home so that developmental issues such as identity must perforce be resolved through dealings with family members rather than friends. Given, too, the fact that such individuals are not usually popular among their age peers, slights received in that setting can generate displaced rancour at home.

Nevertheless, even such an extension of the usual developmental view lacks something from the standpoint of the clinician. The affect and cognitive capacities of the aggressive individual, his immediate social setting and the qualities of the victim should be taken into account too. Aggressive teenagers are not aggressive all the time to everybody. In some instances of chronic aggression or belligerence directed towards another individual such as a sibling or step-parent, the hostility, envy or provocation within the relationship becomes the appropriate focus of clinical interest. Similarly, there may be situational variables such as certain qualities of the victim which can perpetuate aggressive behaviour (Berkowitz & Geen 1967) so that generalisations derived from a broad developmental theory of aggression are found to be weak when applied to the individual case.

This need to be specific in the individual instance is acute when the aggressive behaviour is seen as having a recent onset (Type 3). Changes in the overall situation or in the individual can precipitate aggressive behaviour, hitherto not particularly evident. Often these changes or developments are obvious and can readily be seen to have overwhelmed or side-tracked an individual's capacity to cope by using more civilised forms of behaviour. When this is not the case, it is important to consider:

— depression (irritability is quite common as an associated affect)

— obsessional preoccupations

— guilt or fear of discovery, imagined or real (self-blame for parental divorce on one hand, drug abuse on the other)

— unsuspected sensitivity over a specific issue such as appearance, homosexuality or educational failure

— psychosis, as in the instance of an explosive reaction to paranoid perceptions.

Management

In the face of a chronically aggressive style of behaviour, psychiatric involvement is usually fruitless. Among Type 1a adolescents there are those whose aggressive behaviour is mainly a problem in conflicts with authority figures, particularly within the home, and who may benefit from tuition in negotiation, a skill which they nearly always lack, having experienced and witnessed predominantly aggressive ways of resolving conflicts between people. In this respect, the package described by Kifer et al (1974) is useful: the teenager learns to assess the Situation, lists

Options available to him, and considers the likely Consequences of each option (S-O-C). This can be learned by role-play simulation, preferably involving parents since they, too, usually lack relevant skills.

The Type 1b aggressive adolescent who lacks enough self-esteem to risk what might be seen as loss of face in negotiation will be hard to engage in direct psychiatric treatment in any case. His family and teachers may be encouraged to pay attention to his poor self-confidence by the use of pointed praise for achievements, by refining expectations to avoid excessive exposure to failure, or by the use of techniques such as "earshotting" whereby parents make audible positive comments about his qualities when he believes (erroneously) that they are unaware that he can overhear. Unfortunately, most young people with poor self-esteem have parents whose self-esteem is also low (Coopersmith 1967) and whose involvement with treatment is often tenuous.

Type 2 aggressive adolescents are unlikely to give up their position within the family power structure on their own initiative, even though they are likely to feel more comfortable should they do so. Where parental resources are sufficient, a family therapy approach (commonly on structural lines) may enable change to occur in the whole system of family relationships. It is probably wise to emphasise to parents that asserting their authority is helpful in promoting the adolescent's personal development even when it gives rise to disagreements. Some adolescents from liberally-minded homes where parents fudge issues of authority will behave outrageously in order to provoke confrontations, thereby testing their own strength and learning where limits lie. Parents can respond to such a challenge by withdrawing their own authority even further, thereby exacerbating the situation.

In the cases of aggressive behaviour of recent onset (Type 3), an adequate formulation is a prerequisite for treatment. Perhaps the commonest precipitant is a change in family structure through divorce or remarriage. Such circumstances call for the use of a whole-family approach, buttressed where appropriate by individual counselling, so long as this can be framed in such a way that the adolescent does not feel blamed, or identified inappropriately as ill. Some adolescents whose aggressive outbursts are essentially uncontrolled rage may be able to use cognitive strategies of anger control (Novaco 1975) though the overall success rate with such approach is not, in the author's experience, very sizeable.

REFERENCES

Adams S 1961 The PICO project. In: Johnstone N et al (eds) The Sociology of Punishment and Conviction. Wiley, New York

Alexander J F, Parsons B V 1973 Short term behavioral intervention with delinquent families: impact on family process and recidivism. Journal of Abnormal Psychology 81: 219–225

Alexander J F, Barton C, Schiavo R S, Parsons B V 1976 Systems-behavioral intervention with families of delinquents: therapist characteristics, family behavior and outcome. Journal of Consulting and Clinical Psychology 44: 656–664

Baldwin J 1975 British areal studies of crime: an assessment. British Journal of Criminology 15: 211–226

Bebbington P, Hill P 1985 A Manual of Practical Psychiatry. Blackwell Scientific, Oxford

Belson W A 1968 The extent of stealing by London boys. Advancement of Science 25: 171–184

Belson W A 1975 Juvenile Theft: The Causal Factors. Harper and Row, New York

Belson W A 1978 Television Violence and the Adolescent Boy. Teakfield, Farnborough

Berg I 1985 The management of truancy. Journal of Child Psychology and Psychiatry 26: 325–331

Berg I, Consterdine M, Hullin R, McGuire R, Tysers 1978 The effect of two randomly allocated court procedures on truancy. British Journal of Criminology 18: 232–244

Berkowitz L 1973 Control of Aggression. In: Caldwell B, Ricciuti A N (eds) Review of Child Development Research vol 3. University of Chicago Press, Chicago

Berkowitz L, Geen R G 1967 Stimulus qualities of the target of aggression: a further study. Journal of Personality and Social Psychology 5: 364–368

Bottoms A E, McClintock F H 1973 Criminals Coming of Age. Heinemann Educational, London

Bowlby J 1969 Attachment and Loss. Vol 1. Attachment. Hogarth Press, London

Bowlby J 1973 Attachment and Loss. Vol 2. Separation: Anxiety and Anger. Hogarth Press, London

Bowlby J 1980 Attachment and Loss. Vol 3. Loss. Hogarth Press, London

Burt C 1925 The Young Delinquent. London University Press, London

Cawson P 1985 Intermediate treatment. Journal of Child Psychology and Psychiatry 26: 675–681

Central Policy Review Staff 1978 Vandalism. HMSO, London

Conger J J, Miller W C 1966 Personality, Social Class and Delinquency. Wiley, New York

Coopersmith S 1967 The Antecedents of Self-Esteem. Freeman, San Francisco

Craft M, Stephenson G, Granger C 1964 A controlled trial of authoritarian and self-governing regimes with adolescent psychopaths. American Journal of Orthopsychiatry 34: 543–554

Crowe R R 1974 An adoption study of antisocial personality. Archives of General Psychiatry 31: 785–791

Davidson W S, Robinson M J 1975 Community psychology and behavior modification: A community based program for the prevention of delinquency. Corrective and Social Psychiatry 21: 1–12

Davies J G V, Maliphant R 1971 Autonomic responses of male adolescents exhibiting refractory behaviour in school. Journal of Child Psychology and Psychiatry 12: 115–127

Davies J G V, Maliphant R 1974 Refractory behaviour in school and avoidance learning. Journal of Child Psychology and Psychiatry 15: 23–31

Davies M, Sinclair I A C 1971 Families, hostels and delinquents: an attempt to assess cause and effect. British Journal of Criminology 11: 213–229

Davitz J 1952 The effects of previous training on postfrustration behavior. Journal of Abnormal and Social Psychology 47: 309–315

Douglas J W B, Ross J M, Simpson H R 1968 All Our Future. Peter Davies, London

Duck S W 1973 Similarity and perceived similarity of personal constructs as influences on friendship choice. British Journal of Social and Clinical Psychology 12: 1–6

Empey L T, Erickson M L 1972 The Provo Experiment: Evaluating Community Control of Delinquency. Heath, Lexington Mass

Empey L T, Lubeck S G 1971 The Silverlake Experiment: Testing Delinquency Theory and Community Intervention. Aldine, Chicago

Eron L D, Huesmann L R, Leficowitz M M, Walder L O 1974 How learning conditions in early childhood — including mass media — relate to aggression in late adolescence. American Journal of Orthopsychiatry 44: 412–423

Eysenck H J 1964 Crime and Personality. Routledge and Kegan Paul, London

Eysenck H J, Nias D K 1978 Sex, Violence and the Media. Temple Smith, London

Farrington D P 1977 The effects of public labelling. British Journal of Criminology 17: 112–125

Farrington, D P 1978 Family backgrounds of aggressive youths. In: Hersov L, Berger M, Shaffer D (eds) Aggression and Anti-Social Behaviour in Childhood and Adolescence. Pergamon Press, Oxford

Farrington D P, Osborn S, West D J 1978 The persistence of labelling effects. British Journal of Criminology 18: 277–284

Ferguson T 1952 The Young Delinquent in his Social Setting. Oxford University Press, Oxford

Gath A 1985 Chromosomal anomalies. In: Rutter M Hersov L (eds) Child and Adolescent Psychiatry: Modern Approaches. 2nd edn. Blackwell Scientific, Oxford

Gath D, Cooper B, Gattoni I F, Rockett D 1975 Child Guidance and Delinquency in a London Borough. (Institute of Psychiatry: Maudsley Monographs No. 24) Oxford University Press, London

Gibbs J C 1977 Kohlberg's stages of moral development: a constructive critique. Harvard Educational Review 47: 43–61

Glueck S, Glueck E T 1950 Unraveling Juvenile Delinquency. Commonwealth Fund, New York

Grant J D, Grant M Q 1959 A group dynamic approach to the treatment of nonconformists in the Navy. Annals of the American Academy of Political and Social Science 322: 127–135

Hare R D 1978 Electrodermal and cardiovascular correlates of psychopathy. In: Hare R D, Schalling D. (eds) Psychopathic Behaviour: Approaches to Research. Wiley, London

Hargreaves D 1967 Social Relations in a Secondary School. Routledge & Kegan Paul, London

Hartshorne H, May M A 1928 Studies in Deceit. Macmillan, New York

Heard D 1987 The relevance of attachment theory to child psychiatric practice: an update. Journal of Child Psychology and Psychiatry 28: 25–28

Hill P 1983 Aggro, theft and grumpiness. Update 27: 543–549

Hill P 1986 Child psychiatry. In: Hill P, Murray R, Thorley A (eds) Essentials of Postgraduate Psychiatry. 2nd edn. Grune and Stratton, London

Hindelang M J, Hirschi T, Weis J G 1979 Correlates of delinquency: the illusion of descrepancy between self report and official measures. American Sociological Review 44: 995–1014

Hirschi S 1969 Causes of Delinquency. University of California Press, Berkeley

Hoefler S A, Bornstein P H 1975 Achievement Place: an evaluation review. Criminal Justice and Behavior 2: 146–168

Hoffman M L 1970 Conscience, personality and socialization techniques. Human Development 13: 90–126

Hoghughi M S, Forrest A R 1970 Eysenck's theory of criminality: an examination with approved school boys. British Journal of Criminology 10: 240–254

Hudgins W, Prentice N M 1973 Moral judgement in delinquent and non delinquent adolescents and their mothers. Journal of Abnormal Psychology 82: 145–152

Hutchings B, Mednick S A 1974 Biological and adoptive fathers of male criminal adoptees. In: Major Issues in Juvenile Delinquency. World Health Organization, Copenhagen

Jensen G F 1972 Parents, peers and delinquent action: a test of the differential association perspective. American Journal of Sociology 78: 562–575

Jephcott A P, Carter M P 1954 The Social Background of Delinquency. Nottingham University Press, Nottingham

Jesness C F 1962 The Jesness Inventory: Development and Validation. California Youth Authority Research Report No. 29, Sacramento.

Jesness C F 1963 Redevelopment and Revalidation of the Jesness Inventory. California Youth Authority Research Report No. 35, Sacramento.

Jesness C F 1975 Comparative effectiveness of behavior modification and transactional analysis programs for delinquents. Journal of Consulting and Clinical Psychology 43: 758–779

Johnson A M 1949 Sanctions for superego lacunae of adolescents. In: Eissler K (ed) Searchlights on Delinquency. International Universities Press, New York

Kahn J, Carter W, Dernley N, Slater E 1969 Chromosome studies in remand home and prison populations. In: West D J (ed) Criminological Implications of Chromosome Abnormalities. Institute of Criminology, Cambridge

Kifer R E, Lewis M A, Green D R, Phillips E L 1974 Training predelinquent youths and their parents to negotiate conflict situations. Journal of Applied Behavior Analysis 7: 357–364

Knight B J, West D J 1977 Criminality and welfare dependency in two generations. Medicine, Science and the Law 17: 64–67

Kohlberg L 1976 Moral stages and moralization: the cognitive-developmental approach. In: Lickona T (ed) Moral Development and Behaviour. Holt, Rinehart and Winston, New York

Landau S F 1981 Juveniles and the police. British Journal of Criminology 21: 27–46

Lewis D O 1981 Vulnerabilities to Delinquency. MTP Press, Lancaster

Lewis D O, Shanok S S, Pincus J H 1981 The neuropsychiatric status of violent male juvenile delinquents. In: Lewis D O (ed) Vulnerabilities to Delinquency. MTP Press, Lancaster

Liberman R P, Ferris C, Salgado P, Salgado J 1975 Replication of the Achievement Place model in California. Journal of Applied Behavior Analysis 8: 287–299

Lipton D, Martinson R, Wilks J 1975 The Effectiveness of Correctional Treatment: A survey of Treatment Evaluation Studies. Praeger, London

McCord W, McCord J 1959 Origins of Crime. Columbia University Press, New York

McGuffin P, Gottesman I 1985 Genetic influences on normal and abnormal development. In: Rutter M, Hersov L (eds) Child and Adolescent Psychiatry: Modern Approaches. Blackwell Scientific, Oxford

Mallick S K, McCandless B 1966 A study of catharsis of aggression. Journal of Personality and Social Psychology 4: 591–596

Massimo J L, Shore M F 1963 The effectiveness of a comprehensive, vocationally-oriented psychotherapeutic program for adolescent delinquent boys. American Journal of Orthopsychiatry 33: 634–642

Mayhew P, Clarke R, Sturman A, Hough J 1976 Crime as opportunity London: HMSO

Mays J B 1954 Growing Up in the City. Liverpool University Press, Liverpool

Mednick S A 1981 The learning of morality: biosocial bases. In: Lewis D O (ed) Vulnerabilities to Delinquency. MTP Press, Lancaster

Milgram S 1963 Behavioral study of obedience. Journal of Abnormal and Social Psychology 67: 371–378

Milgram S 1965 Some conditions of obedience and disobedience to authority. Human Relations 18: 57–76

Novaco R 1975 Anger Control. Lexington Books, Lexington, Mass

Olweus D 1979 Stability of aggressive reaction patterns in males: a review. Psychological Bulletin 86: 852–875

Palmer T B 1973 Matching worker and client in corrections. Social Work 18: 95–103

Palmer T 1974 The Youth Authority's Community Treatment Project. Federal Probation 38: 3–14

Patterson G R 1982 Coercive Family Process. Castalia Press, Eugene, Oregon

Persons R W 1967 Relationship between psychotherapy with institutionalized boys and subsequent community adjustment. Journal of Consulting Psychology 31: 137–141

Phillips E L, Phillips E A, Fixsen D L, Wolf M M 1971 Achievement Place: modification of the behaviors of pre-delinquent boys within a token economy. Journal of Applied Behavior Analysis 4: 45–59

Piaget J 1952 The Moral Judgement of the Child. Routledge & Kegan Paul, London

Power M J, Alderson M R, Phillipson C M, Schoenberg E, Morris J N 1967 Delinquent schools? New Society 10: 542–543

Power M J, Benn R T, Morris J N 1972 Neighbourhood, school and juveniles before the courts. British Journal of Criminology 12: 111–132

Riddle M, Roberts A H 1977 Delinquency, delay of gratification, recidivism and the Porteus Maze Tests. Psychological Bulletin 84: 417–425

Robins L N, Lewis R G 1966 The role of the antisocial family in school completion and delinquency: a three generation study. Sociology Quarterly 7: 500–514

Rutter M 1966 Children of Sick Parents. Oxford University Press, London

Rutter M 1981 Maternal Deprivation Reassessed. 2nd edn. Penguin, Harmondsworth

Rutter M, Giller H 1983 Juvenile Delinquency. Penguin, Harmondsworth

Rutter M, Madge N 1976 Cycles of Disadvantage: A Review of Research. Heinemann Educational, London

Rutter M, Maughan B, Mortimore P, Ouston J, Smith A 1979 Fifteen Thousand Hours: Secondary Schools and their Effects on Children. Open Books, London

Sarason I G 1978 Verbal learning, modeling and juvenile delinquency. American Psychologist 23: 254–266

Seidman E, Rappaport J, Davidson W S 1980 Adolescents in legal jeopardy: initial success and replication of an alternative to the criminal justice system.

In: Ross R R, Gendreau P (eds) Effective Correctional Treatment. Butterworths, Toronto

Shaffer D, Meyer-Bahlburg H, Stokman C 1980 The development of aggression. In: Rutter M (ed) Scientific Foundations of Developmental Psychiatry. Heinemann, London

Shore M F, Massimo J L 1973 After ten years: a follow-up study of comprehensive vocationally oriented psychotherapy. American Journal of Orthopsychiatry 43: 128–132

Sinclair I A C, Clarke R V G 1982 Predicting, treating and explaining delinquency: the lessons from research on institutions. In: Feldman P (ed) Developments in the Study of Criminal Behaviour. Vol. 1. The Prevention and Control of Offending. Wiley, Chichester

Stott D H, Wilson D M 1977 The adult criminal as juvenile. British Journal of Criminology 17: 47–57

Sullivan C, Grant M Q, Grant J D 1957 The development of interpersonal maturity: applications to delinquency. Psychiatry 20: 373–385

Sutherland E H 1939 Principles of Criminology. Lippincott, Philadelphia.

Wadsworth M E J 1976 Delinquency, pulse rates and early emotional deprivation. British Journal of Criminology 16: 245–256

Wahler R G 1976 Deviant child behavior within the family. In: Leitenberg H (ed) Handbook of Behavior Modification and Behavior Therapy. Prentice Hall, Englewood Cliffs NJ

Wallerstein J S, Kelly J B 1980 Surviving the Breakup. Grant McIntyre, London

Wallis C P, Maliphant R 1967 Delinquent areas in the county of London: ecological factors. British Journal of Criminology 7: 250–284

Warren M Q 1969 The case for differential treatment of delinquents. Annals of the American Academy of Political and Social Science 381: 47–59

Warren M Q 1977 Correctional treatment and coercion: the differential effectiveness perspective. Criminal Justice and Behavior 4: 355–376

Weeks H A 1958 Youthful Offenders at Highfields. University of Michigan Press, Ann Arbor, Michigan

West D J, Farrington D P 1977 The delinquent way of life. Heinemann Educational, London

Weinreich-Haste H 1979 Moral development. In: Coleman J C (ed) The School Years. Methuen, London pp. 46–78

Weiss G, Hechtman L, Milroy T, Perlman T 1985 Psychiatric status of hyperactives as adults: a controlled prospective 15-year follow-up of 63 hyperactive children. Journal of the American Academy of Child Psychiatry 24: 211–220

West D J 1982 Delinquency: its Roots, Careers and Prospects. Heinemann Educational, London

West D J, Farrington D P 1973 Who Becomes Delinquent? Heinemann Educational, London

9

Depression

Some of the problems that dog the discussion of depression in childhood continue to present difficulties in the consideration of depression in adolescence. Young teenagers may lack the inclination to disclose their feelings at interview or may lack the vocabulary with which to discuss them and this means that the interviewing professional has to resort to inference with the risk of unreliability or error. As with younger children, the problem seems to arise most seriously with the less intelligent and unforthcoming individuals (Rutter & Graham 1968). Unfortunately, parental report does not help resolve the problem since parents are quite likely to be unaware of even severe depressive feelings in their teenage offspring (Cytryn et al 1980, Rutter et al 1976).

There are also difficulties in conceptualisation. "Depression" is a term that may be used colloquially as a synonym for anergia, unhappiness, misery or despair. It may be used descriptively without reference to whether the mood is idiopathic and autonomous or secondary to unpleasant experiences and understandable empathically. In professional use, it is a term only to be used when the dysphoric mood state is virtually pervasive and accompanied by adverse effects upon cognition, motivation and physiological processes such as sleep and appetite. According to user, the term may refer to understandable reaction, symptom, syndrome or primary disorder.

In addition, there is the obligation to take a developmental perspective (see Rutter 1986), particularly with respect to the manner in which depression may be influenced by immaturity in various domains: cognitive, emotional or social. There are also effects on prevalence: the prevalence of depressive symptomatology increases remarkably at puberty and the sex distribution

126

alters dramatically to yield a post-pubertal female predominance by middle adolescence.

Not surprisingly, there are disagreements between authorities as to the form and extent of depression in adolescence. Much of this disagreement stems from definition problems and, quite clearly, any account of depression in adolescence is going to have to define its terms and consider various issues separately.

Depressive feelings

Feelings of depression, however unpleasant, may not be associated with impaired personal or biological functioning. In such circumstances they are likely to be part but not the whole of the depressive syndrome. Nor are they specific to depression as shown by Pearce's (1978) study: one-third of children and adolescents with morbidly depressed feelings, sadness, unhappiness or tearfulness had more in common with youngsters judged not to have the full syndrome of depression than with those considered depressed.

The affect of depression is more than sadness (Izard & Schwartz 1986) and the emotional components include hostility, irritability, guilt and anxiety as well as a sense of emotional unresponsiveness and mental emptiness. There may also be distress caused by accompanying physical sensations such as heaviness or pain in the chest and head. Cognitive aspects such as negative evaluation of self and the future are associated with pessimism and hopelessness. Nevertheless, sadness is central and the pattern of the associated emotions and cognitions varies between subjects and situations. General clinical usage assumes that depressive feelings are likely to follow loss (of a loved person or of previous nurturance) but can be distinguished from grief by the presence of negative cognitions such as self-reproach or self-depreciation. Following such an assumption, the findings of Horowitz et al (1980) suggest that adults may display four different types of depressive state following loss: 1. fear and helplessness; 2. rage at others or self; 3. shame and loss of self-esteem; 4. withdrawn numbness.

This illustrates the range of depressive feeling around a core of sadness and negative cognitions and certainly all of these types may be seen in adolescence. There are grounds for thinking that there are sex differences in response. For instance, anger and

127

antisocial behaviour with outwardly directed hostility are more commonly found in boys reporting depressed feelings, whereas depressed girls report more shame and fear and thus resemble adults in the profile of their constituent emotions (Izard & Schwartz 1986).

The presence of suicidal ideation is variable and is discussed elsewhere (Ch. 10) though its presence enables further differentiation of depressive feelings from mere sadness. Like suicidal thoughts, depressive feelings show a dramatic increase at puberty (Rutter 1986). In the Isle of Wight follow-up study on 14–15-year-olds (Rutter et al 1976), 41.7% of boys and 47.7% of girls reported appreciable misery or depressive feelings. This would not necessarily be synonymous with depression in its full complexity yet 19.8% of boys and 23% of girls expressed feelings of self-depreciation. It would appear that depressive feelings are not uncommon among young teenagers though this is not to say that depression is as prevalent since most Isle of Wight youngsters who complained of depressed feelings or appreciable sadness did not show evidence of impaired personal functioning. Those who did (and therefore were diagnosed as having depression) were much fewer: the prevalence rate for pure depression among 14–15-year-olds in the study being 0.45%, and for mixed affective disorder (anxiety and depression) 1.3%, with twice as many girls affected as boys overall.

Depression (depressive syndrome)

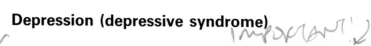

One obvious issue in the study of depression in adolescence is to determine whether depression in adolescence is different clinically and nosologically, from depression in adulthood. In view of the parlous state of classification in adult depression it is sensible to try and simplify matters and assume that depression is a unitary condition in both adolescence and adult life. Unfortunately, even then the exercise is compromised by the lack of consensus as to the nature, status and form of depression in adulthood.

The fundamental concern in such an endeavour is the nature of the clinical presentation of depression in terms of observed behaviour and self-report. On this basis various operational criteria for depression in adults have been proposed and accepted, particularly in North America, and have been used as the basis of case identification in a number of studies of depression in children and young adolescents. There has usually been little attempt to modify these for use with children, but a number of children and adolescents have been found to fulfil for example, DSM-III criteria for major depression. Other standards such as the Research Diagnostic Criteria (Spitzer et al 1978) have also been similarly employed. Various self-report schedules and semi-structured interviews (see Kazdin & Petti 1982, Costello 1986) have been employed to elicit information from children and young adolescents but there has been only fair agreement between different sets of criteria and some doubt expressed as to whether certain items in interview schedules accurately probe for phenomena included in such criteria (Cantwell 1983). Nevertheless it can be taken as confirmed that a number of adolescents display depressive features isomorphic with adult depression.

Whether there are more ways to be depressed in early adolescence than such schedules can cover is more contentious and depends upon the boundaries of the condition. What constitutes depression is a topic for debate in the absence of specific biological markers. It is generally accepted that these do not exist at a high level of specificity in adolescence. The dexamethasone suppression test, for instance, will be abnormal in perhaps half of all adolescents with major depression by DSM-III criteria (Extein et al 1982, Robins et al 1982) but it can also be abnormal, albeit less frequently, in association with other psychiatric pathology so that its specificity is imperfect, as is the case with adults (see Abou-Saleh 1985). Studies of growth hormone response and sleep architecture which show abnormalities in depressed adults are inconsistent in young adolescents because such biological features show an interaction with maturation which makes their interpretation in the young unreliable (Puig-Antich 1986).

An alternative strategy is to inspect the relatives of known cases of depression in adulthood. There seems to be good evidence for an increased rate of depression in children and young adolescents in such a group and, furthermore, a generally similar clinical picture to that found in adults (see e.g. Cytryn et al 1982). This may be taken in parallel with follow-up studies of children considered to be depressed (Poznanski et al 1976, Kovacs et al 1984) and of depressed adolescents followed up in adult life (Zeitlin 1986) to indicate that the clinical constellation of depressive features is generally similar in adults and adolescents. The burgeoning of North American research into childhood depression which assumes isomorphism in depression across childhood, adolescence and adulthood and uses the operational criteria derived from adult psychiatry would thus appear to be based on reasonable assumptions even though the developmental viewpoint (Rutter 1986) has not yet been fully taken into account.

The idea that depression may present with non-depressed behaviour in the young so that certain psychiatric pictures are "depressive equivalents" is now largely discarded since, historically speaking, it had become overused to the point of meaninglessness. Unhappiness and poor self-esteem are common symptoms in many psychiatric disorders but an underlying depression is not the only reason for their presence. Little was to be found in common between youngsters with depression according to operational criteria and those with conditions such as enuresis which had been claimed to be depressive equivalents (Pearce 1978).

A more realistic problem is that depressive features are overlooked by the clinician even though they are likely to be present and can be revealed with further interviewing or more specific questioning. Rather similarly, they may be detected but given insufficient weight in formulation. Evidence that this is so exists in Zeitlin's (1986) study and it is likely that Puig-Antich's (1982) finding of a high rate of conduct disorder in association with depression in prepubertal boys (and remitting with treatment of the depression) would also apply to young adolescent males. The presence of antisocial behaviour may inhibit exploration of the affective domain by an assessing psychiatrist because it appears to be the most obvious and pressing clinical feature. It thus masks because it distracts the psychiatrist rather than actually concealing depression.

The safest position, pending further research on family studies or biological markers, is to assume that depression can be identified in the adolescent according to criteria that are generally similar to those used in adults and that the case for depressive equivalents or a radically different form of presentation on account of developmental factors is as yet unproven. This does not contradict the above observation that in adolescent boys, antisocial behaviour may be associated with identifiable depressive affect.

Classification

There are no clear indications that any distinct form of depression affects adolescents rather than adults, so that the attempts to classify depression in adults (Andreasen 1982) can reasonably be extended to cover adolescence. Unfortunately no scheme for classifying adult depression has pre-eminence so that the apparent advantage in so doing cannot be exploited. Nor is there any universally accepted classification scheme that can be extended up the age range from middle childhood, though Carlson & Garber (1986) consider that there is sufficient consensus among authorities on childhood depression to propose a scheme which with minor modification would seem to have face validity for depression in adolescence. It comprises three categories, detailed below.

Endogenous type (Kendell type A; Kendell 1976): depression with morbid guilt, delusions, hallucinations and psychomotor retardation certainly occurs as an episodic illness even in apparently robust personalities in adolescence, either in unipolar or bipolar form (Carlson & Strober 1978).

Depression in association with marked symptoms of anxiety or antisocial behaviour is recognised as a separate category by some authorities (Frommer 1968) and is loosely comparable to neurotic or Kendall type B depression in adults, subsuming Paykel's (1971) "anxious" and "hostile" groups.

Chronic depression associated with privation or deprivation of parental affection or with other causes of low self-esteem and vulnerability is recognised as a separate group by a number of writers and corresponds to Paykel's "personality disorder" type.

Whether these suggested types are dimensions rather than categories is unknown. Whilst offering a convenient framework for the recognition of common variants of the clinical picture, they are not obviously mutually exclusive and their validity will ultimately depend upon whether they do in fact carry different clinical information in terms of variables such as response to treatment and prognosis.

Clinical presentation

Bearing the above in mind and assuming a general isomorphism with depression in adult life, it is appropriate to detail those features which do seem to be especially prominent in depression in the young generally and adolescence in particular. In the absence of satisfactory controlled studies, anecdotal report is the only source of information in this area and caution should be exercised accordingly.

Separation anxiety which re-appears in adolescence. This may be the mechanism for the well-recognised presentation of acute adolescent depression as school refusal (see Ch. 19, and Kolvin et al 1984).

Antisocial behaviour within and outside the home, principally in boys. Again, this should be shown to have an onset in adolescence to avoid confusion with demoralisation or low self-esteem in youngsters with long-standing conduct disorder. As with Puig-Antich's (1982) somewhat younger depressed children with associated conduct disorder, antidepressant treatment appears to have a beneficial effect upon the antisocial behaviour as well as the depressive features.

A falling off of school performance in both academic and social areas is determined by a number of mechanisms. The youngster may blame his "poor memory" but closer assessment reveals poor concentration rather than a memory problem.

Apathy, boredom and the loss of ability to experience pleasure in anything is one of the few spontaneous complaints which the average depressed adolescent is likely to make.

Hallucinations are commoner than generally believed since they are often not inquired for sufficiently closely. Chambers et al (1982), using a semi-structured interview (KIDDIE-SADS) in a prospective study, found a higher rate of mood-congruent hallucinations in childhood depression than the retrospective studies of Garralda (1984) and Burke et al (1985) on general child psychiatry patients would suggest. It seems likely that the same holds true for adolescents.

Running away from home which, as in childhood, is usually understood to be virtually a suicidal equivalent when serious or repetitive. This may be an overstatement and certainly the studies of youngsters who run away suggest that they are a mixed bunch from a psychopathological view (Russell 1981).

Hypochondriacal ideas, and pain or heaviness in the chest

(Kashani et al 1982) appear relatively commoner complaints than among depressed adults. It may be clear to the interviewing psychiatrist that what is being described is the subjective experience of the psychophysiological concomitants of high arousal, particularly when there are anxiety symptoms evident. The propensity for adolescents to develop somatic and dysmorphophobic preoccupations is an understandable extension of the experience of bodily changes at puberty and the capacity to think about the thoughts and perceptions of others (see Ch. 3).

Conversely, loss of libido, loss of appetite, fatigue, subjective slowing of thought, and persecutory delusions seem less common among depressed adolescents than among adults (Hudgens 1974, Inamdar et al 1979). Weight loss is less common than in adult depression, presumably because it is masked by continuing growth and is replaced by the phenomenon of slowing of normal weight gain.

Clinical assessment

The core of adequate clinical appraisal in a case of suspected depression is a detailed mental state (see Table 9.1). This requires questioning and discussion with the adolescent of topics which are painful or alarming. Given this, and the fact that many teenagers do not in any case participate willingly in the diagnostic process for the reasons outlined in Chapter 2, it should not be expected that all will be revealed in the first interview.

Only an individual interview with the patient is likely to elicit a full picture of personal psychopathology. Some teenagers are not prepared to confess the depth of their despair in the presence of their parents and siblings, especially when they are morbidly guilty. A whole-family interview is a useful adjunct to assessment but should not substitute for separate interviews with adolescent and parents. From time to time the author's clinical practice groans under the weight of second referrals of families with depressed youngsters who have been seen at hard-line family therapy clinics where individual interviews are apparently taboo and the clinical management has underestimated the severity of their suffering.

A number of semi-structured interview schedules which have been designed for research use with children such as the CAS (Hodges et al 1982), the KIDDIE-SADS developed by Puig-

Table 9.1 Abnormalities in the mental state of depression

Mood	Sadness, misery, despair
Cognition	Poverty of ideation Poor concentration (complaint of poor memory)
Thought content	Preoccupation with painful topics Circular rumination Separation anxiety Hypochondriasis Suicidal ideation Delusional beliefs
Self-evaluation	Worthlessness Self-reproach, guilt
Motivation	Loss of interest Inability to initiate activities
Perception	Dulled sensitivity Depersonalisation, derealisation Misperceptions, hallucinations
Motor activity	Retardation Agitation
Somatic	Sleep disturbance Altered appetite Weight gain or loss Local sensations of pain or heaviness

Antich, or the Interview Schedule for Children (ISC) developed by Kovacs (neither of which has been published in a journal) may also be used with young adolescents but there is no indication for their routine use in clinical practice.

A self-report questionnaire (see Costello (1986) and Kazdin & Petti (1982) for a discussion of those which can be used with young adolescents) can yield a useful baseline against which to gauge progress and may yield information not obtained at interview. Some normative data has been obtained for The Beck Depression Inventory (Beck & Beamesderfer 1974) when given to American 14–17-year-olds (Teri 1982). Such questionnaires must not be used as substitutes for clinical interview since they are not usually validated against adolescent subjects and may well have different cut-off scores for pathology from those relating to either adult or child samples.

Physical examination should be carried out not merely to exclude intracranial or metabolic pathology, important though that is, but to reassure the teenager with hypochondriacal concerns that his physical symptoms are not lethal. The physical examination can also be an extension of the interview:

A 15-year-old girl noted by her parents and school to have been increasingly withdrawn and listless was referred for assessment. At interview she was monosyllabic and unforthcoming. During a simple physical examination, the psychiatrist noticed superficial, recent scars on her throat, possibly self-inflicted, which had been previously covered by the high neck of her sweater. At this point she wept softly and explained that she could not bring herself to tell anyone how awful she felt and that she had known that, if examined physically, such scars would be seen: "I knew they would, you know, tell you how I feel".

It is doubtful whether routine physical investigations are helpful in the absence of leads from history or investigation, though diabetes, hypokalaemia secondary to (undisclosed) diuretic use for premenstrual irritability, uraemia, and hypothalamic tumour have all been seen by the author to present with apparent depression in adolescence. Routine psychometric assessment is equally unnecessary though it can be crucial in instances such as the assessment of depressive demoralisation following head injury when poor academic performance may be due to protracted absence from school as well as to the effects of brain damage.

Treatment

Reliance on a single mode of treatment is likely to be unnecessarily parsimonious. Parents and teachers will need advice on how the young person is to be managed if he or she is to be treated as an out-patient. The adolescent deserves straightforward explanation and reassurance, whatever else is offered. Persisting environmental adversity should be corrected as far as possible. It seems likely that, as with adults, a combination of measures is superior to their use singly (DiMascio et al 1979). According to circumstances, relatively more emphasis may be placed on one particular form of intervention.

Although not proven scientifically, it would seem that this choice of principal treatment intervention is logically determined by the classification suggested above. Major depression with disturbance of biological functions and morbid guilt arising in a previously adequate personality is seen by many as an indication for medication. Most psychiatrists would consider a cyclic antidepressant the drug of first choice but would add that results are not always encouraging. While there are no grounds for preferring one drug within this large group to any other, there is reason to think that a larger dose than considered conventional may be necessary. For instance, Puig-Antich et al (1979) in a study of major depression in prepubertal children found that a significant clinical response was only obtained with plasma levels of imipramine and desmethylimipramine (combined) over 155 ng/ml. Ambrosini & Puig-Antich (1985) draw on this finding to provide explicit guidelines for imipramine dosage with increasing doses up to 5 mg/kg/day or plasma levels of 200 ng/ml unless ECG abnormalities (which they specify) supervene. The problem with such enthusiasm is that the relationship between drug therapeutic effect and plasma level was only seen within the drug-treated group; the placebo group obtained just as impressive remission rates. Given this, it would seem premature to recommend such heroic dosages. Nevertheless it is a counterblast against pharmacotherapeutic timidity, and one interpretation of the results of these studies is that low doses of imipramine are counter-therapeutic. Ambrosini & Puig-Antich state (1985, p 188): "In our experience all nonpsychotic children who had adequate serum levels responded to tricyclics" and imply that such experience applies to young adolescents. The author's experience, using common tricyclic or tetracyclic antidepressants in doses equivalent to imipramine in the 150–200 mg dose range, has been that with Kendell type A depression in 14–18-year-olds a good response can be expected in the majority of non-suicidal outpatients. It is good practice, but not absolutely essential, to monitor ECG and plasma levels with such dosages, particularly as there is often a poor relationship between oral dose and plasma level. At higher dosage, ECG monitoring is mandatory and such patients should probably be admitted for treatment.

Although there is no logical reason for withholding ECT, convention holds that its use is avoided in school-age adolescents. The basis for this is sentiment and it can, admittedly on rare occasions, be apparently life-saving. With young adolescents in particular, there is a tendency to minimise the issues by ascribing serious psychopathology to "adolescence" or by compromising with parents' fears and not pressing for admission to hospital when suicidal intent is apparent.

Psychotherapy

Acute depression which is a reaction to stress is generally

managed by psychotherapeutic means. Although there is no hard evidence to support this practice, it is logical in that it should promote the development and deployment of coping mechanisms in the adolescent and his or her family. The temptation for the inexperienced is to move rapidly to a formal interpretative mode when it is often wiser to use a supportive model with sensitive use of explanation and guidance. Whether individual or family approaches are preferred is a matter for judgement and therapist availability in the absence of evidence for comparative superiority. Although there are excellent short accounts of the principles of individual psychotherapy with depressed adolescents (Weiner 1975), there is a dearth of publications on family and group treatment of depression in adolescents. This is surprising in view of their wide use.

The central component of an individual psychotherapeutic approach is the location of perceived loss, whether this is the love of an important figure, of self-worth or a sense of mastery, or the respect of others. The sensation of loss requires exploration by mutual discussion and is to be shared empathically and demonstrably. The therapist will have a greater vocabulary and ability to link those mental components of suffering which the adolescent experiences as puzzling or frightening because they do not make sense to her or him. Similarly the therapist will be able to make assumptions, albeit tentatively, about feelings that are only imperfectly acknowledged. For some teenagers, their depressive symptoms are threats to their developing sense of independence because they are inexplicable and overwhelming. The provision of meaning by explanation can assist the healing process by siding with the individual's attempt to retain mastery by developing understanding. At the same time, the therapist can suggest how the patient can take their own recovery further by setting tasks such as talking about certain topics to parents, making lists of future plans, or practising initiative and assertion.

It is evident from the above that it is possible to unify a traditional psychotherapeutic stance with interventions derived from a cognitive approach to depression. While there has been no direct work on the efficacy of cognitive therapy in adolescent depression, the author's experience has been that methods used with adults such as those described by Beck et al (1979), and components of stress inoculation (Meichenbaum 1975), rational emotive therapy (RET) (Ellis 1962), and rational restructuring (Goldfried & Goldfried 1975) also have general application with

137

Construction [handwritten]

depressed teenagers. Those who are chronically depressed and have low self-esteem tend to attribute failure to their own short-comings, and here a learned helplessness model (Dweck 1977, Seligman & Peterson 1986) becomes useful. In these circum-stances, such "cognitive" methods come into their own but should be used in concert with support and environmental manipulation to correct persisting adversity and exploit to the full any opportuities for success and pleasure. In chronically depressed patients, the support of a medium-term therapeutic group for adolescents can be invaluable. Some will need direct tuition in social skills since longstanding depression may have led them into habits of social avoidance and self-effacement which diminish the number of opportunities to learn such skills.

Prognosis

The long term outlook for adolescents who present with depression is curiously obscure. A proportion of those who were depressed in childhood and seen by psychiatric services then seem likely to continue to be depressed in young adult life (East-gate & Gilmour 1984, Poznanski 1981, Zeitlin 1986).

Depressive feelings in older children and young adolescents seem to carry an appreciable risk of developing into full depression; two-thirds of the cases described by Kovacs et al (1984) did so within five years.

For those who first develop depression in adolescence, the long-term prognosis is unknown, though clinical experience suggests that the short-term prognosis is quite good, given adequate treatment. The exception is bipolar manic-depressive disorder which is highly likely to continue as a lifelong problem; adults with bipolar disorder, the first episode of which was in adolescence, have a worse prognosis than those with a later onset (Olsen 1961, Welner et al 1979).

Aetiology

IMPORTANT! [handwritten]

The cause of depression in adolescence is unknown, hence the relegation of this section to the end of this chapter. There are a number of models for which some supporting evidence exists. These are well expounded in a book edited by Rutter et al (1986) but the extent to which they inform clinical practice is variable. Some of the component ideas of such models and mechanisms are useful in formulation or management: learned helplessness, competence and vulnerability, loss and attachment theory, the role of shame, psychobiological pathology, genetics, and the role of family support systems are all commonly referred to in formulation. It cannot be said that they fall into any unified model of causation.

The studies by Dweck (Dweck & Bush 1976, Dweck et al 1978) suggest that a learned helplessness paradigm is useful in accounting for gender differences in the frequency of depressive feelings and depression. When they are told they are doing badly, girls are more likely than boys to blame their failure on their own shortcomings and to give up rather than redouble their efforts. Teachers, although more critical of boys than girls, express this in a more diffuse way to boys whilst being quite specific about girls' intellectual shortcomings. Encouragement, conversely, is specific for boys but vague for girls. The outcome of repeated exposure to such pointed criticism, uncorrected by effective praise might be thought to engender a style of helplessness and resignation.

Kagan (1984, p. 182) points out that helplessness or hopelessness depends upon an evaluation of all possible strategies of coping with a challenge and a realisation that all have been exhausted, a cognitive exercise which depends in turn upon the capacity for thinking in formal operational terms (Ch. 3). Given that formal operational thought is not achieved to any great degree until adolescence, this provides one hypothesis for the increase in prevalence of depressive affect and depression at and around puberty. An alternative explanation in terms of endocrine influence is more traditionally invoked and parallels are drawn with the increase in psychological symptomatology associated with the puerperium, the pre-menstrual period and oral contraception. Other possible explanations include the possibility that more social stressors occur at puberty, that adolescents are more vulnerable in terms of (for instance) family support because they are thought to be moving out of the family orbit, or that relevant genetic susceptibilities only come into play at this phase of development. It is not possible to choose between these models in the present state of knowledge and it can be argued that none explain adequately why the increase in depression at puberty applies to both boys and girls, albeit differentially, nor why mania also first appears as a psychopathological entity at the same developmental stage.

Bipolar manic-depressive disorder

For practical purposes, mania does not occur before puberty. It seems highly unlikely that it exists in an altered form, since Dahl's (1971) follow-up study of children attending a child psychiatric clinic yielded no cases of manic-depressive disorder. The situation changes remarkably in adolescence. About one-third of cases of manic-depressive disorder have their first episode in adolescence (Loranger & Levine 1978, Perris 1966, Winokur et al 1969).

The mental state during an acute episode of either mania or depression in an adolescent is comparable to the classical picture described in adults. In Carlson & Strober's (1978) small but systematically described series, expansive euphoria, overactivity, pressure of speech, hypersexuality, irritability and distractibility were the commonest features of mania in adolescence, with grandiosity, sleep loss and flight of ideas rather less frequent. Delusions of self-reference or grandiosity were quite frequent, as was formal thought disorder, so that it was unsurprising that an initial diagnosis of schizophrenia had commonly been made.

Similarly, the clinical picture of depression in a depressive episode is closely comparable to the adult picture. Depressive mood often associates with psychomotor retardation or agitation, and poor concentration, listlessness and self-reproach with suicidal ideation are all frequently seen. Delusions of persecution, guilt or somatic disorder are moderately frequent.

It seems at least possible that many of the earlier descriptions of psychogenic or reactive psychosis would be reclassified by contemporary criteria as manic-depressive disorder. The same may also be true of schizo-affective disorder in adolescence (Carlson & Strober 1978) though this is more contentious. The issue is clinically relevant because of the value of prophylactic lithium and the importance of accurate prognosis. Steinberg (1985) points out how difficult it can be to form a view on prognosis in adolescence on account of the complexity of the interactions of external and developmental factors which may be seen as relevant. In ascribing relative weight to such factors in formulation the possibility arises that "external stresses (may divert) attention from endogenous factors in the disorder" (Steinberg 1985, p 569). There is also the problem of atypical forms of clinical presentation, though one of the most striking aspects of manic-depressive disorder in adolescence is how very much it is like the standard descriptions of the condition and how little its phenomenology is affected by adolescent developmental concerns.

Differentiation of bipolar from unipolar disorder is always somewhat tentative when depression alone presents. The presence of a family history of bipolar disorder is usually considered a reasonable guide, as is the development of a manic swing in response to antidepressant medication (Strober & Carlson 1982). Some teenagers experience recurrent episodes of mania without intervening depression, though overall it seems that mania and depression are about equally common throughout adolescence among individuals ultimately shown to have bipolar disorder. An early onset has a bad prognosis, both for further episodes and for rapid cycling between mania and depression (Carlson 1983, Olsen 1961).

In terms of clinical management, an episode of mania or depression in an adolescent with bipolar affective disorder will require admission for the sake of the youngster's safety. The general principles of treatment are similar to those applicable to adults although ECT is much less often used (rightly or wrongly). Lithium prophylaxis is reasonably well established in adolescence (Steinberg 1980) though some adolescents will require large doses and others will demonstrate an exacerbation of EEG abnormalities, though the significance of this is unknown (Berg et al 1974, Brumback & Weinberg 1977).

REFERENCES

Abou-Saleh M T 1985 Dexamethasone suppression tests in psychiatry: is there a place for an integrated hypothesis? Psychiatric Developments 3: 275–306

Ambrosini P J, Puig-Antich J 1985 Major depression in children and adolescents. In: Shaffer D, Ehrhardt A, Greenhill L (eds) The Clinical Guide to Child Psychiatry. Collier Macmillan, London

Andreasen N 1982 Concepts, diagnosis and classification. In: Paykel E (ed) Handbook of Affective Disorders. Guilford Press, New York

Beck A T, Beamesderfer A 1974 Assessment of depression: The depression inventory. Psychological Measurements in Psychopharmacology 7: 151–169

Beck A T, Rush A J, Shaw B F, Emery G 1979 Cognitive Therapy of Depression: a Treatment Manual. Guilford Press, New York

Berg I, Hullin R, Allsopp M, O'Brien P, MacDonald R 1974 Bipolar manic-depressive psychosis in early adolescence. British Journal of Psychiatry 125: 416–417

Brumback R A, Weinberg W A 1977 Mania in childhood. II. Therapeutic trial of lithium carbonate and further description of manic-depressive illness in children. American Journal of Diseases in Children 131: 1122–1126

Burke P, Delbeccaro M, McAuley E, Clark C 1985 Hallucinations in children. Journal of the American Academy of Child Psychiatry 24: 71–75

Cantwell D P 1983 Depression in childhood: Clinical picture and diagnostic criteria. In: Cantwell D, Carlson G (eds) Affective Disorders in Childhood and Adolescence: an Update. MTP Press, Lancaster

Carlson G 1983 Bipolar affective disorders in childhood and adolescence. In: Cantwell D, Carlson G (eds) Affective Disorders in Childhood and Adolescence: an Update. MTP Press, Lancaster

Carlson G, Garber J 1986 Developmental issues in the classification of depression in children. In: Rutter M, Izard C, Read P (eds) Depression in Young People. Guilford Press, New York

Carlson G A, Strober M 1978 Manic-depressive illness in early adolescence. Journal of the American Academy of Child Psychiatry 17: 138–153

Chambers W, Puig-Antich J, Tabrizi M, Davies M 1982 Psychotic symptoms in prepubertal major depressive disorder. Archives of General Psychiatry 39: 921–931

Costello A 1986 Assessment and diagnosis of affective disorders in children. Journal of Child Psychology and Psychiatry 27: 565–574

Cytryn L, McKnew D H, Bunney W E 1980 Diagnosis of depression in children: a reassessment. American Journal of Psychiatry 137: 22–25

Cytryn L, McKnew D, Bartko J, Lamour M, Hamovit J 1982 Offspring of patients with affective disorders. Journal of the American Academy of Child Psychiatry 21: 389–391

Dahl V 1971 A follow-up study of child psychiatric clientele with special regard to manic-depressive psychosis. In: Annell A L (ed) Depressive States in Childhood and Adolescence. Almqvist and Wiksell, Stockholm

Dimascio A, Weissman M M, Prusoff B A, Neu C, Zwilling M, Klerman G L 1979 Differential symptom reduction by drugs and psychotherapy in acute depression. Archives of General Psychiatry 36: 1450–1456

Dweck C S 1977 Learned helplessness: a developmental approach. In: Schulterbrandt J, Raskin A (eds) Depression in Childhood: Diagnosis, treatment and Conceptual Models. Raven Press, New York

Dweck C S, Bush E S 1976 Sex differences in learned helplessness. I. Differential debilitation with peer and adult evaluators. Developmental Psychology 12: 147–156

Dweck C S, Davidson W, Nelson S, Enna B 1978 Sex differences in learned helplessness. II. The contingencies of evaluative feedback in the classroom. III. An experimental analysis. Developmental Psychology 14: 268–276

Eastgate J, Gilmour L. 1984 Long-term outcome of depressed children: a follow-up study. Developmental Medicine and Child Neurology 26: 68–72

Ellis A 1962 Reason and Emotion in Psychotherapy. Lyle Stuart, New York

Extein I, Rosenberg G, Pottash A, Gold M 1982 The dexamethasone suppression test in depressed adolescents. American Journal of Psychiatry 139: 1617–1619

Frommer E 1968 Depressive illness in childhood. In: Coppen A, Walk A Recent Developments in Affective Disorders. (British Journal of Psychiatry Special Publication No. 2)

Garralda M E 1984 Hallucinations in children with conduct and emotional disorders. I. The clinical phenomena. Psychological Medicine 14: 589–596

Goldfried M, Goldfried A 1975 Cognitive change methods. In Kanfer F, Goldstein A (eds) Helping People Change. Pergamon, Oxford

Hodges K, Kline J, Stern L, Cytryn L, McKnew D 1982 The development of a child assessment interview for research and clinical use. Journal of Abnormal Child Psychology 10: 73–189

Horowitz M, Wilner N, Marmar C, Krupnick J 1980 Pathological grief and the activation of latent self-images. American Journal of Psychiatry 137: 1157–1162

Hudgens R W 1974 Psychiatric Disorders in Adolescents. Williams and Wilkins, Baltimore

Inamdar S C, Siomopoulos G, Osborn M, Bianchi E C 1979 Phenomenology associated with depressed moods in adolescents. American Journal of Psychiatry 136: 156–159

Izard C, Schwartz G 1986 Patterns of emotion in depression. In: Rutter M, Izard C, Read P (eds) Depression in Young People. Guilford Press, New York

Kagan J 1984 The Nature of the Child. Basic Books, New York

Kashani J, Lababidi Z, Jones R 1982 Depression in children and adolescents with cardiovascular symptomatology: the significance of chest pain. Journal of the American Academy of Child Psychiatry 21: 187–189

Kazdin A E, Petti T A 1982 Self-report and interview measures of childhood and adolescent depression. Journal of Child Psychology and Psychiatry 23: 437–457

Kendell R E 1976 The classification of depressions: a review of contemporary confusion. British Journal of Psychiatry 129: 15–28

Kolvin I, Berney T, Bhate S 1984 Classification and diagnosis of depression in school phobia. British Journal of Psychiatry 145: 347–357

Kovacs M, Feinberg T L, Crouse-Novak M, Paulaskas S L, Pollock M, Finkelstein R 1984 Depressive disorder in childhood. II. A longitudinal study of the risk for a subsequent major depression. Archives of General Psychiatry 41: 643–649

Loranger A W, Levine P M 1978 Age at onset of bipolar affective illness. Archives of General Psychiatry 35: 1345–1348

Mash E J, Hammerlynck L A, Handy L C (eds) 1976 Behavior Modification and Families. Brunner/Mazel, New York

Meichenbaum D 1975 Self-instructional methods. In: Kanfer F, Goldstein A (eds) Helping People Change. Pergamon, Oxford

Olsen T 1961 Follow-up study of manic-depressive patients whose first attack occurred before the age of 19 years. Acta Psychiatrica Scandinavica, Supplement 162: 45–51

Paykel E S 1971 Classification of depressed patients: A cluster analysis derived grouping. British Journal of Psychiatry 118: 275–288

Pearce J B 1978 The recognition of depressive disorders in children. Journal of the Royal Society of Medicine 71: 494–500

Perris C 1966 A study of bipolar (manic-depressive) and unipolar recurrent depressive psychoses. Acta Psychiatrica Scandinavica, Supplement 194: 9–189

Poznanski E 1981 Childhood depression: the outcome. Acta Paedopsychiatrica 46: 297–304

Poznanski E, Krahenbuhl V, Zrull J 1976. Childhood depression: a longitudinal perspective. Journal of the American Academy of Child Psychiatry 15: 491–501

Puig-Antich J 1982 Major depression and conduct disorder in prepuberty. Journal of the American Academy of Child Psychiatry 21: 118–128

Puig-Antich J 1986 Psychological markers: effects of age and puberty. In: Rutter M, Izard C, Read P (eds) Depression in Young People. Guilford Press, New York

Puig-Antich J, Perel J M, Lupatkin W et al 1979 Plasma levels of imipramine and desmethylimipramine and clinical response in prepubertal major

143

depressive disorder. A preliminary report. Journal of the American Academy of Child Psychiatry 18: 616–627

Robins D R, Alessi N E, Yanchyshyn G W, Colfer M 1982. Preliminary report on the dexamethasone suppression test in adolescents. American Journal of Psychiatry 139: 942–943

Russell D H 1981 On running away. In: Wells C, Stuart I (eds) Self-Destructive Behavior in Children and Adolescents. Van Nostrand Reinhold, New York

Rutter M 1986 The developmental psychopathology of depression: issues and perspectives. In: Rutter M, Izard C, Read P (eds) Depression in Young People. Guilford Press, New York

Rutter M, Izard C, Read P (eds) 1986 Depression in Young People. Guilford Press, New York

Rutter M, Graham P 1968 The reliability and validity of the psychiatric assessments of the child. I. Interview with the child. British Journal of Psychiatry 114: 563–579

Rutter M, Graham P, Chadwick O, Yule W 1976 Adolescent turmoil: fact or fiction? Journal of Child Psychology and Psychiatry 17: 35–56

Seligman M, Peterson C 1986 A learned helplessness perspective on childhood depression: theory and research. In: Rutter M, Izard C, Read P (eds) Depression in Young People. Guilford Press, New York

Spitzer R L, Endicott J, Robins E 1978 Research Diagnostic Criteria (RDC) for a Selected Group of Functional Disorders. 3rd edn. New York State Psychiatric Institute, New York

Steinberg D 1980 The use of lithium carbonate in adolescence. Journal of Child Psychology and Psychiatry 21: 263–271

Steinberg D 1985 Psychotic and other severe disorders in adolescence. In: Rutter M, Hersov L (eds) Child and Adolescent Psychiatry: Modern Approaches. 2nd edn. Blackwell Scientific, Oxford

Strober M, Carlson G 1982 Bipolar illness in adolescents with major depression. Archives of General Psychiatry 39: 549–55

Teri L 1982 The use of the Beck Depression Inventory with adolescents. Journal of Abnormal Child Psychology 10: 277–284

Weiner L B 1975 Depression in adolescence. In: Flach F F, Draghi S C (eds) The Nature and Treatment of Depression. Wiley, New York

Welner A, Welner Z, Fishman R 1979 Psychiatric and adolescent in-patients: eight–ten year follow-up. Archives of General Psychiatry 36: 698–700

Winokur D, Clayton P J, Reich T 1969 Manic Depressive Illness. Mosby, St. Louis

Zeitlin H 1986 The Natural History of Psychiatric Disorder in Children. Oxford University Press, Oxford

10

Suicidal behaviour

Suicidal thoughts

The concept of death changes with age. Small children imagine death as a monster and, with further maturation, as something associated with separation or bodily injury. By the age of 10 or so children come to understand death as something which is universal and might thus happen to them at some stage (Childers & Wimmer 1971). The progress of such conceptual development is often understood in terms of Piaget's ideas (see Anthony 1940), so the acquisition of formal operational thought in the teens as described in Chapter 3 is seen as crucial in developing a mature view of death. It enables the formation of ideas about death which may be treated hypothetically in reflective thought or discussion. Adolescents become able to consider their own mortality, and thus their own life and its value for themselves and others in terms of the consequences of personal choices or events. They can become philosophical.

Should this capacity combine with pessimism or anger they may then ruminate on the purpose of their own lives in a manner which is alarming to another person who becomes aware of it. Parents who secretly read their teenage children's diaries, or teachers who are presented with poems or pictures of morbid content, are likely to be concerned that the adolescent in question is suicidal. What weight should be placed upon thoughts of suicide? The status of suicidal ideas in private writings is unexplored but the position concerning suicidal thoughts expressed at interview is a little clearer.

There are no grounds for thinking that suicidal ideation is very common. Paykel et al (1974) in a general population study of adults found that only 13% of their subjects reported having had suicidal feelings at any stage of their life. Those who did so tended to have other psychiatric symptomatology. Herjanic and Welner (1980) interviewed children and young teenagers attending psychiatric and paediatric clinics and found that 25% of black and 35% of white children had suicidal thoughts. Rather similarly, Connell (1972) found that 27% of a sample of seriously antisocial youngsters aged between 8 and 17 years old had experienced suicidal ideas, mostly very mild and amounting to reflecting on whether life was worth living. Frequent suicidal ideation was found to be confined to children aged over 10 in a study by McIntyre et al (1972).

Suicidal ideas were reported at interview by 7.6% of Isle of Wight 14-year-olds (Rutter et al 1976) with no appreciable difference between boys and girls. No other epidemiological information is available but the inference can be drawn that suicidal thoughts in early adolescence are by no means common. Nevertheless, such figures suggest that they occur much more frequently than parasuicide, and very much more frequently than suicide; in most instances it is unlikely that they will be followed by suicidal behaviour. That is not to say that such ideas should not be taken seriously but it implies that they are not usually dangerous.

This should not breed complacency. Stevenson et al (1972) compared adolescent psychiatric patients who had threatened or attempted suicide with adult patients who had done likewise. The similarity between the two groups was striking. In both teenagers and adults, suicidal intent was linked in time to episodes of psychiatric illness and was communicated to close relatives on several occasions. Within a psychiatric population, then, it appears that the implications of suicidal ideation in adolescence and in adulthood are similar. Probably the best guideline in assessing the risk of suicide is to be suspicious of expressed suicidal ideation in an adolescent who is not otherwise symptomatic, and to take suicidal ideas increasingly seriously with age in adolescents who have psychiatric symptoms. It is obvious that the coexistence of multiple depressive symptoms with suicidal ideation in the older teenager is likely to indicate a need for admission yet, since the suicide rate is appreciably less among younger adolescents, they may be treated as out-patients if adequate supervision is available at home. Black (1986) suggests that the recognition of possible depression in the individual and the existence of a disturbed family background, family history of psychiatric illness, and previous or current child abuse, are elements which should lead to psychiatric referral as a preventive measure. This is sound advice but the psychiatrist receiving such a referral will have little else in terms of evidence from scientific studies to guide him in ascertaining suicidal risk in the individual case.

Suicide

Although suicide rates rose during the late 1970's, this increase was not especially marked within the adolescent age group (McClure 1984a), most of the increase being due to suicides amongst 25–44-year-old men. A more detailed inspection of the official figures for England and Wales by McClure (1984a, b) reveals the following:

— no recorded suicides below the age of 10 between 1950 and 1980

— in the 6 years between 1975 and 1980, only 36 suicides in the 10–14 age group

— little overall change in the suicide rate for 10–14-year-olds between 1941 and 1980 but, within the overall figures, an increase among girls and a decrease among boys.

— an near-doubling of the suicide rate among 15–19-year-olds during the years 1950–1980 (Fig. 10.1)

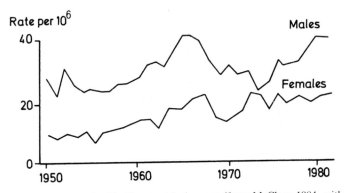

Fig. 10.1 Suicide rate for 15–19-year-olds, by year (from McClure 1984, with permission)

— a fairly constant finding that boys outnumbered girls by 2 or 3 to 1 in the 15–19 age group

— an increase in the suicide rate for each year of age within the teenage years (Fig. 10.2).

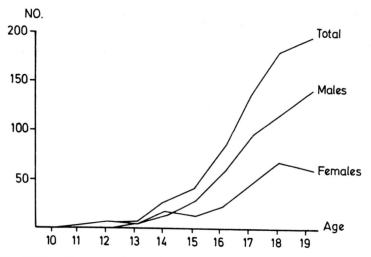

Fig. 10.2 Suicide and age in young people (total suicides for the period 1975–1980) (from McClure 1984, with permission)

This suggests that the suicide figures for the United Kingdom are not as alarming as rumour sometimes has it, presumably a confusion arising from the dramatic rise in parasuicide rates in the last twenty years or so. Nevertheless, suicide is the third commonest cause of death among adolescents and young adults (after accidents and cancer) in the UK (Wilkinson 1985) and the third commonest among adolescents in the USA (after accidents and homicide, Holinger 1979).

Shaffer and Fisher (1981) examined suicide rates among American children and adolescents with essentially similar findings: a very small rate of increase among 10–14-year-olds and a sizeable increase among 15–19-year-olds over the years 1964–1977 with an excess of males in each age group.

Both McClure (1984a) and Shaffer and Fisher (1981) examine the possibility that suicide in adolescents may be commoner than the official figures suggest because it might be recorded as accidental death or the cause of death recorded as "undetermined" with respect to motive. They conclude that it seems likely that the number of suicides misclassified in such a way is small and would not affect the overall conclusion that suicide is uncommon in adolescence. Nevertheless, it is likely that proportionally more suicides are misclassified according to cause of death as accidental or undetermined among the younger age groups (McClure 1984b). If this possibility were to be taken into account, the negligible increase in rate over time in the 10–14 age group when official suicide rates are considered would become translated into a more substantial increase. In terms of UK figures, this notional increase in rate among younger adolescents and older children then becomes comparable to the rise in rate among 15–19-year-olds obtained from official figures, though the overall rate for younger adolescents still remains well below that for older teenagers. It is important to note that the increase in suicide rates is not an artefact of more adolescent deaths being reclassified as suicide rather than accidental, since the rate of accidental death has also risen over the years.

The methods used by adolescents to kill themselves vary by country, culture, race, sex and age. Hanging or self-strangulation, eating or drinking poisonous substances, intentional overdoses of drugs, jumping off high places and firearms (particularly in the USA) are the commonest methods.

Shaffer (1974) examined available records for a group of 30 12–14-year-olds, i.e. all the children aged under 15 who killed themselves intentionally in England and Wales during the years 1962–1968 inclusive. On the basis that this group represents a total population of young suicides, the following individual characteristics of suicidal young adolescents are listed:

— male gender bias (21 boys, 9 girls)

— an excess representation of very high and very low intelligence (17 known to be outside the likely range of one standard deviation from IQ 100)

— tall for age (18 known to be above 50th percentile for height)

— presence of psychiatric symptomatology: antisocial in 5, mixed antisocial and affective in 17, affective only in 4. Only 4 youngsters had no symptoms recorded. Psychiatric disorder was present in 15.

— anticipated disciplinary action by court or school, or parents due to be informed of misdemeanour detected by school (11 cases)

— previous suicidal threat, discussion or attempt (14 cases)

— absence from school (8 cases, 3 of which were chronic school refusers

— existence of a family member who had been treated for psychiatric problems (16 cases) or drank excessively (9 parents) or who had attempted suicide (4 cases). In 3 cases, suicide was consequent upon the difficulties of living with a psychotic parent.

The importance of prediction is obvious, particularly since suicidal threats or gestures account for about 10% of referrals to child and adolescent psychiatrists (e.g. Lukianowicz 1968). Nevertheless, only 14 of the above 30 cases were known to have made such threats or attempted suicide previously (there may have been more cases whose threats were unrecorded). Treating the features listed above as formal predictors of suicide is not likely to be of much use within a group of adolescents since the above elements are neither rare or exclusive to pre-suicidal individuals. No feature was found to be present in all instances. They are of some use in considering suicidal risk in a given clinical case.

It is important to note that suicide in this age range is not likely to be impulsive. Most of the young teenagers in Shaffer's (1974) study had planned their suicide, sometimes going to remarkable lengths. Nor is suicide obviously due to inwardly-directed aggression which could have been externalised. Half of the notes left by Shaffer's (1974) youngsters expressed hostility but in most (5 out of 7) of these the direction of the hostility was outward rather than inward. An association with antisocial behaviour was slightly commoner than with depressive affect in the same study, and the marked association with disciplinary crises and fights with other youngsters as precipitants suggests that excessive inhibition of hostility is not related to suicide in adolescence. If anything, the conclusion suggested by the findings is that suicide is likely to be a violent remedy for a disturbed and socially isolated young person who finds himself unable to communicate his predicament effectively to those who might alleviate it and who sees no other recourse open to him.

Overdoses

Most overdoses taken by adolescents are not fatal. Indeed, to save words "overdose" is used here as shorthand for "non-fatal overdose".

The term "parasuicide" (Kreitman et al 1970a), meaning a deliberate act which mimics the act of suicide without having a fatal result, is often used in connection with teenage overdoses. Although the concept was introduced in order to overcome the difficulties provoked by the older terms "attempted suicide" and "deliberate self-poisoning" (Kessel 1965), there is now a risk that all overdoses which do not result in death are classified clinically as parasuicide rather than failed suicide. Undoubtedly parasuicide and suicide are different phenomena on epidemiological grounds, yet the issue with the individual case is the determination of true suicidal intent or other motive and until this is done the overdose remains a piece of human behaviour which is dangerous and requires explanation.

General characteristics of overdoses

Studies which explore subgroupings within the group of teenagers who take overdoses suggest two main categories: attempted suicide using a method with high lethality, and self-poisoning with less overtly dangerous means as a reaction to an interpersonal crisis (Henderson et al 1977, Choquet et al 1982). The former group are more likely to have other psychiatric pathology, more adverse social factors and be older. In several respects they resemble adolescents who successfully commit suicide (compare Garfinkel et al 1982 with Shaffer 1974).

Nevertheless, in virtually all studies of teenage overdoses this distinction is not made, and the phenomenon has been treated as essentially homogeneous. This means that it is possible to make statements about teenage overdoses as a whole, but the information obtained is obviously derived from the study of groups and its clinical application to individual cases is compromised by the importance of motive: the issue which group studies nearly always ignore.

Cases of adolescent overdoses have increased at a rapid rate over the last forty years, though there is some evidence that a plateau has been reached as far as female overdoses are concerned and there may even have been a decline since 1977 in the UK (Alderson 1985). Girls outnumber boys by about two to one in the 15–19 age group (see Wells 1981). Overdoses are exceptional before puberty but thereafter the rate has been found to increase with age (more rapidly in girls) to a peak in the mid-twenties in most though not all studies. In Hawton & Goldacre's (1982) series there was a slight seasonal effect (commonest in spring) and a relative excess of overdoses on and around Mondays, findings generally comparable with adult studies.

The commonest agents taken in overdose by young adolescents are analgesics, though in the late teens psychotropic agents are as commonly used. Alcohol is often drunk as well and may have facilitated the taking of an overdose of tablets as well as potentiating its effect. The overdose is most likely to have been taken at home with a high likelihood of discovery (Garfinkel et al 1982) and there is usually good evidence that the act was unplanned and impulsive (Hawton et al 1982a). Substantial planning so as to avoid discovery is, like substantial self-inflicted violent physical injury, associated with greater suicidal intent (Otto 1972).

Background

Among adolescents who take overdoses, the percentage of broken homes (whether by separation, divorce or parental death) is raised, though not necessarily above the level found among psychiatrically disturbed adolescents (Mattson et al 1969) unless the age at which parental loss occurred is taken into account, since early loss did differentiate overdosers from other adolescent psychiatric patients in Stanley & Barter's (1970) study. Early parental loss has also been found to be associated with suicidal thoughts and actions: in a study of college students (Adam et al 1980) it appeared to be the disruptive consequences of the loss on continuing family life that were significant. When parental loss was followed by a subsequent stabilisation of family life, suicidal trends were minimal. This would buttress the conclusions of Haider (1968) that it is overt disturbance in current family relationships which is crucial rather than identification with the dead or departed parent (as suggested by e.g. Zilboorg 1937). A poor relationship with the father was noted by Lumsden Walker (1980) and Hawton et al (1982b). Taylor & Stansfeld (1984a) conducted an important study of overdosers aged 8–17 admitted from a defined geographical area to a general hospital. When compared with out-patient psychiatric controls, more frequent disturbances of relationships with both parents were found in the overdose group. Inspection of Taylor & Stansfeld's figures reveals that a disturbed relationship with the father was of particular note. In the same study, a lack of emotional warmth within the families of overdosers was striking (60% as compared with 8% of controls) and was associated with a documented history of physical ill-treatment in 20%. The authors suggest that "the lack of a supportive network of relationships was more apparent than any more subtly deviant qualities of the network" and, when compared to psychiatric controls, found no excess of such variables as low socio-economic status which differentiate overdosers from normal controls (e.g McIntyre & Angle 1973).

A family history of suicidal behaviour is often obtained (Hawton et al 1982b) and, certainly as far as children are concerned, is more common than among other psychiatric cases (Pfeffer et al 1979, 1980). Two possible explanations suggest themselves: the unwitting demonstration by an adult relative of a method of communicating distress to others (Kreitman et al 1970b), or a genetic predisposition. As far as the latter possibility is concerned, Buchsbaum et al (1977) found suicidal behaviour to be commoner in the families of college students who had low platelet monoamine oxidase levels. Rather against the latter hypothesis is the fact that mental illness was no commoner in the parents of Taylor & Stansfeld's (1984a) overdosing adolescents and children than in psychiatric controls. Certainly the idea that an overdose is to many desperate adolescents a recognised way of letting others know of the intensity of their despair has clinical face value; it has a familiar ring to the ears of the experienced adolescent psychiatrist.

Precipitants

Most overdoses follow a quarrel or similar upset, typically with a parent or boy- or girl-friend. The altercation may be relatively minor but it often occurs in a setting of isolation within a family which is judged by the youngster, correctly or otherwise, to be unsympathetic or uncomprehending. Parents may be unreceptive to attempts to communicate distress or the adolescent may judge that only an overdose will provide an adequate statement of their plight, either to family or friends. A few find themselves in a predicament which they feel unable to communicate to their parents: pregnancy, incest or the realisation that they are homosexual. The high rate of physical illness among adolescents who take overdoses is puzzling; the prevalence of somatic symptoms in such a group studied by Garfinkel et al (1982) was even higher than in a control group of paediatric emergencies which were not overdoses. Chronic ill-health may draw parents into a preoccupation with physical rather than psychosocial issues, some youngsters may do the same themselves and then experience difficulty in coping with psychological stresses caused by their illness. It is as if they have invested so much in physical issues and development that their experience of resolving psychosocial problems is minimal; by comparison they are naïve and inexperienced in such matters. Alternatively, somatic symptomatology may arise in depression and the overdose result either from despair in association with the morbid mood or from hypochondriasis fuelled by subjective physical symptoms and associated with an assumption that a fatal outcome was inevitable. Fears of impending insanity (very occasionally justified) can be seen similarly as arising out of an interaction between morbid changes in mood, judgement and thinking.

> A 15-year-old boy, chronically alienated from his single-parent mother who had recently declared herself to be homosexual and taken a female partner, became miserable and anhedonic, and began both to truant and run away from home. He was introduced by friends to the illicit use of drugs and took a cocktail of pseudo-ephedrine and benzhexol which produced hallucinations and a temporary shrinkage of his penis. His understanding was that he was going mad and was turning homosexual. Seeing no future for himself, he took a large overdose.

Mental state

Compared with psychiatric controls, youngsters who take overdoses are more likely to be clinically depressed (26% vs. 2% in Taylor & Stansfeld's (1984a) study), and are more hostile (Cohen-Sandler et al 1982). Hawton (1982) suggested that "a minority of adolescents involved in suicide attempts are found to have a psychiatric illness, depression being the usual diagnosis". Yet Taylor & Stansfeld (1984a) in a consecutive series of cases of overdose from a specified local area found 62% to have psychiatric diagnoses. This figure included 36% with emotional disorder and 20% with conduct disorder, leading the authors to conclude that "self-poisoning is not a coherent diagnostic grouping", a conclusion arrived at by Shaffer (1982): overdosing is a non-specific behaviour that can occur in the setting of a number of psychiatric conditions. Young people who take over-doses may not be psychiatrically disordered; when they are, they differ but little from other adolescents with the same diagnosis (see above).

A number of motives underly the taking of overdoses. Several of these may coexist in any individual case; they are not mutually exclusive.

1. A wish to kill oneself out of despair or to obtain permanent relief in death from an intolerable situation or state of mind. Although this is commonly stated by the adolescent, it should not be accepted too readily. It may be offered as a reason because any alternative motive would sound less compelling or arouse parental wrath. Even when confirmed, it is necessary to establish just what the youngster's concept of death is since that may lead to consideration of other motives. Death may be understood to be reversible (see 3 below). Some wish to kill a part, rather than the entirety of themselves but act impulsively and desperately without thinking things through.

2. Revenge. Fantasies of how others will respond to their death ("They'll realise . . . . . they'll be sorry . . . . . they'll say we should have loved her more") include an extreme indifference to the distress their suicide would cause their family. It is as though young people who take overdoses find themselves temporarily unable to hold on to the idea that others can care for them or protect them. In some circumstances it may well be that the reality is that they have not been sufficiently well nurtured and cared for; that there has been insufficient warmth and caring for them to develop the capacity genuinely to care for themselves and others and preserve themselves from self-destructive impulses when their own frustration and anger is aroused.

3. A wish for temporary escape. Death may be viewed as a protracted sleep or there may be a direct statement that the overdose was taken in order to obtain rest or relief in temporary oblivion.

This blends with fantasies of rebirth or re-awakening to a new or radically changed life. The bases for this may include an immature concept of death as reversible, idiosyncratic religious ideas or a notion that one can offer one's present life in barter for a new one.

4. Protest or a cry for help. A teenager may take an overdose in order to draw attention to an intolerable situation such as continuing incest or irreconcilable differences between themselves and their parents as, for instance, in the children of first-generation immigrants who wish to preserve a cultural heritage with standards differing from those that their children are exposed to in school or their peer group. This is clearly a communication which may be directed at a particular person or people but is unlikely to be a cry for help from any specific social agency (unless the adolescent is in the care of a local authority). Indeed, the difficulty in engaging overdosers in psychiatric treatment subsequently is well-known (see Taylor & Stansfeld 1984b).

5. An exploratory gamble. In order to discover whether a particular person loves them, or whether they are meant to live, some young people are prepared to stake their lives on the basis that, if the answer is negative, life would be pointless in any case.

6. Manipulation. Although conscious coercion of others is a motive commonly attributed to overdoses, this was not particularly common within the admitted motives of the group of overdosers, both teenagers and adults, reported by James & Hawton (1985).

7. Demonstration of affection. This may blend with Group 6 since the overdose may take place after desertion or infidelity by a boy- or girl-friend.

8. A wish to contact or be united with dead loved person. In the minds of some young people it seems as though it is possible to take an overdose in order to visit a dead person and then return to life ("I just wanted to see them and say good-bye") though serious grief may produce a wish for permanent union, life without them being intolerable (or even the thought that the dead person's after-life would be intolerable without the company of the adolescent with them in death).

9. Identification with a cult or hero-figure. Sporadic outbreaks of overdosing occur within networks of adolescents and may be provoked by an overdose taken by a media figure or a charismatic local character. This is no new phenomenon: similar outbreaks of suicidal activity have been repeatedly recorded in history.

10. An unwanted effect of sensation-seeking. An overdose of a drug taken for recreational or mood-enhancing purposes may be the result of ignorance or misjudgement.

Management

All adolescents who take an overdose should be admitted to hospital, either to a paediatric or general medical ward (Royal College of Psychiatrists 1982). Psychiatric consultation should be automatic. Hospital admission provides the best opportunity for engaging the parents; their motivation to become involved diminishes with their daughter's discharge. Once she has left hospital, the temptation to gloss over the threatening fact that she tried to kill herself becomes irresistible for many families who wish only to forget the whole episode. It follows that a meeting with the parents should be arranged as soon as possible whilst their daughter is still in hospital. This may include the adolescent: if so, the decision needs to be taken as to whether she requires an additional separate interview (particularly to establish motive), in order to establish whether serious depression is present, and assess suicidal intent, matters which are difficult to clarify in a whole-family interview. The suicidal patient requires admission to an adolescent unit.

In most instances though, this initial assessment will lead to an offer of out-patient treatment following discharge, and this will normally be carried out by members of the psychiatric team. Typically it will be psychotherapeutic in approach and draw upon elements of crisis intervention theory. Whereas it is usual for treatment to be a psychiatric affair, other agencies can be called in to help alleviate psychosocial stress or provide supervision, support, counselling and the like, particularly when they are already involved. They may welcome consultative support from psychiatric services. Where sexual or physical abuse within the family has occurred it is necessary to ensure the adolescent's safety and the Social Services department will usually need to be informed.

Within a psychotherapeutically inspired approach, whether individual- or family-centred, some principles seem sensible even though comparative studies of interventions with adolescents who take overdoses are not available and only anecdotal support is offered in justification. The following components are suggested:

1. Establishing with patient and family that an overdose can be

fatal. Adolescents may have concepts of death which are immature or distorted (see above). They can easily underestimate the dangerousness of their overdose, particularly when this is seen by them as a way of communicating or responding to stress (Parker 1981); a respite function quite different from committing suicide. Similarly, they may be unaware of the danger of an overdose of aspirin or paracetamol.

2. Assisting adequate and clear communication. The overdose can provoke discussion of the hitherto undiscussed and the psychiatric contribution may be to facilitate this.

3. Exploration of anger and guilt. Taking the teenager through her fantasies of the funeral that would have followed in the event of her death ("Who would have been sorry? what would they have been saying? who would have cried?") enables the ramifications of anger and guilt to be explored. Tying this in with an idea of getting rid of psychic discomfort by projection allows an opportunity for the adolescent to accept that a measure of personal responsibility and guilt belongs to her. Both steps are advised: demonstration by the psychiatrist of covert anger together with a refusal to accept that the act, itself uncaring, was justified.

4. Balancing fears of dependency with autonomy and a wish to be cared for. An overdose can fulfil a number of wishes: for power, for recognition of the adolescent's loneliness or helplessness, for escape from persecution and so forth. The theme of independence–dependence conflict can often be uncovered and will be accentuated by any requirement to remain in treatment. The use of a problem-solving model (Hawton & Catalan 1982) has obvious appeal given such considerations. Within the family, the result of the overdose may be an increase in supervision and a restriction of social opportunity which is the opposite of what the adolescent wished. Parental anger may be concealed beneath a cloak of apparent caring, the message received by the adolescent being: "We think that if you're going to do silly things like take overdoses then you aren't mature enough to look after yourself". This may, of course, be true.

5. Resisting defensive omnipotence. In order to counteract feelings of helplessness, the overdoser may attempt to render the psychiatrist helpless by threatening suicide. A vein of self-satisfaction at being able to put herself beyond treatment or help can frequently be observed. It may develop into malicious triumph at professional impotence: "You can't stop me killing myself" to which may sometimes be added ". . .and you're going to get into trouble when I'm dead". It is wise to say to her that one cannot prevent her killing herself and indeed that she may have a secret plan to do so if things do not improve; that her suicide will not result in "trouble" for the psychiatrist though it will elicit his concern. Openly labelling an overdose as a weapon defuses some of its power as a secret weapon. The connection with the adolescent's need to maintain a defensive omnipotent stance should also be made so that the focus can be kept on their feelings of helplessness.

6. Denying the rationality of the overdose. At the point of the overdose, the individual has made a choice. The consequence is an attack on herself and, if there is suicidal intent, a denial that hope and caring exist. The future seems hopeless and there is "an emergence of fantasies wherein death is seen as providing the gratifications that the world withholds" (Morse 1973). These fantasies override rational judgement. It may be painful for the teenager to return to the state of mind in which she took a suicidal overdose and the fantasies precipitating it may be too threatening to consider consciously without therapeutic support. A number of teenagers will claim amnesia for the moments during when they took the overdose in order to steer clear of the affect and fantasies present at the time. The danger is that if these are not confronted they may recur and precipitate a repetition.

Prognosis

A number of studies suggest that the overall rate of repeat among parasuicides of all ages is about 20–25% in the next year (see e.g. Gardner et al 1977) with the highest risk for repetition being in the first three months. Adolescents may have a somewhat lower repetition rate: Hawton's (1982) review estimated that 10% would repeat within a year and noted that repeaters have higher rates of: drug and alcohol abuse, living away from home, associated of psychiatric disturbance, long-term problems, poor peer relationships, and earlier parental loss.

In a classification study, Hawton et al (1982c) argued that a simple typology based on the duration of problems (less or more than one month, and, in the latter group, with or without behaviour problems) had predictive value. Group I included adolescents with a history of problems lasting less than one month. Little distinguished the teenagers in this category from those in the general population; they were all girls, had transient problems and were unlikely to repeat. Group II youngsters had chronic problems, usually with family or friends as a whole, and were typically lonely and isolated. Similarly, they were unlikely to repeat. Group III contained those with long-standing problems and behaviour difficulties such as stealing, fighting, habitual drunkenness, conflict with school, employer or social services and a distinct likelihood of being in local authority care (one-third of cases). This group, which contained about a quarter of all overdosers aged between 13 and 18, was most likely to repeat (7 out of 12 cases within 13 months).

The eventual suicide of teenage overdosers is an unusual event. Nevertheless, Otto (1972) in a 10-year follow-up of nearly 2000 Swedish children and adolescents who had attempted suicide showed an eventual suicide rate of about 4% (10% of boys, 3% of girls), with the highest risk in the first two years after the first suicidal act. The prediction of eventual suicide is imprecise, to say the least, though an extension of the intent scales developed with adult parasuicides (e.g. Pierce 1981) would seem logical in spite of their high false-positive rate. Shaffer (1985), well aware of such limitations, suggests the following markers of high risk on the grounds of comparison with successful suicide amongst the young:

— male

— white

— significant depression

— high intelligence

— antisocial behaviour

— habitual use of drugs or alcohol

— family history of suicidal behaviour

— concealment of act

— highly lethal method

— significant premeditation *or* impulse under influence of drugs or alcohol.

Wrist-cutting

The phenomenon of wrist-cutting has been poorly studied. No figures are available to indicate an incidence rate among a general population of teenagers and information is confined to that gained from clinical reports, usually on in-patients and usually by psychiatrists. In some studies of self-injury the distinction has not been made between cutting of the anterior aspect of the wrist using a sharp edge such as a razor blade or broken glass, and the self-injurious behaviour seen in some mentally handicapped and autistic young persons. The latter usually takes the form of biting or hitting oneself, hardly ever cutting except incidentally during the smashing of a window. It is obvious that the two types of self-injury are qualitatively different.

More typical wrist-cutting may itself be subdivided:

1. A suicidal bid with true intent to kill oneself ("coarse cutting"). Often a deep single cut in each wrist is employed. Most characteristically this type is seen in older males, conforming to the classical suicidal stereotype, though it can be seen in young depressed women who may successfully kill themselves thereby. For some of these unfortunate individuals, the difference between suicide and an attack on their bodies arising out of self-hatred becomes blurred in the anguish of the moment; it is not enough for the psychiatrist merely to rule out suicidal intent in the narrow sense of a wish to die.

2. As a component of self-mutilation secondary to psychotic phenomena such as instructing voices or an attempt to produce crucifixion stigmata

3. A communication of despair or threat, comparable to other forms of parasuicide such as some overdoses.

4. Copycat cutting within communities such as schools, psychiatric wards, adolescent units or prisons (see Verduyn & Hoefkens 1986). There is often a competitive flavour, each cutter trying to equal the expressed despair of others. An element of social attention-seeking may be suspected.

5. Classical wrist-slashing or cutting, to which the rest of this section is devoted. Pao (1969) who coined the term "coarse cutting" (1, above), called this type "delicate self-cutting", referring to the precision sometimes employed by experienced cutters.

Description

The classical wrist-cutter (5, above) is a young woman in her late teens or early twenties. Young men hardly ever cut their wrists in the same way unless they are in prison, and even then the pattern is more likely to correspond to that listed in 3 or 4 above. The few young men who do so outside prison are commonly of inadequate personality or are strikingly effeminate with sexual and gender orientation difficulties. Cuts are multiple, fine incisions, made on the anterior aspect of the wrist and forearm, though they may also be made on other areas of the body such as the genitals and face. The habit of cutting always starts after puberty and often in the mid-teens. The individuals quite often elicit positive descriptions such as attractive or talented (Raine 1982, Simpson 1976) though this is obviously not always the case. A surprisingly large minority have medical connections. As a rule they have had a disturbed and "deprived" childhood for a variety of reasons, and rates of divorce, parental death, privation of emotional warmth, early admission to hospital and parental rejection are all higher among classical wrist-cutters as a whole than in control groups (see e.g. Rosenthal et al 1972, Waldenberg 1972).

The psychopathology of wrist-cutters overlaps that of other diagnostic groups so that little consensus obtains, although borderline state (borderline personality disorder) is commonly invoked as a diagnosis. Within various clinical samples, the following associations are found with surprising consistency:

— about one-half of cases abuse alcohol or drugs

— roughly one-third have an eating disorder, particularly bulimia

— menstruation is often irregular and viewed with disgust

— sexual orientation or gender identity problems affect rather more than half of all cases. Extremes of promiscuity or virginal abhorrence are common.

— low self-esteem and disgust at one's own body are extremely frequent

— difficulty explaining feelings in words is experienced by a majority

— all cases have severe difficulties with personal relationships

— rapid and unpredictable mood swings are very common

— comparatively high scores on the obsessionality scales of various questionnaires.

(See e.g. Graff & Mallin 1967, Gruenbaum & Klerman 1967, Gardner & Gardner 1975, Pao 1969, Rosenthal et al 1972, Simpson 1975.)

The cutting episode

Several studies have noted an apparent precipitation of an episode of cutting by a threat of abandonment, subjectively perceived by the cutter (e.g. McKerracher et al 1968, Rosenthal et al 1972). This is not always the case and there may be other difficulties in personal relationships that are seen as insoluble and which bring about powerful emotions that the girl cannot verbalise or share. Being thus unable to resolve her distress, she becomes increasingly despairing and frustrated. The result is mounting tension which increases over a period of hours. A seasoned cutter will start to plan her cut during this period and begin to withdraw socially. A state of depersonalisation supervenes as tension increases to unbearable levels. The girl seeks privacy and cuts secretly in a self-absorbed state of mind, oblivious to the responses of others. She makes one or more delicate cuts until blood is produced. The sight of blood welling up in the wound, its red colour contrasted against the pale skin, and (for some) the sight of the subcutaneous tissue beneath the skin bring a feeling of warmth and comfort which floods into the mind of the cutter. This terminates the numbness and emptiness of depersonalisation dramatically and results in an intense feeling of pleasure and relief. Pain is not usually felt and the subsequent reactions of staff, whether hostile or sympathetic, are tolerated with some detachment initially though the bandage or plaster may later be flaunted for peer approval.

The accounts of deprived and unhappy early childhoods provided by so many cutters suggest that emotional distance, lack of physical contact and geographical separation from their parents seem to have resulted in a lasting unease about their own bodies, their own worth and their own psychological solidity. The childhood experience of being emotionally distant from parents with a lack of ever having felt emotionally understood and accepted appears to result in pessimism about ever being able to share their feelings with others without subsequent rejection and psychological annihilation. At the same time, their sense of self-worth and security is tenuous and fragile: they lack faith in themselves and in others. Lacking trust and a sense of personal boundaries, they readily lapse into fear, anger and despair at the threat of abandonment. Unable to seek comfort from others, increasing mental tension triggers a depersonalisation reaction which defensively dampens unpleasant affect before it becomes overwhelming. Yet this saving response brings feelings of emptiness and deadness which are supremely threatening in their own right to a girl who has not been filled with approval and affection to the extent that would produce self-worth, secure identity and pride. The sight of her own blood has extraordinary impact in providing reassurance and, as it were, parental love ("I felt life coming back into me", "It was warm and beautiful . . . . like a caress would be"). Simpson (1980) and Kafka (1969) cite numerous similar quotes and suggest that blood serves as a transitional object. Classical wrist-cutting is thus primarily a disorder of attachment rather than a suicidal act or one primarily motivated by a desire for attention. In fact the search for privacy before cutting and the wish for a relief from a sensation of deadness militate strongly against either alternative; cutting is solitary and life-seeking.

One classical cutter can, nevertheless, socially exploit the wound later and provoke an outburst of imitative cutting by others motivated by attention-seeking. This will often be accompanied by a polarising of staff attitudes into sympathy and rejection which can have disastrous consequences for the patient's relationships and staff cohesion, a situation brilliantly described by Main (1957).

Treatment

Wrist-cutting is difficult to manage. It offends health-care professionals because it is recurrent, self-inflicted, and apparently damaging. Wrist-cutters are presented to psychiatrists (and to emergency services) for treatment of the wound; they appear to need urgent treatment yet their attitude to their own wound is quite often rather dismissive. Although cutters are manifestly disturbed individuals there is nothing definitely in favour of admission to hospital, particularly if it is to be followed by discharge should the behaviour become contagious. Cutting is not likely to be life-threatening and about one-half of classical wrist cutters will give up the habit though a few (about 10%) will take fatal overdoses in the longer term (Nelson & Grunebaum 1971). Admission would therefore seem to be indicated only when cutting is suicidal rather than classical or when a classical cutter shows suicidal tendencies apart from cutting. Chaos in other areas of life — sexual, eating or substance abuse — may require admission for asylum and education. Simpson (1980) argues that a straightforward, quasi-custodial institution with less than intense personal relationships and firm limit-setting may allow for improvement. Although it might seem from the apparent aetiology of the problem that a psychotherapeutic approach would be indicated, the results of conventional or dyadic psychodynamic psychotherapy are often disappointing (Simpson 1976).

If it is thought that a girl is brewing up for a cut, a hug from a member of staff who can encourage her to find words for her feelings is helpful. Once cutting has happened, a plaster may be all that is needed, but if suturing is required it should be done under local anaesthesia and with a minimum of lecturing. To minimise secondary gain and the learning of a social (rather than a private) habit, no special privileges should ensue. Taking a neutral attitude to the cut may be assisted by a realisation by the staff that it is usually not suicidal in motivation.

For most classical cutters, cutting provides immediate and effective relief from an extremely unpleasant state of mind. If the technique had been discovered by a doctor, it might conceivably have entered the official therapeutic armamentarium. Sometimes it is wise to leave well alone and teach the girl how to look after her own physical wounds while offering persistent supportive psychotherapy over a period of years in an attempt to facilitate the healing of psychological wounds.

REFERENCES

Adam K S, Lohrenz J G, Harper D, Steiner D 1982. Early parental loss and suicidal ideation in university students. Canadian Journal of Psychiatry 27: 275–281

Adam K S, Bouckoms A, Scarr G 1980 Attempted suicide in Christchurch: a controlled study. Australian and New Zealand Journal of Psychiatry 14: 305–314

Alderson M 1985 National trends in self-poisoning in women Lancet i: 974–975

Anthony S 1940 The Child's Discovery of Death. Kegan Paul, London

Black D 1986 Adolescent suicide: preventive considerations. British Medical Journal 292: 1620–1621

Buchsbaum M S, Haier R J, Murphy D L 1977 Suicide attempts, platelet monoamine oxidate and the average evoked potential. Acta Psychiatrica Scandinavica 56: 69–79

Childers P, Wimmer M 1971 The concept of death in early childhood. Child Development 42: 1299–1301

Choquet M, Faly F, Davidson F 1982 Suicide and attempted suicide among adolescents in France. In: Farmer R, Hirsch S (eds) The Suicide Syndrome. Croom Helm, London

Cohen-Sandler R R, Berman R, King R A 1982 Life stress and symptomatology: determinants of suicidal behavior in children. Journal of the American Academy of Child Psychiatry 20: 178–186

Connell H M 1972 Attempted suicide in school children. Medical Journal of Australia 1: 686–690

Gardner A R, Gardner A J 1975 Self-mutilation, obsessionality and narcissism. British Journal of Psychiatry 127: 127–132

Gardner R, Hanka R, O'Brien V C, Page A J F, Rees R 1977 Psychological and social evaluation in cases of deliberate self-poisoning admitted to a general hospital. British Medical Journal ii: 1567–1570

Garfinkel B D, Froese A, Hood J 1982 Suicide attempts in children and adolescents. American Journal of Psychiatry 139: 1257–1261

Graff H, Mallin R 1967 The syndrome of the wrist-cutter. American Journal of Psychiatry 124: 36–42

Grunebaum H, Klerman G 1967 Wrist-slashing. American Journal of Psychiatry 124: 527–534

Haider I 1968 Suicidal attempts in children and adolescents. British Journal of Psychiatry 114: 1133–1134

Hawton K 1982 Attempted suicide in children and adolescents. Journal of Child Psychology and Psychiatry 23: 497–503

Hawton K, Catalan J 1982 Attempted Suicide. Oxford University Press, Oxford

Hawton K, Goldacre M 1982 Hospital admissions for adverse effects of medicinal agents (mainly self-poisoning) among adolescents in the Oxford region. British Journal of Psychiatry 141: 166–170

Hawton K, Cole D, O'Grady J, Osborn M 1982a Motivational aspects of deliberate self-poisoning in adolescents. British Journal of Psychiatry 141: 286–291

Hawton K, Osborn M, O'Grady J, Cole D 1982b Classification of adolescents who take overdoses. British Journal of Psychiatry 140: 118–123

Hawton K, O'Grady J, Osborn M, Cole D 1982c Adolescents who take overdoses: their characteristics, problems and contacts with helping agencies. British Journal of Psychiatry 140: 124–131

Henderson A S, Hartigan J, Davidson J 1977 A typology of parasuicide. British Journal of Psychiatry 131: 631–641

Herjanic B, Welner Z 1980 Adolescent suicide. Advances in Behavioral Pediatrics 1: 195–223

Holinger P C 1979 Violent deaths among the young. American Journal of Psychiatry 136: 1144–1147

James D, Hawton K 1985. Overdoses: explanations and attitudes in self-poisoners and significant others. British Journal of Psychiatry 146: 481–485

Kafka J 1969 The body as transitional object. British Journal of Medical Psychology 42: 207–213

Kessel N 1965 Self-poisoning. I. British Medical Journal ii: 1265–1270

Kreitman N, Philip A E, Greer S, Bagley C 1970a Parasuicide (correspondence). British Journal of Psychiatry 116: 460

Kreitman N, Smith P, Tan E S 1970b Attempted suicide as language: an empirical study. British Journal of Psychiatry 116: 465–473

Lukianowicz N 1968 Attempted suicide in children. Acta Psychiatrica et Neurologica Scandinavica 44: 415–435

Lumsden Walker W 1980 Intentional self-injury in school age children. Journal of Adolescence 3: 217–228

McClure G M G 1984a Trends in suicide rate for England and Wales 1975–80. British Journal of Pyschiatry 144: 119–126

McClure G M G 1984b Recent trends in suicide amongst the young. British Journal of Psychiatry 144: 134–138

McIntyre M S, Angle C, Struempler L J 1972 The concept of death in midwestern children and youth. American Journal of Diseases of Children 123: 527–532

McIntyre M S, Angle C R 1973 Psychological "biopsy" in self-poisoning of children and adolescents. American Journal of Diseases of Children 126: 42–46

McKerracher D W, Loughnane T, Watson R A 1968 Self-mutilation in female psychopaths. British Journal of Psychiatry 114: 829–832

Main T F, 1957 The ailment. British Journal of Medical Psychology 30: 129–145

Mattson A, Leese L R, Hawkins J W 1969 Suicidal behavior as a child psychiatric emergency. Archives of General Psychiatry 20: 100–109

Morse S J 1973 The after-pleasure of suicide. British Journal of Medical Psychology 46: 227–238

Nelson S H, Grunebaum H 1971 A follow-up study of wrist-slashers. American Journal of Psychiatry 128: 1345–1349

Otto U 1972 Suicidal acts by children and adolescents. Acta Psychiatrica Scandinavica Supplement 233

Pao P-N 1969 The syndrome of delicate self-cutting. British Journal of Medical Psychology 42: 195–206

Parker A 1981. The meaning of atttempted suicide to young parasuicides: a repertory grid study. British Journal of Psychiatry 139: 306–312

Paykel E S, Myers J K, Lindenthal J J, Tanner J 1974. Suicidal feelings in the general population: a prevalence study. British Journal of Psychiatry 124: 460–469

Pfeffer C R, Conte H R, Plutchik R, Jerrett I 1979 Suicidal behavior in latency age children: an empirical study. Journal of the American Academy of Child Psychiatry 18: 679–692

Pfeffer C R, Conte H R, Plutchik R, Jerrett I 1980. Suicidal behavior in latency age children: An empirical study II: an out-patient population. Journal of the American Academy of Child Psychiatry 19: 703–710

Pierce D W 1981 The predictive validation of a suicide intent scale: a five-year follow-up. British Journal of Psychiatry 139: 391–396

Raine W J B 1982 Self mutilation. Journal of Adolescence 5: 1–13

Rosenthal R J, Rinzler C, Wallsh R, Klausner E 1972 Wrist-cutting as a syndrome: the meaning of a gesture. American Journal of Psychiatry 129: 1363–1368

Royal College of Psychiatrists 1982 The management of parasuicide in young people under sixteen. Bulletin of the Royal College of Psychiatrists 6: 182–185

Rutter M, Graham P, Chadwick O, Yule W 1976 Adolescent turmoil: fact or fiction? Journal of Child Psychology and Psychiatry 17: 35–56

Shaffer D 1974 Suicide in childhood and early adolescence. Journal of Child Psychology and Psychiatry 15: 275–291

Shaffer D 1982 Diagnostic considerations in suicidal behavior in children and adolescents. Journal of the American Academy of Child Psychiatry 21: 414–415

Shaffer D 1985 Depression, mania and suicidal acts. In: Rutter M, Hersov L (eds) Child and Adolescent Psychiatry: Modern Approaches. 2nd edn. Blackwell Scientific, Oxford

Shaffer D, Fisher P 1981 The epidemiology of suicide in children and young adolescents. Journal of the American Academy of Child Psychiatry 20: 545–565

Simpson M A 1975 The phenomenology of self-mutilation in a general hospital setting. Canadian Psychiatric Association Journal 20: 424–434

Simpson M A 1976 Self-mutilation. British Journal of Hospital Medicine 16: 430–438

Simpson M A 1980 Self-mutilation as indirect self-destructive behavior. In: Farberow N L (ed) The Many Faces of Suicide. McGraw Hill, New York

Stanley E J, Barter J T 1970 Adolescent suicidal behavior. American Journal of Orthopsychiatry 40: 87–96

Stevenson E K, Hudgens R W, Held C P, Meredith C H, Hendrix M E, Carr D L 1972 Suicidal communication by adolescents. Diseases of the Nervous System 33: 112–122

Taylor E A, Stansfeld S A 1984a Children who poison themselves. I. A clinical comparison with psychiatric controls. British Journal of Psychiatry 145: 127–135

Taylor E A, Stansfeld S A 1984b Children who poison themselves. II. Prediction of attendance for treatment. British Journal of Psychiatry 145: 132–135

Verduyn C M, Hoefkens A 1986 Deliberate self-harm in adolescence: contagion effects in an adolescent unit. British Journal of Clinical and Social Psychiatry 4: 87–89

Waldenberg S 1972 Wrist-cutting - a psychiatric injury. M.Phil. Dissertation, London University

Wells N 1981 Suicide and Deliberate Self-harm. Office of Health Economics, London

Wilkinson G 1985 Young suicides (book review). British Medical Journal 290: 309

Zilboorg G 1937 Considerations on suicide with particular reference to that of the young. American Journal of Orthopsychiatry 7: 15–31

11

Anxiety-related disorders

Worries

Perhaps it is obvious that the developmental tasks set by the biological and social changes typical of adolescence can cause anxious preoccupations in the minds of adolescents themselves. As has been noted earlier, the development of formal operational thought allows mental comparisons to be made between what is and what might be. This enables individuals to make judgements about their own shortcomings, comparing their present state with a personal ideal. Since they themselves are changing, they may well not have any clear idea of how others view them, or what their own capacities and characteristics are. Consequently they may doubt their own judgements of themselves or come to the wrong conclusions. At the same time they are becoming aware of the limitations of adults in providing total care and protection. Parents, the source of security, reassurance and comfort in childhood, are now seen to be fallible and there is a general social expectation that adolescents will be less dependent than children upon their families of origin for the resolution of personal distress. In addition, wider horizons of experience and information are accompanied by a perception of dangers (road traffic accidents, AIDS, nuclear war) for which adult protection may not apply.

Not surprisingly, the concerns of adolescents vary according to which culture they are living within, their gender and their age. Porteous (1985) demonstrated the impact of such variables on large groups of normal English and Irish adolescents. In this and an earlier study (Porteous 1979) he confirmed what a number of North American studies have demonstrated over time: the commonest concerns of individuals in mid-adolescence are about educational progress, family relationships, employment prospects, and how they are judged by their peers. However, for each of these, only about one quarter of those surveyed said they had definite concerns in such an area.

The importance of such surveys is twofold. Firstly, the judgement by mental health professionals as to the normality or otherwise of an adolescent's worries. This will depend upon the culture-specific standards of the adolescent and the professional; the two may not concur. What is a common concern among black 14-year-old London girls will not necessarily be common among white 18-year-old boys in Northern Ireland. The experience of an interviewer with one of those two groups will not set valid expectations for the other. Secondly, there is a difference between worries which are quite common among a clinic population and those prevalent in the general teenage population. For instance, worries about:

— physical unattractiveness

— friendlessness

— being rejected by peers

— going mad

— leaving home

— lack of a confidante

— whether it is worth living

— parental favouritism

— parental arguments

— becoming ill

— being bossed around too much

— communication difficulties with parents

were all expressed by less than 10% of the 15-year-olds surveyed by Porteous (1979) even though they are common enough among clinic patients. There is a danger that the clinic-based professional will become accustomed to such complaints and regard them as usual when they are in fact uncommon.

Concern that one's body is too fat was not asked about in the above study, yet would appear to be a common worry amongst girls from mid-adolescence onwards (see Ch. 12).

Fears and phobias

Given that adolescence is an intermediate stage between childhood and adulthood, it is not surprising that the irrational fears reported by young adolescents in the general population are coextensive with those which are most typical of childhood. Thus Bamber (1979) in a review of the literature noted that most studies showed that fears of water, insects and animals, separation from a parent (including their death), the dark and the unknown are all most common in early adolescence and decline in frequency thereafter.

Conversely, the prevalence of fears of bodily injury or disease, social ridicule, the possibility of war, and an abnormal personal appearance (due to body shape or a transient change such as blushing) tends to rise with progression through adolescence. Apart from fears related to the general political situation, all fears are commoner among girls and girls tend to have more fears than boys.

Bamber's own questionnaire study (1979) of over 1000 Northern Irish 12–18-year-olds provides a normative base consistent with a number of other studies, including those from other cultures such as Japan (Abe & Masui 1981). It is a little difficult to interpret the published tables and summarise the data succinctly but among the fears commonly reported across both sexes and throughout the age range were the following:

a social cluster: speaking in public, feeling rejected, being parted from friends, looking foolish; and

a cluster related to tissue damage: dead bodies, insane people, dentists, and having a surgical operation.

These two main categories — social fears and fears related to tissue damage — when taken together accounted for nearly 40% of the variance. A further cluster included fears of animals (bats, insects, snakes, mice) but these were only reported commonly by girls.

Controversy as to the reason for the existence of such fears is likely to continue to swing between three conceptual poles: a symbolic understanding of the feared object or situation, a notion of biological programming, and the effects of experience and learning. There is a plausible ring to Bamber's view (1979, p 212) that "it is doubtful if there can be one all-embracing theory which can adequately explain the variety of underlying fear clusters. Rather, different clusters of fears would seem to require theoretical explanations which may be valid only for the particular cluster in question".

Single-object phobias

A number of adolescents seen clinically for other reasons will give an incidental account of phobias of animals, heights, dentists and so forth. The severity of the fear is often considerable and avoidance of the relevant situation clearly displayed. Curiously, help specifically for such fears is not often sought, possibly because family and friends recognise the germ of such fears in themselves and indulge the affected young person accordingly. In the event of treatment being requested, it is appropriate to base this on behavioural lines and wise to heed the maxim which applies to younger children and ask the parents whether they too have similar fears. If so, there is a litle evidence to suggest that they should be treated first (Windheuser 1977).

School phobia is dealt with in the separate section on school refusal (Ch. 19).

Agoraphobia

Although unknown in childhood, the cluster of agoraphobic fears is a recognised clinical problem in adolescence. It may present as school refusal or be perceived by parents as social withdrawal, even depression. Some mothers recognise their own phobias developing in their daughter (it is exceptional among boys). Overt separation anxiety with clinging or morbid worries about the welfare and whereabouts of parents is rather commoner than in adult patients. Correspondingly, the handicap caused by the fears is likely to fluctuate according to the availability of a parental attachment figure and that individual's attitude to the girl. If she or he is rejecting and impatient, the separation anxiety increases and magnifies the problem.

How far one can trace a continuity with insecure attachment in early childhood seems to vary from case to case. In some teenagers, the characteristic fears of waiting in public places or of open streets and parks seem to develop gradually out of an insecure, clinging, dependent, uncomfortable state of mind which has been a lifelong characteristic. This is not always the case and other girls seem to demonstrate an onset which represents a watershed between an uneventful early development and the present problem. A precipitant for such onsets cannot always be discovered.

The treatment of adolescents with agoraphobia follows the same general principles as in adults. Behavioural approaches are generally considered superior to the use of MAOIs or imipramine and there seems little point in combining the two unless there is evidence of associated depression or panic attacks (Anon 1983). The major difference compared with adult psychiatry is the employment of the girl's family as a therapeutic resource. A combination of family interviews and a systematic programme of prolonged exposure to real situations provides satisfactory results in the author's experience. The purpose of family interviews is to enlist practical support for such a programme, to minimise maladaptive means of coping (especially avoiding going out) and to correct any misunderstandings. For instance, an agoraphobic girl with a mother who is handicapped by similar fears will have formed a view of the outside world based on her observation of her mother's behaviour: the outside world is apparently not a safe place. In some instances it will be necessary to force a metaphorical wedge between a fearful daughter and a fearful mother whose frigidity and helplessness has alienated her from her husband and who finds comfort in the need that her daughter has for her company.

Social phobia

A number of studies in personality identify two factors in shyness (Crozier 1979). One is concerned with fears of social criticism and negative evaluation: looking foolish, being ignored or rejected. The other is to do with social competence: speaking to a large audience, meeting strangers or someone of the opposite sex. Such shyness factors are obviously similar to the fears identified in fear surveys. As a dimension of personality, shyness will interact with the demands of a social situation to produce discomfort or, in extreme cases, avoidance and suffering of phobic degree. Other elements may combine in socially phobic individuals: personal vulnerabilities such as a lifelong gaucheness, a speech impediment, or a previous humiliation can all amplify the threat implied in the situation.

The suggestion that there are two components to shyness (which has not uniformly been demonstrated; a minority of studies find a general social anxiety factor) seems to have a parallel in the forms of clinically significant social phobia among adolescents. There are those who tiptoe through life as if constantly cringeing, excessively wary of the adverse opinions of others and not daring to make the simplest overture to another person. Not uncommonly they are gauche and may sport mannerisms or dress which lead to them being viewed as odd (see Briggs 1987). They may see their problems as complex and deep-seated, resenting the attempts of psychological professionals to deal with the outward form of their social behaviour. It is likely that such individuals have a chronically low opinion of themselves (Nicholls 1974) and are unusually sensitive to the opinions of others (which are often negative). It may be that they survive such field dependence by disqualifying the views of others yet cannot replace these by a more satisfactory self-evaluation. Certainly they habitually underestimate their own social competence (Clark & Arkowitz 1975).

On the other hand there are individuals who can function reasonably well in small groups but are paralysed with fear when having to perform in front of a larger audience or when confronted by strangers, a situation comparable to stage fright. Interviews, eating in front of others, or speaking up in public are situations which cause enormous distress and are thus avoided. An extreme sensitivity to one's own internal autonomic or proprioceptive cues is common in the latter group, perceived tremor or a hesitancy in speech triggered by high arousal causing an escalation of apprehension at the prospect of failure and humiliation. This, in turn, increases the likelihood of further and more noticeable tremor, dysfluency and so forth, and a vicious spiral is established. The fear of blushing which is commonly encountered is a variant of this.

The above dichotomy is based on clinical impression and should not be taken to imply necessarily separate, mutually exclusive categories; a dimensional conceptualisation with contributions from each component may be equally valid. It does, however, appear to suggest different treatment approaches. The adolescents in the first group described above with a general sense of inferiority and sensitivity to the evaluations of others are likely to respond to social skills training, particularly in a group setting (see Marzillier 1977, Twentyman & Zimmering 1979), whereas the second general category with fears related to publicly revealed incompetence may learn to manage as a result of desensitisation or with propanolol taken before an identified social ordeal.

Social fears related to the adolescent's unrealistic ideas about his or her own body may well be qualitatively different from the above. Avoidance of others because of a conviction that one's body smell is unusually offensive is a symptom which should be taken seriously in adolescence in case it is an early manifestation of schizophrenia or depressive illness.

Dysmorphophobia

An apprehension about the way in which others perceive the shape or form of one's own body is common in adolescence and clearly relates in large part to the physical changes which accompany puberty and are ordinarily beyond the adolescent's control. Usually such concern is transient and not handicapping although it may lead to social diffidence. Persistent complaints about a claimed physical abnormality which is not evident to anyone except the patient (who falsely believes it to be noticeable to others and viewed adversely by them) merits the clumsy term dysmorphophobia. This is sometimes thought of as having a more sinister prognosis than a concern about an actual but minimal deformity for which corrective surgery is requested, but there is an overlap between the two categories. Certainly adults who were judged psychologically normal at the time they underwent plastic surgery to the nose for observable cosmetic defects showed a high rate of neurosis (37%) and schizophrenia (10%) on 15-year follow-up compared to those having similar operations following injury, for whom the corresponding rates were 9% and 1% respectively (Connolly & Gipson 1978). Lacey & Birtchnell (1986) suggest that the patients with dysmorphophobia tend to complain about their "deformity" in vague terms, insist that something should be done to correct it, and lack insight. Such criteria, if taken to define dysmorphophobia, would not apply to most teenagers with exaggerated or inappropriate fears or concerns about their appearance; they seem to have a good prognosis and should be managed by reassurance.

Conversely, the teenager who has an obvious deformity which is a focus for teasing such as bat ears, scoliosis or buck teeth should not be denied corrective surgery on the grounds that he or she has ordinary adolescent worries over appearance. The timing of some such operations may hinge upon a balance between waiting for growth to cease and the risk of escalating social anxieties (Cosman 1982). The term "Quasimodo complex" has been applied to the end-stage of social withdrawal promoted by teasing and heightened self-consciousness (Harris 1982). Misjudgement of body size and shape, particularly of hips and thighs, is quite common among mid-adolescent girls and can lead to self-starvation as discussed in Chapter 12.

Anxiety states and panic attacks

The extent to which these two phenomena can be viewed as independent is still unresolved (see Gelder 1986). General experience suggests that most adolescents who experience panic attacks are also chronically anxious, though their anxiety may be justified by their life circumstances and need not be seen as neurotic. If agoraphobia is excluded, most adolescents with generalised anxiety who present to clinical services will have an identifiable stressor such as impending examinations or difficulties in family relationships. They tend to come to notice late, since their anxiety is not usually evident to parents; indeed they may conceal it from them or report it in physical terms such as headache or abdominal discomfort. Not uncommonly the first public manifestation is a panic attack which may result in them being brought to a casualty department.

The presentation of panic in an adolescent is comparable to that in an adult, usually with obvious hyperventilation and consequent paraesthesiae, even tetany. In such circumstances it is hard to miss, though Bartter's syndrome (a rare condition of unknown aetiology in which the kidney fails to conserve potassium with resulting hypokalaemia and hyperkaliuria) is an important differential diagnosis of tetany in adolescence. A number of other symptoms such as light-headedness, weakness, unsteadiness ("giddiness" without rotational vertigo), chest pains and sweating can also follow hyperventilation (Hill 1979).

Rebreathing into cupped hands or a paper bag abolishes the acute symptoms, though it is not always true that the voluntary hyperventilation will reproduce them unless there is considerable acute anxiety as well. Although teaching the patient diaphragmatic breathing would seem to be logical management, a large number of adolescents with panic attacks and hyperventilation can only use their new breathing technique in real-life situations when encouraged to by another person present with them at the time; they lack the poise and independence to manage their own panic alone.

Some teenagers misinterpret the subjective symptoms of high psychophysiological arousal as evidence of impending death and become more anxious, with a consequent escalation of anxiety into panic. Painful tension of the occipito-frontalis muscle in the scalp is understood as the headache of a brain tumour, strained intercostal muscles (from hyperventilation) and a rapid heart rate are signs of a heart attack and so on. As with adults, such young people may be greatly relieved by the use of a beta-blocker which interrupts the vicious spiral.

An acute episode of general anxiety can follow a discovery of an unsuspected quality in a friend, a relative or one's self. The disclosure to an adolescent that his father is not his biological parent or the revelation that a friend is homosexual are typical triggers.

Paul, aged 13, discovered in the showers at school that a friend he had known for some years, was circumcised, unlike himself. He was remarkably shocked, became preoccupied with the observation and could think of nothing else, lying awake at night and reading the accounts of the fate of the uncircumcised in the Old Testament. He began to imagine that circumcision was the sign of inclusion in a powerful clique at the school which included prefects and masters, and that people around him were aware of his uncircumcised state, communicating amongst themselves about it. His anxiety was acute but settled over two weeks with simple supportive counselling.

Chronic anxiety may also present in less dramatic mode such as a decline in educational prowess, complaints of insomnia or pain, or separation difficulties. In such instances it is common to find an interaction between stress in the family, school or peer group and a long-standing tendency to anxiety, perhaps best understood as a variant of temperament (Hersov 1985), which itself should be understood in terms of a further interaction between constitutional factors, attachment resolution, and experience. The mode of interaction between these various components is less straightforward than might at first appear. It is to enquire about traumatic experiences and sexual abuse in as relating to a failure in anxiety management rooted in turn in a failure to establish secure attachments in infancy. Anxious, insecure attachment is usually thought to result from distortions in the relationship between infant and attachment figure and likely to be a response to erratic or anxious handling on the part of the parent. However, Grossman & Grossman (1983) demonstrated a continuity between irritability in the neonatal period and insecure attachment at the age of one. The suggestion is therefore that genetic factors may be more influential in the genesis of handicapping anxiety than is ordinarily acknowledged and may breed erratic parental handling rather than *vice versa*. Such a notion might be supported by the intriguing finding of Shaffer et al (1985) that soft signs (minor incoordination, tremor, mirror movements etc.) previously detected and recorded at the age of 7 years were strongly associated with anxiety disorders at the age of 17. Only a minority of children with an excess of soft signs became anxious adolescents, but all female and most male adolescents with anxiety disorders had been found to have excess soft signs at the age of 7.

In order to account for the fact that the continuity is less than complete it is necessary to invoke intervening variables such as personal experience and family life. In assessment it is important to enquire about traumatic experiences and sexual abuse in particular.

The management of anxiety in adolescence follows well-recognised principles. An underlying depression must be excluded. Coincident stress should be relieved when possible. If the stressor is acute and short-lived (such as an examination) and the previous personality is robust, there may be a role for a benzodiazepine in full (adult) doses. Supportive psychotherapy is the usual therapeutic recourse on individual, group or family lines. Biofeedback using a relaxometer can be utilised by a number of adolescents though many seem to have difficulty generalising their learned relaxation to real-life settings. Cognitive therapy appears to suffer the same drawback, perhaps because younger adolescents look to their parents for relief (and older ones regress to this position) rather than assuming responsibility for their symptoms themselves. For such reasons, the management of anxiety in teenagers needs to involve their parents.

Depersonalisation

The term "depresonalisation" is here used as shorthand for various complaints involving a sense of unreality, whether of the self or the surroundings. As Ackner (1954) pointed out, the term is applied somewhat loosely yet the experiences included share a common core, namely a sense that one's body feels dead and unresponsive or a perception of the outside world as strangely flat and still. Such an experience is distressing and may be a primary or secondary complaint, having been described in association with a number of conditions. Roth's observations, conveniently summarised in Slater & Roth (1969), suggest that a close functional relationship exists between mounting anxiety and depersonalisation, the latter being a specific form of constriction of consciousness triggered by panic and serving to limit its damaging effects upon the body and behaviour. A celebrated case reported by Lader & Wing (1966) demonstrated this link between increasing panic and supervening depersonalisation very clearly, with psychophysiological indices of high arousal falling to normal once depersonalisation occurred. It is therefore not surprising that depersonalisation has been reported in association with a number of psychiatric conditions including phobias, depression and early schizophrenia, and the author has known several chronic cases following heavy abuse of LSD. The key mechanisms involved would seem to be located in the temporal lobes since these organise and integrate perceptions.

Although most clinical instances of depersonalisation seem to be accounted for by such an explanation, there remain at least two other groups of young people with depersonalisation which deserve a different explanation. One is composed of adolescents and young adults who episodically depersonalise in common situations such as fatigue or excitement. They can often predict this and do not usually present as patients. The second group consists of shy teenagers who seem to have immature personalities, are ruminative and introverted, lack an easy ability to make friends, and impress as socially naïve. Their depersonalisation has an onset but is not associated with any defined psychiatric disorder; it is primary. They are often distressed by the thought that they are going mad and may present with self-harming behaviour. Presumably they are coextensive with those young women who develop the habit of slashing their wrists in order to terminate acute depersonalisation yet, as a group, those with primary depersonalisation seem to possess less chaotic personalities and experience chronic, unyielding depersonalisation rather than an episodic experience.

The treatment of primary depersonalisation in adolescence can be remarkably difficult. It is usual to prescribe a monoamine oxidase inhibitor but this is not always effective. The recommendation in older texts that a course of thiopentone injections may prove beneficial is to be espoused with caution:

> A young pupil nurse was referred following a suicidal attempt. She complained of chronic depersonalisation, derealisation, intermittent visual distortions and hallucinations of old people's faces. A shy, timid and immature girl with a sheltered home background, she thought she was going mad and was frightened but had no other psychiatric pathology. No precipitant for the depersonalisation could be identified and it was judged to be primary. The male registrar involved in her care gave her a course of slow intravenous injections of thiopentone (without any attempt to abreact her). This had no effect on her depersonalisation though she fairly rapidly developed a phantom pregnancy, of which she claimed the father to be the registrar.

Therapeutic impotence in resistant cases may lead to talk of ECT but various authors have commented that this is ineffective in primary instances and the author's experience concurs with this. Sometimes all that can be done is to reassure that serious insanity is not a consequence of well-established depersonalisation, and to arrange support and rehabilitation with an expectant outlook.

Obsessive-compulsive disorder

About half of all adult patients with obsessional disorder experience their first symptoms before the age of 20 (Kringlen 1970, Pollitt 1957). Clinical experience suggests that there are also some adolescents who have obsessional symptoms in their teenage years but who do not develop a chronic or repeatedly relapsing disorder extending into adult life. It is an uncommon clinical picture; the point prevalence rate among American adolescents in the general population was estimated at 0.33% by Rapoport and her colleagues (Rapoport 1986). Estimations of prevalence are bedevilled by a blurring of nosological boundaries since distinctions between obsessions, tics, rituals, phobias and hypochondriacal fears are difficult to specify.

One aspect of this is the controversy over the diagnostic importance of internal resistance, initially emphasised by Aubrey Lewis (1935). This cannot be demonstrated clearly in a number of adolescents with what otherwise looks remarkably like an obsessional disorder.

> Two unrelated adolescents, a boy of 15 and a girl of 14, were admitted to hospital on separate occasions since it had become virtually impossible to prise them out of the lavatory at their (different) homes.
>
> Both spent hours defaecating and wiping their bottoms in order to ensure that their rectums were empty and no trace of faeces remained on their anal rings. Ritualisation with inspection by mirrors and counting of sheets of lavatory paper used was common to both. Neither would agree that their behaviour or concern was irrational; neither struggled against it; both agreed that it stopped them doing other things and made some attempt to conceal it but that was the nearest to resistance that could be demonstrated. The practices involved in defaecation were extremely difficult to modify and a protracted hospital admission resulted in each case.

Stern & Cobb (1978) have suggested that resistance is not universally demonstrated among adults with obsessional disorder and could be replaced by notions of absurdity or alienation. However, this position would make the distinction between obsessions and the tics and rituals associated with Tourette's syndrome (Ch. 15) extremely difficult, and ignores the fact that many individuals with phobias regard their fear as irrational, even absurd. A blurring of phenomenological boundaries between obsessional disorder and such other conditions becomes unavoidable. Thus the clinical intuition — to infer that the ideas or actions involved are "alien and absurd . . . and . . . are reluctantly performed" (Stern & Cobb 1978) — is at odds with the requirement to make a tight diagnosis which would standardise samples suitable for academic study.

Most obsessional symptoms in adolescence fall within the general categories of checking, cleaning and rumination (Apter et al 1984, Bolton et al 1983, Rapoport et al 1981). Boys seem particularly prone to fears of accidental insemination or seminal contamination. Anxiety and depressive symptoms are common at first evaluation. It can be difficult to obtain a full account of symptoms since many obsessional adolescents are remarkably secretive. No consistent premorbid personality emerges either from published series or general experience, neither is there any consistent pattern of family relationships or family psychopathology. Although an association with neurological damage is quite often discovered (Kettl & Marks 1986, McKeon et al 1984) this is neither constant nor of a definable pattern (Rapoport 1986).

In most ways, the phenomenonolgy of obsessional disorder in adolescence is directly comparable to the clinical picture in adult life. There is an impression that resistance may be not infrequently absent and that accompanying anxiety or depressive symptoms are commoner in younger patients. The chronic picture familiar to adult psychiatric clinics of an individual with rituals established over many years is, of course, not seen in adolescence. Primary obsessional slowness is generally thought to be uncommon but has been described among the most severe cases (Apter et al 1984). The most obvious distinguishing feature of the disorder in adolescence is the involvement of family members in rituals and the inclusion of feelings towards them in ruminations. Quite commonly, anxiety associated with obsessional fears activates attachment behaviours, a turning to attachment figures for the relief of distress. Obsessional rituals become bound up in this mechanism so that the involvement of a parent in a cleansing or good-night ritual serves to maintain their proximity to the distressed adolescent.

It follows that involvement of parents in behavioural treatments, particularly response prevention, becomes necessary. Bolton et al (1983) discuss the impact of such an intervention, pointing out that it provides the adolescent with the experience that disaster does not follow a failure to carry out a ritual, it enhances parental control and thus the young person's sense of security (though he may protest at the time), and it specifies what are the normal expectations of the adolescent's behaviour. Response prevention needs to be buttressed with self-monitoring, modelling, task-setting, and general attention to concomitant anxiety. A number of teenagers need specific and determined encouragement to fill their leisure time actively, rather than allow it to be taken over by rituals.

Using such a regime as the principal approach with a combination of out-and in-patient settings, Bolton et al (1983) achieved symptom remission in half of their cases and substantial improvement in most of the remainder. In contrast, Apter et al (1984) found it impossible to carry out response prevention because of the opposition of the patients, which makes the point that a substantial measure of nursing or parental vigour is required. Nevertheless, half of their patients also improved on a combination of interventions including, variously, milieu management, systematic psychotherapy, supportive interviews and clomipramine. Given such findings and the fact that the course of the condition is typically relapsing and remitting in adolescence (Pollitt 1957), it is hard to be confident that response prevention is the key intervention.

Clomipramine has been shown to have an effect greater than placebo in a group study (Flament et al 1985) within which high doses were used (a mean of 141 mg/day). The presence of depressive symptoms at the commencement of treatment did not affect the result, a finding in accord with informal experience, which differs from results obtained in adult studies, suggesting that the effect on serotonin is the key activity, rather than an antidepressant action (Rapoport 1986). In the author's experience, lower doses than those employed in Flament's study usually suffice. What group studies obscure is that some adolescents respond completely and others not at all. The practical implication is that a trial of clomipramine is nearly always a worthwhile first step, though if a positive result is obtained, prescription may need to be for many months. It can (and should) be sensibly combined with family therapy, the aim being to re-establish parental authority and an appropriate balance of family relationships.

REFERENCES

Abe K, Masui T 1981 Age-sex trends of phobic and anxiety symptoms in adolescents. British Journal of Psychiatry 138: 297–302

Ackner B 1954 Depersonalisation. II. Clinical syndromes. Journal of Mental Science 100: 854–872

Anon 1983 Management of agoraphobia. Drug and Therapeutics Bulletin 21: 61–63

Apter A, Bernhout E, Tyano S 1984 Severe obsessive compulsive disorder in adolescence: a report of eight cases. Journal of Adolescence 7: 349–358

Bamber J H 1979 The Fears of Adolescents. Academic Press, London

Bolton D, Collins S, Steinberg D 1983 The treatment of obsessive-compulsive disorder in adolescence. British Journal of Psychiatry 142: 456–464

Briggs R 1987 Unlucky Wally. Hamish Hamilton, London

Clark J V, Arkowitz H 1975 Social anxiety and self-evaluation of interpersonal performance. Psychological Reports 36: 211–221

Connolly F, Gipson M 1978 Dysmorphophobia — a long-term study. British Journal of Psychiatry 132: 568–570

Cosman B 1982 Cosmetic surgery for the disabled child. In: Downey J, Low N (eds.) The Child with Disabling Illness. Raven Press, New York

Crozier W R 1979 Shyness as a dimension of personality. British Journal of Social and Clinical Psychology 18: 121–128

Flament M, Rapoport J, Berg C et al 1985 Clomipramine treatment of childhood obsessive compulsive disorder. Archives of General Psychiatry 42: 977–983

Gelder M 1986 Panic attacks: new approaches to an old problem. British Journal of Psychiatry 149: 346–352

Grossman K, Grossman K E 1983 Cited in Kagan J The Nature of the Child, pp 59–62. Basic Books, New York

Harris D 1982 The symptomatology of abnormal appearance: an anecdotal survey. British Journal of Plastic Surgery 35: 312–332

Hersov L A 1985 Emotional disorders. In: Rutter M, Hersov L A (eds) Child and Adolescent Psychiatry: Modern Approaches. 2nd edn. Blackwell Scientific, Oxford

Hill O W 1979 The hyperventilation syndrome. British Journal of Psychiatry 135: 367–368

Kettl P A, Marks I M 1986 Neurological factors in obsessive compulsive disorder. British Journal of Psychiatry 149: 315–319

Kringlen E 1970 Natural history of obsessional neurosis. Seminars in Psychiatry 2: 403–419

Lacey J H, Birtchnell S A 1986 Body image and its disturbances. Journal of Psychosomatic Research 30: 623–631

Lader M, Wing L 1966 Physiological Measures, Sedative Drugs and Morbid Anxiety (Maudsley Monograph No. 14) Oxford University Press, London

Lewis A 1935 Problems of obsessional illness. Proceedings of the Royal Society of Medicine 29: 325–336

McKeon J, McGuffin P, Robinson P 1984 Obsessive compulsive neurosis following head injury. British Journal of Psychiatry 144: 190–192

Marzillier J 1977 Outcome studies of skills training: a review. In: Trower P, Bryant B, Argyle M (eds) Social Skills and Mental Health. Methuen, London

Nicholls K A 1974 Severe social anxiety. British Journal of Medical Psychology 47: 301–306

Pollitt J 1957. Natural history of obsessional states. British Medical Journal i: 194–198

Porteous M A 1979 A survey of the problems of normal 15-year-olds. Journal of Adolescence 2: 307–323

Porteous M A 1985 Developmental aspects of adolescent problem disclosure. Journal of Child Psychology and Psychiatry 26: 465–478

Rapoport J 1986 Childhood obsessive compulsive disorder. Journal of Child Psychology and Psychiatry 27: 289–295

Rapoport J, Elkins R, Langer D et al 1981 Childhood obsessive-compulsive disorder. American Journal of Psychiatry 138: 1545–1554

Shaffer D, Schonfeld I, O'Connor P A et al 1985 Neurological soft signs. Their relationship to psychiatric disorder and intelligence in childhood and adolescence. Archives of General Psychiatry 42: 342–351

Slater E, Roth M 1969 Clinical Psychiatry. 3rd edn. Bailliere, Tindall and Cassell, London

Stern R S, Cobb J 1978 Phenomenology of obsessive compulsive neurosis. British Journal of Psychiatry 132: 233–239

Twentyman C T, Zimmering R T 1979 Behavioural training in social skills: a critical review. In: Herson M, Eisler R, Miller P (eds) Progress in Behaviour Modification. Vol. 7. Academic Press, New York

Windheuser H J 1977 Anxious mothers as models for coping with anxiety. Behaviour Analysis and Modification 2: 19–32

12

Eating disorders

Anorexia nervosa

The behavioural and physical manifestations of anorexia nervosa
are a consequence of an abnormal attitude to normal body shape,
size and weight. Self-starvation in an attempt to control body
shape results in both physiological and psychological abnormalities. Understanding anorexia nervosa hinges upon an appreciation of the mechanisms involved.

Paramount among the features of the condition is an insistence
upon avoiding fatness. Anorectics perceive themselves as fat or
in imminent danger of becoming so, even when clearly emaciated
in the eyes of an observer. Typically, they judge themselves as
fat around the thighs and hips. Such fatness disgusts them and
they starve themselves in order to lose it. As a consequence of
doing so they become preoccupied with food, their weight and
the achievement of slimness generally.

Such a concern with fatness is determined by cultural and
developmental factors. Contemporary Western culture prizes
female slimness and this is commercially supported and exploited
by the manufacturers of slimming foods, the publishers of slimming magazines and the purveyors of a bewildering number of
devices, treatments and procedures intended to help people lose
weight and change shape. No teenage girl can avoid the message
that, according to such conventions, physical attractiveness is
linked to a slim body and fatness is considered ugly. Coupled
with this is the fact that a majority of normal adolescent girls
(but only a few boys) overestimate their body width and depth,
experiencing themselves as fatter than they really are (Huenemann et al 1966, Nylander 1971, Halmi et al 1977). This percep-

tual distortion is most evident at the age of about 17–18. Not surprisingly, dieting to lose weight is endemic among late teenage girls. The practice may be intensified and perpetuated by a number of other influences.

For instance, it has been hypothesised that for each individual there are critical weights at which different developmental phases of puberty are initiated by the hypothalamus. In their exploration of this, Frisch & Revelle (1970) found the mean weights for triggering the growth spurt and menarche in girls to be 31 kg and 48 kg respectively. A more sophisticated version of this theory posits a certain critical weight-for-height ratio which acts as a threshold for initiating menstrual cycles and similarly, there are findings to support this (Frisch & McArthur 1974). In fact, this ratio reflects the proportional amount of fat in the body, something which increases during puberty and up until the age of 18 when body composition stabilises. The threshold for menarche can be crossed in both directions and if weight (or fat proportion) falls below it, pubertal maturation is halted or even reversed; a biological regression with consequent amenorrhoea or, in the male, loss of libido. Such a cessation or reversal of development may allow a girl to avoid growing up into a woman if this is an uncomfortable process for her. The conflicts provoked by developing sexuality and independence which can accompany adolescence are thus avoided by self-starvation, enabling a retreat into simpler pre-pubertal life. This theory has been well articulated by Crisp (1980) on the basis of extensive clinical experience with hospital patients. It may not always apply to the simpler, milder cases managed in primary care settings.

There is some evidence that the distorted perception of bodily depth and width mentioned above increases with weight loss. Casper et al (1979) were able to show that the most severely emaciated anorectics overestimated their body size to the greatest extent and had the worst response to treatment. The thinner a girl becomes, the more she loses sight of how thin and wasted she is. In one experimental study, anorectics judged themselves fatter immediately after a carbohydrate meal (Crisp & Kalucy 1974). Paradoxically an improvement in the accuracy of self-perception accompanies recovery of normal body weight (Slade & Russell 1973). It can be shown to be responsive to suggestion; Crisp & Kalucy (1974) encouraged anorectics to "drop their guard for a moment", whereupon their previously demonstrated overestimations lessened. The perpetuation of misjudgement therefore rests upon a vicious cycle wherein increasing weight loss results in greater proportional overestimation of size and consequent redoubling of efforts to lose weight. Fear of fatness provides an emotional and cognitive basis for maintaining defensive guard and sustaining the most extreme perceptual exaggeration. Nevertheless, not all anorectics are prey to such perceptual misjudgement and some will underestimate their bulk (Casper et al 1979, Touyz et al 1984) so it seems unlikely that the mechanism operates universally.

The manner in which self-starvation and weight loss may become ways in which to express autonomy by thus exercising a measure of control over a life previously sacrificed to the ideal of pleasing parents and others has been given prominence by Hilde Bruch (1974). A parallel theme of self-sacrifice pervades the thinking of a number of family therapists who suggest that families containing an anorectic girl have rigid, over-close and mutually contradictory modes by which family members relate to each other (Minuchin et al 1975, Selvini-Palazzoli 1978). Certainly many families with anorectic children seem to be free of overt conflict, self-sufficient, close and avowedly happy (Heron & Leheup 1984) and the suggestion prompts itself that independence may be hard to win for an adolescent growing up in such a setting. Nevertheless, such mechanisms are largely untested scientifically and where controls have been selected for contrast, they have not been well chosen. The universality or specificity of any particular pattern of family relationships in association with anorexia nervosa has not been demonstrated and the direction of causation remains undetermined. To what extent the patterns of relationships are themselves consequences of having a loved daughter who is intent on starving herself is unexplored. Although it is occasionally found to be the case that a girl will continue with her starvation because this distracts her parents from open disagreements with each other, clinical experience suggests that this mechanism is more often a preoccupation of the therapist than of the girl or family.

It is striking how many anorectics have been tidy, neat, conscientious perfectionists as younger children. Generally compliant and conforming, they strive for high standards of school work, appearance and behaviour, seeking approval on their parents' terms rather than according to their own. The impression is of young people who are already setting themselves high personal standards and struggling with issues of self-control before the onset of anorexia nervosa. Various authorities have described or demonstrated how anorectics mistrust their own proprioceptive cues and rely excessively on the judgements of others of their appearance or use objective, external measures such as weight (e.g. Bruch 1974, Russell et al 1975). In such circumstances, the conflict between dependence upon others for a sense of self-worth and a search for personal confidence and autonomy becomes acute since one's own judgements are displaced by those of others, exacerbating a deep sense of passivity and ineffectual helplessness. To what extent such a personality derives from patterns of family relationships and how much it arises independently and then interacts with them is a moot point. On first principles, it seems unlikely that family dynamics alone provide a sufficient aetiological explanation for anorexia nervosa (not all sisters in a family with an anorectic will be affected) but that they interact with certain individual vulnerabilities, as yet poorly understood.

Clinical presentation

The features of the condition derive from a "relentless pursuit of thinness" (Bruch 1974), the consequence of a horror of normal mature body shape. Ordinary body build is, for the anorectic, fat and thus loathsome; a mark of self-indulgence, shame and failure in her own terms. A rigid attitude towards eating and fatness dominates the girl's life and swamps any rational appraisal of the result of protracted starvation. She will not allow herself to eat normally but stringently avoids carbohydrates and fats, restricting herself to tiny quantities of food and a minimal calorie intake. This is often accompanied by overactivity, general bustle, or vigorous calisthenics; an apparent attempt to burn up calories and avoid the deposition of fat.

As a result of starvation, hunger supervenes and elaborates into a preoccupation with food. This torments the girl who, in spite of having anorexia nervosa, is far from exhibiting anorexia if this means lacking appetite (Garfinkel 1974) though she may deny hunger in order to deceive herself or her helpers. Whilst terrified of putting on weight and becoming fat, her self-starvation induces thoughts and dreams of food. Preparing food for others, reading recipe books, window shopping in food stores, planning meals and counting calories become endlessly absorbing. Warding off the temptation to eat in the face of such preoccupation tests self-control to the limit. Only those with a considerable amount of obsessionality in their pre-morbid personalities can engage in the struggle and become anorectic; sloppier souls give in.

It is no surprise, then, that food preparation, eating and weighing become activities suffused with ritual and obsession. Similarly the whole issue of control over eating and body shape comes to be shot through with primitive morality: fatness is bad, thinness good; people are either friends or enemies. Polarisation between extremes of triumph and failure, elation and despair, pride and a sense of personal annihilation is common, though usually secret. The battle for control is fought privately at first, though it rapidly spreads to involve other family members once they notice what is going on. In its early phases, the loss of weight goes unobserved by the girl's caretakers and indeed may start away from home at boarding school or college, a fact overlooked by those who place their faith in an exclusively intrafamilial model of causation.

When the deviousness, secrecy and persistence of the anorectic are considered, it is hard to gainsay the importance of a wish to discover and retain a sense of autonomy. It is remarkable that an issue of such import to a young teenager should be pursued single-handed with no request for help from her parents. On the contrary, great lengths are gone to in order to conceal a reduced intake from them: complaints of allergy to particular foods, excuses of routine dieting, leaving meals because of a rush to get to school, having to eat in private because of revision pressures, dumping food in kitchen bins and so on. Bulky clothes may be chosen to conceal thinness. Under pressure to eat, a stubbornness is revealed which often surprises the parents of erstwhile compliant children; they may describe it as willpower but it is more likely to be a desperate stance struck by an individual who fears their own self-esteem or sense of antonomy threatened.

At the same time, excuses may be offered for excessive exercising and activity. The early morning waking which accompanies the weight loss (Lacey et al 1975) is explained away to others in terms of feelings of health and energy, which tends to reassure the rest of the family that nothing serious is amiss. Amenorrhoea, which may be a comparatively early sign if selective carbohydrate restriction is closely pursued, usually goes unremarked upon and is easily shrugged off if questioned about.

Self-induced vomiting is discovered as a method of weight control by about half of anorectics known to hospital clinics (Casper et al 1980, Garfinkel et al 1980). Although it tends to be commoner among established and chronic adult anorectics, it can occasionally be seen in those as young as 12 or 13. Laxative and diuretic abuse is much more likely to be seen in young adults than adolescents.

At the time of referral the girl is emaciated and usually weighs between 35 and 40 kg. She will not be a willing patient, protesting that she feels well or that there are special considerations which mean that she is the right weight for her height. On examination, her emaciated body belies her protestations of health. A somewhat submissive, but ultimately stubborn, stance is characteristic. Reasons given for starting to diet are often banal and may camouflage the beliefs and attitudes which maintain the situation, and a careful distinction in formulation between precipitating and perpetuating factors is wise.

It is not uncommon to find that low mood and social isolation, together with a loss of interest in matters other than food and issues such as the achievement of perfection in schoolwork, suggest that depression may be the primary diagnosis. The central preoccupation with food, weight and eating is not found in depression, nor is there a phobia of normal body weight and shape except in anorexia nervosa.

Physical evidence of starvation is immediately evident on inspection. The face is pinched with prominent cheekbones, limbs are spindly, chest and buttocks flat. Pubic hair is preserved and a fine downy (lanugo) hair may be seen over the face, upper back and forearms. There may be a yellowish skin secondary to carotenaemia if the girl's diet largely consists of root vegetables. Hands and feet are cold from poor cardiovascular perfusion and postural hypotension is likely. The slow heart rate and the finding that tendon reflexes are slow to relax can provoke thoughts of hypothyroidism though the overactivity and common tolerance of cold are quite untypical of myxoedema. Nevertheless, the blood T3 (and sometimes T4) levels may be found to be low, a result of the general state of lowered metabolic rate akin to hibernation (Crisp 1980) which is secondary to starvation. To confuse matters further, a high blood cholesterol may be seen, particularly if the girl has been eating large amounts of cheese. Because of the risks of thyroxine addiction, it is important not to be drawn into a mistaken diagnosis of hypothyroidism.

Amenorrhoea secondary to weight loss or gross carbohydrate restriction is accompanied by low and non-cyclical blood and urine LH and FSH levels. Prolactin activity is normal though HGH and cortisol levels are high (see Isaacs 1979).

Hypokalaemia is common and will be severe if laxatives or diuretics are abused. Drinking large amounts of water before being weighed yields a spuriously high weight which can fool clinical staff but carries the risk of water intoxication, even seizures.

Chronic anorectics with years of sparse food intake are likely to develop gastric atrophy and constriction which results in early feelings of fullness during a meal and can yield a flat glucose tolerance curve.

Prevalence

On the basis of various studies it is believed that anorexia nervosa is on the increase (Jones et al 1980, Kendell et al 1973, Theander 1970) though it is a little difficult to be precise in view of heightened clinical awareness and differing diagnostic criteria. It is generally agreed that the condition is commoner among socially advantaged groups. For example, Crisp et al (1976) demonstrated a prevalence rate of 1% of girls aged 16 and over attending English independent (fee-paying) schools but only one case among nearly 3000 girls attending ordinary comprehensive state schools, a figure which pro-rates to one in 550 girls aged 16 and over in that setting.

Such figures are not very different from those obtained by Nylander (1971): an overall rate of 0.75% in a general population study of 14–19-year-old girls in a Swedish town.

These studies used stringent criteria and it is apparent that milder forms of anorexia nervosa are commoner. For instance, 5% of English college students were found by Mann et al (1983) to have some, but not all, of the features of anorexia nervosa, and Hill (1977) has asserted that 4% of female teenagers in the UK will show enough self-induced weight loss to cause amenorrhoea.

There is a general consensus that the modal age of onset is 17–18 years and that the overwhelming number of cases (90–95%) are female, hence the use of the female pronoun in this section.

Differential diagnosis

The essential features of anorexia nervosa vary in detail according to the criteria used by different centres but generally assume:

1. The presence of abnormal attitudes to normal body shape, weight and eating.
2. Substantial loss of weight (e.g. 25% of premorbid body weight) as a result of self-starvation.
3. Amenorrhoea over several (e.g. 3) cycles.

Confusion is most likely to arise over differentiation from depression (see above). It should be possible to make a distinction between the two conditions by adequate interviewing and observation. A recourse to the use of over-simple operational criteria is likely to cause a muddle. There should be no confusion with panhypopituitarism since this does not cause weight loss. Organic causes of substantial weight loss such as diabetes, tuberculosis, malignancy and AIDS should be readily distinguishable by clinical history, examination and appropriate investigation (though anorexia nervosa can certainly coexist with diabetes). The organically-minded tyro may consider whether the girl has hypothyroidism because of low blood levels of T3 and T4 with a high cholesterol, but a wider clinical perspective usually rules this out. The response to TRH is decisive.

More substantial difficulties arise over the presence of bulimic symptoms in a girl with fluctuating body weight. These supervene, sooner or later, in about half of all cases (Garfinkel et al 1980); the girl giving way to the temptation to gorge and then induce vomiting in a guilty or planned attempt to rid herself of the ingested food. The distinction from the primary bulimic syndrome is most easily made by the normal body weight found in the latter but wide fluctuations in body weight can obscure this straightforward distinction.

Treatment

Most units which deal with anorexia nervosa have a treatment regime which can be tailored to the individual patient yet which ensures a minimum of manipulation by a young anorectic who is likely to be ambivalent about treatment. Specialist anorexia units will have to deal with a wider age-range than adolescent units but it is still possible, on the basis of personal experience and the published literature, to distill a mainstream approach applicable to teenage anorectics.

The aims of the first interviews need to go beyond diagnosis and include engagement of the anorectic and her family in further treament. To this end the psychiatrist should demonstrate that he has an understanding of the subjective experience of anorexia nervosa whilst avoiding being led into bargains which would compromise effective treatment. Niceness alone is insufficient; there is a responsibility to inform the girl and her parents of the risk to life presented by continued starvation. It is generally agreed that a target weight should be selected though there are various views as to how this should be done. Crisp (1980) advocates an average weight (Kemsley 1953/4) for the girl's age when she first developed the condition, thus inviting her to resume growth in all modalities. Dally (1981) suggests around 90% of ideal weight for current age and height, whilst Russell (1985) refers to a premorbid "healthy" or "optimal" weight achieved following puberty but before the onset of self-starvation. The latter approach tends to be complicated by the fact that a number of anorectics have been somewhat plump during puberty and it may have been an insensitive remark about this which precipitated the disorder. There is also the problem that a desperate anorectic will lie about her weight, present or previous, and her parents may not know enough to correct her account.

Weight gain is a necessary though not necessarily a sufficient component of treatment. While starvation persists, the girl will be unable to think of anything but food and attempts at psychotherapy will founder. Until she achieves the weight threshold at which puberty is initiated and maintained, the developmental tasks of adolescence can be shirked. Bearing in mind that the ultimate goal of treatment is likely to be the establishment of a healthy sense of autonomy, it is wise to ensure that she does not feel herself so obliterated by "force-feeding" that she no longer has any control over her destiny. Medical impatience with the rate of weight gain may need to be tempered accordingly, though without colluding in the morbid wish for unattainable, ideal thinness.

A number of young adolescents with anorexia nervosa can be treated as out-patients. Under such circumstances, either they or their parents will have to assume responsibility for their putting on weight. An interim target can be set of a rate of gain of no less than 500 g a week. The help of a dietician is invaluable in buttressing the idea that it is controlled weight gain that is being pursued. Joining the family for a meal at home or in the clinic is an important opportunity to support parents in their efforts to get their daughter to eat. Weighing to assess progress should be done at the clinic to minimise the risks of parents being hood-winked by altering the zeroing of the scales, taking the opportunity to read off the weight to a parent whose view of the scale is curiously obscured by a smear of soap and so forth. The crucial issue is weight gain, not food intake, so that protracted discussion of exactly how much is being (or not being) eaten is unnecessary. Gentle praise for gains in both weight and appearance are in order, as is congratulation for the improved control over healthy weight.

The ultimate sanction is admission for in-patient treatment. This may be urgently necessary at any time if physical health is at risk but is also commonly used if out-patient management fails. Deciding what constitutes failure is not always straightforward since many young anorectics will test out the threat of admission by not quite managing to meet their target rate of weight increase. The author's preference is to stick to targets that have been set and allow no leeway, if only because this cuts short protracted exploration of limits and the degree of trust that can be placed in someone who fails to keep agreements (including that which says the patient will not be allowed to get fat). Agreement with the family in advance that this will be the course of action allows a visit to the unit beforehand so that there is the minimum fuss over admission should this be needed. Parents need considerable support to allow their daughter to be admitted in the face of her threats that they will never be forgiven or that she would rather die. Emphasis must be given to the fact that it is her dread of loss of control over her eating which is the central issue and reassurance given that she will not be allowed to become fat in the eyes of others.

If in-patient management is required in order to obtain a satisfactory rate of weight gain, then the core feature becomes good nursing management. This includes supervision and encouragement during meals as well as support in dealing constructively with ward life and relationships with peers and parents. Ward staff may reassure the girl that any post-prandial fullness, ankle swelling or abdominal distension is temporary. Nothing should detract from the constant message that it is necessary for the girl to gain her health through achieving her target weight. It is probable that behaviour therapy, in awarding privileges in exchange for achieving particular weights, supports consistency in management. It is undeniably effective (Kellerman 1977) but it is not clear whether it adds anything to good nursing care. Eckert et al (1979) were unable to demonstrate its superiority over ward milieu therapy in a randomised trial.

An initial diet of 1500–2000 calories a day should be increased to 3000 calories after a few days. Since a caloric intake of this magnitude is substantially more than normal, a balance needs to be struck between an inadvertent education in overeating (which will result in the girl turning to bulimia) and protracting the experience of the anorectic state of mind with its encouragement of morbid attitudes and habits. A number of older anorectics submit to admission, knowing that they are able to "eat their way out" and rapidly return to their earlier anorectic ways. Hospital admission needs to avoid this trap of a crash diet, passively accepted, whilst taking care that a protracted admission does not create a professional patient. A rate of weight gain around 1 kg a week should be maintained, with food being taken only at specified meal- or snack-times and supervised individually by a nurse. The girl will not be allowed to leave the table until her food is eaten and cannot bargain with her nurse about how much she will eat next time. Any covert food disposal is dealt with by straightforward confrontation.

The addition of medication probably adds little to the above regime although a number of agents have been claimed to be effective: chlorpromazine, sulpiride, pimozide, lithium, antidepressants, cyproheptadine, and metoclopramide (see Vandereycken 1984).

Restoration of adequate weight enables preoccupations with food, a labile or depressed mood, and obsessionality to be considerably alleviated. It now becomes possible to use a variety of psychotherapeutic techniques in order to promote adaptive coping strategies, modify attitudes and encourage personal growth by the anorectic and her family. A number of texts describe the implementation of this (Bruch 1982, Crisp 1980, Garner et al 1982, Minuchin et al 1978). Dally (1981) makes the apposite comment that "it is better to concentrate on psychic synthesis rather than analysis of psychological defences". Bruch (1982) points out that a traditional psychotherapeutic setting replicates "the transactional patterns that have pervaded their whole lives, namely that someone else 'knew' what they felt but they themselves did not know or feel it".

It follows that the central task to be promoted is one of psychological maturation, specifically that of discovery of their essential self, personal validity and individual competence. To enable this to occur, a number of characteristic stances need to be overcome: the assertion that everything is perfect, that appearances are all-important, that others are dismissive of them (except in their misplaced concern about their weight), that recognisable achievement in school or sport is an absolute standard of worth, or that oppositional negativism is necessary for survival but compliance earns love. There is no good evidence that any single therapeutic mode — individual, group or family — is superior to any other and many centres will use these in creative combination. Irrespective of modality, the emphasis will be on the here-and-now.

Provision of insight is a well-recognised trap for the novice therapist since his interpretations are likely to be accepted with good grace yet are put to no use. Becoming a "good" patient within a relationship that does not hinge upon eating is no hardship for many anorectics; it replicates the relationship they have with their parents. More profitable for the young anorectic is to establish with her an understanding of how she can exist as herself in the company of other teenagers without a descent into anorectic attitudes and behaviours, and how her standing with her teachers and parents can be altered to hinge upon who she is rather than solely on her success at tangible achievements.

Within family interviews, the aim is initially to enable the parents to take back the power over their daughter's eating so that in good time it may be transferred back to her, shorn of its acquired attributes of imposition and blind resistance. For many parents who only "want her back as she was before all this" a period of mourning for their erstwhile over-compliant daughter may be required since her discovery of herself is likely to be associated with more appropriately assertive style of relating to them. They, too, may need to discover ways of sustaining their own self-esteem without their daughter providing it for them directly by her being "good" or vicariously through her achievements at school. If her invalidity (an ambiguous term) provides her with attention instead of being taken for granted, or otherwise has a functional impact upon family relationships such as a diversion of attention away from a precarious marriage, then this provides a further focus for therapy. Some families appear to contain parents whose own sense of self-worth and potency depends upon their daughter's capacity to gratify them and provide, through being a "perfect" child, satisfaction for them in their roles as good parents. In such ways they may reflect their daughter's pathology and become intertwined in her condition by, for instance, acceding to her demand not to be admitted as an in-patient even when her physical state requires it because they fear the loss of her affection. They thus resemble the stereotype suggested by Minuchin et al (1978) of the enmeshed, mutually-overinvolved family unable to resolve disagreement, though it seems on the grounds of clinical experience that such a constellation is neither universal among nor confined to families containing an anorectic youngster.

In a pre-pubertal girl, self-starvation can delay the onset of puberty, including the growth spurt, and can result in short stature (Pugliese et al 1983). This makes it important to monitor endocrinological maturation during the treatment of the very young adolescent. Blood LH and FSH levels should rise and then fluctuate cyclically. This normally occurs within 6 months of achieving target weight. If it does not occur, clomiphene may be indicated (Russell 1985). External physical development can by assessed by systematic recording of Tanner staging. Provided that the girl is younger than 18, some further growth in both stature and breast development can be anticipated.

Prognosis

Most cases of anorexia will respond to the above regime in terms of weight gain, resumption of menstruation and attitude change, though treatment, whether out- or in-patient, needs to be continued for a few months at least. A synthesis of the findings from the major follow-up studies (Hawley 1985, Hsu et al 1979, Morgan & Russell 1975, Morgan et al 1983, Steinhausen & Glanville 1983, Sturzenberger et al 1977, Swift 1982, Theander 1970) suggests the following:

— outcome is best at the first presentation, repeated relapses carry a correspondingly poorer prognosis

— age of onset probably has no effect on prognosis once chronicity is taken into account

— about half of all patients recover completely, one-quarter have persisting minor problems with eating or psychosexual adjustment, and a further quarter run a chronic course

— within the chronic group, an appreciable mortality rate (about 5% of all anorectic cases described in hospital series), usually from suicide, occasionally from metabolic chaos, secondary infection or hypothermia

— poor response to treatment if bingeing and vomiting are present

— poor outcome if a marked immaturity of personality is evident

— parental psychiatric disorder, rigid parental attitudes, intra-familial conflict all signify a poor outcome

— boys do worse than girls.

The bulimic syndrome

The terminology applied to episodic overeating accompanied by the use of self-induced vomiting to control weight gain is confused. "Bulimia nervosa" as used by Russell (e.g. 1985) refers to such behaviour when it occurs as a late sequel of anorexia nervosa. However, DSM III indicates that "bulimia" is quite separate from anorexia nervosa. Furthermore, a number of obese women will use vomiting to lose weight.

The core symptom of bulimia is the rapid consumption of vast amounts of food in a short time; so-called binge-eating. It is a secret, furtive behaviour with much associated guilt. Not surprisingly it is commonly followed by self-induced vomiting, a sense of shame or depressed mood, and a burst of dieting with carbo-hydrate restriction. The latter leads to a craving for carbohydrate which is resisted at first but then overwhelms ordinary self-restraint which collapses dramatically with an eating binge. This is not just overeating at a meal and does not arise out of ordinary hunger (Lacey 1982) but is often planned as a private indulgence, frequently with a preparatory ritual which is followed by an escalation into voracious gorging of rich, sweet carbohydrate foods, sometimes accompanied by other forms of self-gratification such as masturbation and terminated by painful abdominal distension. Self-induced vomiting may then be used to gain physical and psychological relief. Laxatives, appetite suppressants and diuretics may all be recruited into the effort to lose weight gained by overeating.

The bulimic syndrome as described above may occur as a development of anorexia nervosa, either at low or normal body weight. This generally happens as a comparatively late complication and is unusual in adolescent anorectics, though when it does occur it can only be dealt with by admission to hospital for the re-establishment of a regular eating programme with an appropriate proportion of carbohydrate in the diet.

When associated with normal body weight and no previous history of anorexia nervosa, the bulimic syndrome is hard to detect. It is a condition that, for practical purposes, only affects women. The modal age of onset is 17–18 (Lacey, personal communication) and the initial manifestation is dietary chaos, with self-induced vomiting following after two years or so. It should thus be on the diagnostic agenda of an adolescent psychiatrist although the vast majority of cases will present in their twenties to adult psychiatrists.

Bulimics are characteristically secretive about their eating and the diagnosis is commonly made only after the observation of certain signs leads to questioning or confrontation. These include: livid stretch marks around the umbilicus or on the flanks; swollen submandibular and parotid salivary glands; and irregular or absent periods.

Frequent self-induced vomiting can give rise to: hoarse voice; erosion of dental enamel on the inner aspect of the incisors; calluses on the backs of the fingers; leaving the table during meals or visiting the lavatory immediately afterwards.

Investigation may reveal unexplained hypokalaemia.

Following a binge, the girl will appear flushed, sweaty, with a thick neck and distended abdomen. She may lie immobile, curled up and resent intrusion.

Not all girls who practice self-induced vomiting or who binge-eat will have the full bulimic syndrome. For instance 21% of female attenders at a family planning clinic reported binge-eating (Cooper & Fairburn 1983), a figure somewhat greater than the 14% of younger female university students surveyed by Clarke & Palmer (1983) who said that they went on eating binges at least "often". The latter figure is likely to be a minimal rate as a postal survey was employed with only a 76% response rate. Self-induced vomiting was less often admitted to in this study (1.3%

of respondents) than in the surveys of female students by Button & Whitehouse (1981) and Halmi et al (1981) who report 2.7% and nearly 12% respectively admitting to self-induced vomiting. The very discrepancy between these results suggest that there is no clear cut-off between normal healthy eating practices and behaviours which combine to yield the full bulimic syndrome.

Aetiology

It follows that those girls who demonstrate the full clinical picture will be more disturbed than those who only show isolated features. Those for whom a cycle of gorging and dieting combines with vomiting and purging to disrupt ordinary eating, weight and emotional stability are likely to show other evidence of person-ality disturbance: poor impulse control, low self-esteem, and little self-confidence in themselves as women. Many will present a superficially capable, sociable exterior. In such a group the binge-eating seems often to be used to control mood and defend against depressive feelings which may surface following treatment (Lacey 1983).

Rather less common a pattern of personality disorder is that with associated impulsivity, stealing, wrist-cutting, alcohol and drug abuse, sexual promiscuity, relationships that swing between intense dependency and superficiality, a labile affect and a pervasive sense of emptiness. Not surprisingly these girls are often regarded as having borderline personality disorder.

The comments made about the importance of body shape and size in the earlier section on anorexia nervosa are of obvious relevance to understanding the bulimic syndrome, whether or not this is associated with a previous history of anorexia nervosa. Just under half of all bulimics were premorbidly obese (Johnson-Sabine & Wakeling 1983) and a sizeable minority of massively obese women fulfil the criteria for bulimia (Lacey 1982), though these would not normally be regarded as typical of the bulimic syndrome since the term is usually applied to those of near-normal (though often widely fluctuating) weight. A sense of failure as a woman seems remarkably common in adult patients who displace this onto their figure and seek a compensation in maintaining a lithe body. The carbohydrate restriction imposed by dieting to achieve this promotes craving and eventual surrender with guilt at failure. This provokes further attempts to achieve normal body weight by dieting to get rid of the psychological and physical effects of over-eating. A cycle is thus established.

Management

It is unlikely that the adolescent psychiatrist will be involved with the treatment of the bulimic syndrome at normal body weight because the likely age of presentation is several years after onset. In adults, cognitive techniques, behavioural strategies and insight-directed psychotherapy may be combined in various packages in an attempt to assist regaining control over chaotic eating and assist more realistic self-appraisal and coping strategies (Fairburn 1983, Lacey 1983).

REFERENCES

Bruch H 1974 Eating Disorders. Routledge & Kegan Paul, London
Bruch H 1982 Anorexia nervosa: therapy and theory. American Journal of Psychiatry 139: 1531–1538
Button E J, Whitehouse A 1981 Subclinical anorexia nervosa. Psychological Medicine 11: 509–516
Casper R C, Halmi K A, Goldberg S C, Eckert E D, Davis J M 1979 Disturbances in body image estimation as related to other characteristics and outcome in anorexia nervosa. British Journal of Psychiatry 134: 60–66
Casper R C, Eckert E D, Halmi K A, Goldberg S C, Davis J M 1980 Bulimia: its incidence and clinical importance in patients with anorexia nervosa. Archives of General Psychiatry 37: 1030–1035
Clarke M G, Palmer R L 1983 Eating attitudes and neurotic symptoms in university students. British Journal of Psychiatry 142: 299–304
Cooper P J, Fairburn C G 1983 Binge-eating and self-induced vomiting in the community: a preliminary study. British Journal of Psychiatry 142: 139–144
Crisp A H 1980 Anorexia Nervosa: Let Me Be. Academic Press, London
Crisp A H, Kalucy R S 1974 Aspects of the perceptual disorder in anorexia nervosa. British Journal of Medical Psychology 47: 349–361
Crisp A H, Palmer R L, Kalucy R S 1976. How common is anorexia nervosa? a prevalence study. British Journal of Psychiatry 128: 549–554
Dally P 1981 Treatment of anorexia nervosa. British Journal of Hospital Medicine 25: 434–440
Eckert E D, Goldberg S C, Halmi K A, Casper R C, Davis J M 1979 Behaviour therapy in anorexia nervosa. British Journal of Psychiatry 134: 55–59
Fairburn C G 1983 The place of a cognitive behavioural approach in the management of bulimia. In: Darby P et al (eds) Anorexia Nervosa: Recent Developments in Research. Alan Liss, New York
Frisch R E, McArthur J W 1974 Menstrual cycles: fatness as a determinant of minimum weight for height necessary for their maintenance or onset. Science 185: 949–951

Frisch R E, Revelle R 1970 Height and weight at menarche and a hypothesis of initial body weights and adolescent events. Science 169: 397–398

Garfinkel P E 1974 Perception of hunger and satiety in anorexia nervosa. Psychological Medicine 4: 309–315

Garfinkel P E, Moldofsky H, Garner D M 1980 The heterogeneity of anorexia nervosa: bulimia as a distinct subgroup. Archives of General Psychiatry 37: 1036–1040

Garner D M, Garfinkel P E, Bemis K M 1982 A multidimensional psychotherapy for anorexia nervosa. International Journal of Eating Disorders 1: 3–47

Halmi K A, Goldberg S, Cunningham S 1977 Perceptual distortion of body image in adolescent girls: distortion of body image in adolescence. Psychological Medicine 7: 253–257

Halmi K A, Falk J R, Schwartz E 1981 Binge eating and vomiting: a survey of a college population. Psychological Medicine 11: 697–706

Hawley R M 1985 The outcome of anorexia nervosa in younger subjects. British Journal of Psychiatry 146: 657–660

Heron J M, Leheup R F 1984 Happy families? British Journal of Psychiatry 145: 136–138

Hill O W 1977 Epidemiological aspects of anorexia nervosa. Advances in Psychosomatic Medicine 9: 48–62

Hsu L K G, Crisp A H, Harding B 1979 Outcome of anorexia nervosa. Lancet i: 62–65

Huenemann R L, Shapiro L R, Hampton M C, Mitchell B E 1966 A longitudinal study of gross body composition and body conformation and their association with food and activity in a teenage population. American Journal of Clinical Nutrition 18: 325–338

Isaacs A J 1979 Endocrinology. In: Dally P, Gomez J, Isaacs A J(eds) Anorexia Nervosa. Heinemann, London

Johnson-Sabine E, Wakeling A 1983. Anorexia nervosa and related eating disorders. Hospital Update (December), pp. 1341–1353

Jones D J, Fox M M, Babigian H M, Hutton H E 1980 Epidemiology of anorexia nervosa in Monroe County, New York: 1960–76. Psychosomatic Medicine 42: 551–558

Kellerman J 1977 Anorexia nervosa, the efficacy of behaviour therapy. Journal of Behavior Therapy and Experimental Psychiatry 8: 387–390

Kemsley W F F 1953/4. Annals of Eugenics 16: 316–334 Reprinted in Crisp 1980 (pp. 189–190)

Kendell R E, Hall D J, Hailey A, Babigian H M 1973 The epidemiology of anorexia nervosa. Psychological Medicine 3: 200–203

Lacey J H 1982. The bulimic syndrome at normal body weight: reflections on pathogenesis and clinical features. International Journal of Eating Disorders 2: 59–66

Lacey J H 1983 Bulimia nervosa, binge-eating and psychogenic vomiting: a controlled treatment study and long-term outcome. British Medical Journal 286: 1609–1613

Lacey J H, Crisp A H, Kalucy R S, Hartmann M K, Chen C N 1975. Weight gain and the sleeping EEG; study of the patients with anorexia nervosa. British Medical Journal 4: 556–559

Mann A H, Wakeling A, Wood K, Monck E, Dobbs R, Szmukler G 1983. Screening for abnormal eating attitudes and psychiatric morbidity in an unselected population of 15-year-old schoolgirls. Psychological Medicine 13: 573–580

Minuchin S, Baker L, Rosman B L, Liebman R, Milman L, Todd T C 1975 A conceptual model of psychosomatic illness in children. Archives of General Psychiatry 32: 1031–1038

Minuchin S, Rosman B, Baker L 1978 Psychosomatic Families. Anorexia Nervosa and Diabetes in Context. Harvard University Press: Cambridge, Mass

Morgan H G, Russell G F M 1975 Value of family background and clinical features as predictors of long-term outcome in anorexia nervosa: four-year follow-up study of 41 patients. Psychological Medicine 5: 355–371

Morgan H G, Purgold J, Welbourne J 1983. Management and outcome in anorexia nervosa. A standardised prognostic study. British Journal of Psychiatry 143: 282–287

Nylander I 1971 The feeling of being fat and dieting in a school population. Acta Sociomedica Scandinavica 3: 17–26

Pugliese M T, Lifshitz F, Grad G, Fort P, Marks-Katz M 1983 Fear of obesity: A cause of short stature and delayed puberty. New England Journal of Medicine 309: 513–518

Russell G F M, 1985 Anorexia and bulimia nervosa In: Rutter M L, Hersov, L A Child and Adolescent Psychiatry: Modern Approaches. Blackwell Scientific, Oxford

Russell G F M Campbell P G, Slade P D 1975 Experimental studies on the nature of the psychological disorder in anorexia nervosa. Psychoneuroendocrinology 1: 45–56

Selvini-Palazzoli M, Self-starvation: from Individual to Family Therapy in the Treatment of Anorexia Nervosa. Jason Aronson, New York

Slade P D, Russell G F M 1973 Awareness of body dimensions in anorexia nervosa: cross sectional and longitudinal studies. Psychological Medicine 3: 188–199

Steinhausen H C, Glanville K 1983 Editorial: Follow-up studies of anorexia nervosa: a review of research findings. Psychological Medicine 13: 239–249

Sturzenberger S, Cantwell D P, Burroughs J, Salkin B, Green J K 1977 A follow-up study of adolescent psychiatric in-patients with anorexia nervosa. The assessment of outcome. Journal of the American Academy of Child Psychiatry 16: 703–715

Swift W J 1982 The long-term outcome of early onset anorexia nervosa. A critical review. Journal of the American Academy of Child Psychiatry 21: 38–46

Theander S 1970 Anorexia nervosa: a psychiatric investigation of 94 female patients. Acta Psychiatrica Scandinavica Supplement 214

Touyz S W, Beumont P J V, Collins J K, McCabe M, Jupp J 1984 Body shape perception and its disturbance in anorexia nervosa. British Journal of Psychiatry 144: 167–171

Vandereycken W 1984 Neuroleptics in the short-term treatment of anorexia nervosa: a double blind placebo-controlled study with sulpiride. British Journal of Psychiatry 144: 288–292

13

Sexual aspects

Normal sexual development

Although sexual curiosity exists in childhood, lust and sexual activity are very much a consequence of sexual maturation at puberty. The normal course and nature of sexuality in adolescence has not been very thoroughly documented in the last two decades, the last major study being that of Schofield (1968) who organised interviews with English 15–19-year-olds and whose results are considered in some detail below.

It is generally accepted that sexual behaviour always develops in a characteristic sequence, though the rate of progression through that sequence will vary between individuals. Schofield suggested five stages:

1. Little or no contact with the opposite sex beyond going out on a date; has never kissed
2. Kissing and breast fondling through clothing only
3. Sexual intimacy short of intercourse
4. Sexual intercourse with one partner
5. Sexual intercourse with more than one partner.

Across all 15–19-year-olds in his sample, Schofield found the following percentages at each stage: (Table 13.1):

Table 13.1 Stages of sex experience (Schofield 1968)

Stage no.	Boys (%)	Girls (%)
1	16	7
2	35	46
3	29	35
4	5	7
5	15	5

A slightly different breakdown by mean age (in brackets) and activity with a partner yields the following percentages (Table 13.2):

Table 13.2 Sex experience (%) of 16 and 18-year-olds (Schofield 1968)

	Boys (16)	Girls (16)	Boys (18)	Girls (18)
Dating	78	91	93	96
Breast fondling through clothes	49	60	74	79
Breast fondling under clothes	36	38	63	61
Genital stimulation	24	22	51	44
Sexual intercourse	11	6	30	16

Girls begin to date earlier than boys and their relationships with boyfriends last longer. Boys have more casual partners and appear to prefer diversity: adventure rather than security. Early starters tend to be the more experienced at each age level and girls are ahead of boys in the early stages. Dating and kissing are likely to start between 13 and 15 (though only one-half of 14-year-old boys will have been on a date) and by 16 about half of both boys and girls were indulging in kissing and breast stimulation through clothing.

Across the age range only 20% of boys and 12% of girls had experienced sexual intercourse. Girls were rather more likely than boys of the same age to have indulged in sexual activities other than intercourse but were somewhat less likely to have had intercourse itself. Unlike boys, they were inclined only to have intercourse in the setting of deep and more permanent relationships.

First sexual intercourse is not likely to be very satisfying for both partners: shame and fear being common responses among girls and disappointment among boys. Of those who expressed an opinion, over a third of boys and nearly two-thirds of girls were disenchanted with their first experience.

Although not explicit, the implication of Schofield's findings is that the difference between sexes is less at each age than the differences within each sex. The sexually experienced among both boys and girls are less involved with their parents and less supervised by them. They are more mature physically, morally tolerant, lively and gregarious. Experienced boys are more likely to be delinquent but their offences are mild and "the result of thoughtless verve and liveliness", whereas girls are prone to antipathy towards their families, which are more likely to contain marital problems and strained relationships between girl and parents.

The obvious problem with Schofield's findings is whether they continue to apply twenty years later. A survey of Canadian teenagers by Meikle et al (1985) found that one-third of 13–18-year-olds claimed to have had sexual intercourse (17% of 13-year-olds and 67% of 18-year-olds), figures comparable to Vener and Stewart's (1974) study of American teenagers aged 13–17, 28% of whom reported having sexual intercourse. It is difficult to draw conclusions from studies in different countries, particularly as some would claim that North American teenagers are more sexually advanced than their English counterparts, but in Vener and Stewart's figures there was a small but significant increase in the proportion of teenagers reporting sexual intercourse between 1970 and 1973. Meikle et al (1985) cite a number of studies, not widely available, which indicate that larger numbers of teenagers are sexually active than in previous years but the increase over time is nowhere near that assumed by phrases such as "sexual revolution".

For the sake of comparison, an exercise in adjusting Vener and Stewart's American figures to conform roughly with Schofield's staging yields the following percentages (Table 13.3):

Table 13.3 Sex experience (%) of US teenagers in Vener & Stewart's survey (1974) (stages according to Schofield 1968)

Stage	Boys		Girls	
	1970	1973	1970	1973
3	57	59	50	51
4	28	33	16	22
5	14	19	6	9

It would seem reasonable to assume that teenagers in the United Kingdom are sexually active at an earlier age than their predecessors but that the magnitude of this change is not overwhelming.

That there are changes over time in the rate of development of sexual behaviour among adolescent suggests that the factors influencing sexual behaviour are not merely endocrine. Ausubel et al (1977), in a survey of adolescent sexual development across cultures, argue that cultural influences are remarkably important.

Even though the urgency and intensity of the sexual drive in adolescence represents a qualitative break with prepubertal development, the expression of sexual feelings and impulses is regulated by social pressures. Western culture is likely, it is argued, to produce muddle in that a natural urge is denied social expression until marriage and a common assumption is that moral pressure can conquer libido. It is said that the legacy of this is a high rate of sexual problems: certainly one-half of Schofield's 1968 sample, when followed up into young adult life had a sexual problem (Schofield 1973).

In order to place the progression of heterosexual behaviour in a wider developmental context for a particular individual, it may be helpful to think in terms of:

a) the management of intense sexual interest within social encounters and in concert with social expectations.
b) the assumption of sex-roles
c) achieving physical gratification.

The topic of normal sexual development cannot be explored further in this book; it is dealt with in a number of texts (e.g. Feldman & MacCulloch 1980).

Schoolgirl pregnancies

Between about 1950 and 1980 there was a marked increase in the number of pregnancies and births in girls under the age of 16 (Russell 1983). Having peaked in 1980, the birth rate now seems to be falling amongst teenagers generally (Walker 1984), though the number of schoolgirls having abortions doubled between 1977 and 1983 (see Black 1986).

Shaffer et al (1978) reviewed earlier studies and concluded, on the basis of somewhat incomplete evidence, that pregnancy in this age group was likely to occur more often in girls of low social class from large families and was unduly prevalent among black girls. No characteristic psychopathology was demonstrated and there was no evidence that most girls intended to become pregnant or intentionally avoided contraception. Ignorance about contraception and sexual functioning generally is still widespread among teenagers, a significant factor in most teenage pregnancies is being caught contraceptively unprepared, particularly as contraceptives are hard to obtain for most young teenagers.

Positive intent to become pregnant does occur among schoolgirls but is unusual. In one study (Perez-Reyes & Falk 1973), a positive wish to have a baby was expressed by the more disturbed girls but they were a minority. Most girls want (and get) a termination even though they are likely to delay seeking help (Russell 1983). For most of them, pregnancy is unwanted and something about which they feel unhappy and ashamed, feelings which do not usually improve in later years (Furstenburg et al 1969) and may contribute to the apparently high subsequent parasuicide rate among those young teenagers who give birth (Gabrielson et al 1970).

There is considerable debate about the adverse consequences for mother and child, should the pregnancy go through to term and beyond. There are higher rates of anaemia and pre-eclamptic toxaemia among the mothers, and low birth weight and low intelligence among the children. The difficulty is that most schoolgirl mothers come from a socially disadvantaged background and continue to live in poverty after the birth. In the relative absence of well-controlled studies, it is impossible to know how far such complications are a function of early pregnancy and how much a product of material circumstances. Be that as it may, the uninspiring outcome for mother and child, and the disruptive effect that pregnancy has on the girl's education, persuade many authorities that termination of pregnancy and an early return to school should be sympathetically considered when requested, that it is likely to have a satisfactory psychological outcome, and that the consequences of allowing the pregnancy to continue include the break-up of the family (Russell 1983, Shaffer et al 1978). A return to education is more important than providing contraceptives in preventing future pregnancies (Klerman & Jekel 1973).

Homosexuality

There is a dearth of literature on homosexuality among contemporary adolescents, presumably because it is illegal for boys under the age of 21 to indulge in homosexual practice, and on account of the enduring prejudice against lesbianism, even though female homosexual practice is implicitly legal over the age of 16 if comparison is drawn with heterosexual practice. Much of what is said here is based on anecdotal experience.

Having homosexual sex is not the same thing as an established homosexual or bisexual orientation, certainly as far as boys are concerned. Boys kept apart from girls in boarding schools and penal institutions will indulge in homosexual sex inside but most will revert to, or acquire a taste for, heterosexual practice when they leave. Some autistic, mentally handicapped or "deprived" boys will sell themselves to older homosexual paedophiles for the sake of shelter, company or cash. Other less handicapped boys will accept a homosexual paedophile's overtures passively out of curiosity, bravado or as a prelude to stealing from him. Homosexual activity seems more widespread in adolescence than in adulthood: Gagnon & Simon (1973), reanalysing the original data of Kinsey et al (1948), estimated that 15% of men had a homosexual experience leading to orgasm before the age of 15 but only 3% of adult men were exclusively homosexual and a further 3% actively bisexual. Schofield's (1968) study did not intend to gather information about homosexuality but incidental replies to preliminary questions indicated a minimal rate of 5% of boys (thought to be a considerable underestimate) and 2% of girls involved in homosexual activity.

The cause of homosexual orientation is just not known, no clear, replicated evidence justifying claims for genetic, endocrine, social learning or family relationship pathology (see Green & Miller 1985).

Clinical experience suggests that for both boys and girls with homosexual preference, the realisation that they are "different" grows gradually during late childhood and early adolescence. They are unlikely to identify with the limp-wristed, mincing stereotype of the male homosexual or the butch lesbian caricature portrayed in television comedy, nor will they see many representations of adolescent gays in the mass media. Nevertheless, at some time between about 15 and 19 they will become aware of their sexual orientation. This is not a decision but a realisation.

A few boys will present with an overdose at this stage, a consequence of a perceived trap: they feel unable to confide in their parents, there may be no other authority with whom to discuss their feelings, they will probably not know any other homosexuals of the same age. As a parallel, there are occasional boys who find themselves drawn to cross-dressing, albeit with heterosexual fantasies, or who are impotent at their first intimate heterosexual encounter and believe themselves to be homosexual.

Others, predominantly boys, will indeed raise the issue with

their parents, whose response seems commonly to be one of
shock and denial. There are possibly more grounds for counselling parents than teenagers and the following parental misap-
prehensions about male homosexuality crop up with remarkable
frequency:

— it is the result of a mistaken decision; the boy has to change
  his mind

— more opportunities to go out with girls will cure it

— the boy will corrupt his brothers

— allowing him to meet other homosexuals will fix his orientation irreversibly; keeping him away from them will allow
  him to forget it

— homosexuals are mainly interested in young boys

— it is the result of too much mother-love

— I (mother or father) caused it because I am sexually
  incompetent

— basically, all adolescents are heterosexual

— I can never feel close to him again

— he will always be lonely and never develop a lasting
  relationship with a partner since all homosexuals are
  promiscuous

— he will get AIDS and die.

Counselling the adolescent requires detailed preliminary questioning rather than simple acceptance of his or her assertion that
they are gay. This should not lead to a dubious or challenging
stance on the part of the psychiatrist who should accept that the
adolescent has to arrive at a realisation of his or her own sexual
preference, but only after the facts have been examined.

Although a minority of male homosexuals can apparently be
converted to heterosexuality (see Green & Miller 1985), this
should not be the psychiatrist's first aim. Rather, the question as
to whether the youngster is homosexual, and to what degree,
needs to be raised and answered. Next is the question of how he
or she and their family (including siblings) can be helped to live
with the problem of being homosexual in a predominantly
heterosexual world where sound role models for being homo-

sexual are generally unavailable, misunderstandings abound and information is hard to obtain. A specialist gay counselling service is probably better equipped than most psychiatrists to deal with such issues, though psychiatric help may be required if there is associated depression or if there is a breakdown in family life. This may occur because the parents threaten violence or the teen-ager provokes his parents unreasonably: leaving copies of Gay News around and bringing boyfriends home for the night. In the latter circumstance, family therapy is likely to be more appro-priate than attempts to treat homosexuality and convert it to heterosexuality.

Flashers and fumblers

A familiar task for adolescent psychiatric services is the provision of a court report on a boy who has been caught exposing himself or attempting to fondle sexually a female stranger. Very little has been written about such youngsters but the consensus of opinion is that the offences which bring them to notice are commonly ill-judged and clumsy sexual overtures, or are attempts to satisfy cravings for both sexual gratification and status recognition when neither is available through conventional social channels.

> Tony was charged with indecent exposure at the age of 17. He had exhibited with his penis both erect and flaccid to a variety of young women and children of both sexes. At interview he appeared more like a 13-year-old in the company of his excessively protective parents. He would masturbate privately to heterosexual imagery which did not include memories of the responses of his 'victims'. His social manner was gauche, immature and apologetic and he had previously attended a school for children with learning difficulties. By his own account, exhibiting his penis (which was very large) to children drew gasps of amazement from them, making him feel proud and nearly powerful enough to brave talking to any woman whom he found sexually inter-esting. If he tried to put this into practice, however, he became over-whelmed with shyness before he could talk and resorted to exposing himself.

Such boys often respond to social skills training which is focussed on their difficulties in social interactions with girls and women. In cases such as the above where restrictive, overpro-tective mothering is evident, it seems that they quite often profit from counselling which is directed at uncovering any resentment which they harbour towards their mother in particular and women in general.

Straightforward experimentation or curiosity account for some (but not all) of the instances wherein a boy is found fondling or examining a younger girl. Simple explanations should be sought before more complex assertions are made. The problem behaviour might well have been considered normal curiosity if a younger boy and girl had been involved; it is wise to consider the social and mental age of the boy concerned. Rather similarly, a sexual assault short of rape on a teenage girl by a teenage boy may have been a clumsy overture or response to a mistaken perception that the girl was encouraging him. Boys can still be told by their peers that when a girl says "no" she means "yes". They may also be encouraged by them.

> Geoff, aged 16, had a severe development disorder affecting his articulation of speech. He was teased or ignored by other boys of his age and kept the company of younger adolescents to whom he used to boast of his fictitious exploits. Accordingly they dared him to kiss the breasts of a girl who happened to be walking by. He had little choice but to accept the challenge and launched himself at the girl, a stranger to him. She was hurt in the ensuing scuffle. Criminal charges followed.

Cross-dressing

The intense sexual drive of the male adolescent can easily lead to experimentation and exploration. Peeping, homosexual mutual masturbation, or fetishistic attempts to embellish solitary masturbation are all common and transient episodes or phases. They do not usually indicate a permanent proclivity. Much cross-dressing among boys should be viewed similarly: an attempt to discover what it is like to be a woman, to create a fantasy woman who is possessed, and to defuse the threat posed by the future demands of active sexual performance.

For some boys this becomes an end in itself, whether because of encouragement by others who get to know, or because it relieves tension and becomes habitual. Although not incompatible with ordinary active heterosexuality it tends to flourish in solitary individuals, and a sensible approach to management is to promote social activities whilst allaying unreasonable fears of homosexuality or transexualism.

A few cross-dressers of both sexes are transsexual, distraught at finding themselves in a body of the wrong gender and harrow-ingly perplexed as to what to do about it. It is likely to remain a private concern until cross-dressing is discovered by the parents or the individual commits a desperate act such as an overdose in order to draw attention to their plight. Perhaps the most helpful approach is to take them seriously and help them form realistic plans for the future. As with adult transsexuals, the prospect of surgical correction and civil reassignment of gender is a pervasive preoccupation. If spurned by official health-care agencies they may turn to prostitution (male and female) or other delinquent acivities in order to raise funds for corrective operations at private clinics overseas. Conversations with adult transsexuals indicate (to the author) that they were all convinced of the incor-rectness of their assigned gender when adolescents but the outcome for teenagers who are likewise convinced is unknown. All of the teenage boys I have seen who have professed a keen desire to be a girl, felt trapped in a body of the wrong gender, and pined for corrective surgery have continued to be transsexual in early adult life. This appears to be less true for the smaller number of girls, who have subsequently become heterosexual, transsexual and homosexual in roughly equal proportions.

Effeminacy in boys which does not include cross-dressing or transexual conviction is hard to evaluate. When pervasive, intense and long-standing throughout childhood, it appears to be quite likely (though not definite) that they will be bisexual or homosexual adults. Two-thirds of the boys studied by Green et al (1987) who showed effeminate behaviour in childhood had such an outcome in adolescence or adulthood.

Klinefelter's syndrome

Boys with the XXY chromosomal configuration tend to be tall with small testes and may develop gynaecomastia in late adolescence. They are likely to be unassertive and timid with less interest in sex than normal controls (Bancroft et al 1982) and have an increased rate of developmental language problems and slight intellectual retardation on verbal subscales (Ratcliffe et al 1982). Significant gender identity disturbance or homosexuality are not obviously any more common than in boys with a normal chromosomal complement (Bancroft et al 1982).

Sexual abuse

Adults may abuse children in a variety of ways which are collectively regarded as sexual, the spectrum ranging from offensively lascivious remarks to sexual intercourse. The perpetrator may be adult or a sexually active teenager though nearly always male. Similarly, the victim (who may be male or female) may be coerced persuasively and affectionately or raped forcibly with other manifestations of physical or emotional abuse. There may have been a single episode or a repeated experience with one or more perpetrators: strangers, family friends, or close relatives. Furthermore, the age of the victim may be anywhere between infancy and the age of consent, the response of the family to disclosure may be hostile, disqualifying or supportive, and the ensuing legal procedures may be sensitively handled or persecutory.

Given such variables, generalisations about sexual abuse of minors are risky, the more so when the methodological shortcomings of most enquiries in this field are taken into account. Various studies indicate that sexually abused children are frequently pre-pubertal but that disclosure may well be delayed until adolescence, particularly among girls (see De Jong et al 1983). Whereas young girls are likely to have been abused by older male family members (particularly fathers, step-fathers or mothers' boyfriends), boys are most often seduced by homosexual paedophiles unrelated to them. Most cases referred to health or welfare agencies are girls and it seems likely that they are more likely to be adversely affected psychologically as a result of the abuse (Finkelhor 1979).

It is hard to know how prevalent significant sexual abuse of minors is. Although Baker & Duncan's (1985) interview survey of a stratified sample of British adults suggested that 10% of children (12% of females and 8% of males) have been sexually abused before the age of 16, their definition of sexual abuse is broad and includes, among other things, "another person, who is sexually mature . . . . showing pornographic material or talking about things in an erotic way", which would include a 15-year-old girl (or boy) being shown a "girlie" magazine by a 17-year-old boy (or girl); not obviously pathogenic. Nevertheless, nearly half of their general population sample reported physical contact as a component of the abuse and 5% reported intercourse. Rather more than half the women and one-third of the men thought the experience was harmful at the time, the more so if the abuse took place within the family, as it did for 13% of boys and 14% of girls who reported abuse. The overall rate of reported incestuous sexual intercourse below the age of 16 was 0.25%, most intra-familial abuse not involving intercourse. Other population studies (see De Jong et al 1983) yield somewhat different figures, much of the variance being accounted for by differing definitions. Nevertheless, many clinicians working in the field consider that it is realistic to estimate that 1% of girls will be subjected to serious intrafamilial sexual abuse before their 16th birthday (see e.g. Bentovim 1987). Whether the problem is becoming more widespread or merely more readily detected is unclear but the rate of referral to treatment agencies has climbed dramatically over the last few years (Wild 1986).

It seems unlikely that all sexual abuse of minors is pathogenic, though it is commonly so with the more serious varieties. Baker & Duncan (1985) report that 51% of their total sample felt the experience to have been harmful (and 3% considered it beneficial). Being female, an early onset of abuse, repeated episodes, and a perpetrator who was a close relative were associated with a negative effect. Other studies add the use of force and genital contact as adverse elements (Browne & Finkelhor 1986).

It is important to distinguish between short-term responses (fear, anxiety, depression, guilt and shame, anger and hostility, sexually precocious behaviour) and long-term consequences. The latter include the following which may affect adolescent girls abused in childhood:

— low self-esteem

— depression

— feelings of isolation and stigma

— educational underachievement

— chronic anxiety or tension (hysterical conversion symptoms in particular)

— substance abuse

— promiscuity or a drift into prostitution

— self-harming behaviour (overdoses and self-mutilation)

— difficulties in distinguishing between sexual and common-place affection.

The correlate of this is that such symptoms in a teenage girl who is being psychiatrically assessed should prompt an enquiry into the possibility of sexual abuse along the lines of "Has anyone interfered with you sexually or got you to do sexual things to them that you thought were wrong?", adding "Not just boyfriends but anyone at home?". It may be wise to add "I always ask about this because I know that people don't usually like to mention it themselves", in case the girl feels suspicious that she may be unwittingly be giving an impression of private sexual misbehaviour.

Occasionally, physical signs may be an indication: vaginal or rectal injury, venereal infection, or pregnancy. In the case of the latter, the true father may be concealed and a spurious boyfriend blamed.

A direct allegation may be made and the psychiatrist will need to consider how valid this is. Accusations by one divorced parent that the young person has been abused by the other parent are particularly problematic since there has often been considerable questioning before the girl is seen by a professional. In the assessment of an allegation, most commonly that of a girl against an older male family member, the following suggest validity:

1. The content of the girl's allegation. An account which is spontaneous, detailed, consistent, and accompanied by obvious distress.

2. The existence of corroborating evidence. Witnesses are rare and physical evidence is said to be obtained in less than 30% of instances (Bentovim 1987).

3. Accompanying psychological symptomatology. This, however, is non-specific (see above).

4. Evidence concerning the alleged perpetrator. Unavailability of normal sexual outlets, sexually abused themselves in childhood, present disinhibiting factors such as alcoholism, dementia etc.

5. Evidence of a family constellation consistent with sexual abuse (when appropriate)

Two particular patterns are anecdotally recorded: in one there is extreme secrecy, avoidance of conflict, and a fear of rejection or separation; in the other there is chaos, neglect and violence. Common to both is a blurring of normal family boundaries and roles, particularly with "parentification" of the abused child towards her mother. Contrary to common assumptions, anger is often expressed by the girl towards her mother rather than the abuser.

In assessment, several issues arise (see also Ch. 2). One is the firmness of the evidence. Allegations of illegal sexual activity which might form the basis of criminal charges require evidence to support a case beyond reasonable doubt and will, of necessity, involve the police. Evidence in child-care cases need only support a case on the balance of probabilities. Psychiatrists can afford to work clinically within a range of certainty from possibility to certainty, but if they are involved in criminal or child-care issues will need to clarify the degree of probability of sexual abuse accordingly. It is particularly important to bear in mind the possibilities of harm to the adolescent caused by repeated questioning and examinations and therefore to exercise some restraint if it is known that a police surgeon and detective will need to examine the girl. Unreasonably precipitate action such as an emergency use of a Place of Safety Order to remove the girl from home may compromise the chances of a full disclosure because of her reasonable fear that she will not subsequently be allowed home, either by social services or her parents. Premature physical examination can prejudice the continuity of evidence so that a police case is sabotaged unwittingly. Because of such difficulties, local procedures for dealing with suspected sexual abuse are currently being established throughout the country and all psychiatrists will need to be conversant with them.

Although there will inevitably be local variations in such procedures, certain common principles will obtain. Firstly, an initial account of the alleged abuse must be obtained. This needs to be sufficiently full for a conclusion of probable abuse to be reached. The girl must be interviewed on her own as well as with a (non-abusing) parent or disclosure will be partial. It is generally worth videotaping the interview though it should be recognised that this may be subsequently used as evidence or as a means of confronting the alleged abuser. A fully detailed account is probably not necessary at this stage, especially if criminal charges seem likely, since the police will want to carry out their own interrogation.

Once abuse is thought likely, a parent must be informed and decisions have to be made as to how detailed a physical examination is needed (usually if abuse has happened within the last week, forensic evidence will be available), and where and by whom it should be carried out. In some areas there will be a special examination room and identified individuals with the necessary expertise, both health service personnel and police surgeons.

The girl's own safety from threats by the alleged abuser and from further abuse must be considered and contact with the social services department is therefore commonly appropriate. The safety of the girl and her protection from further abuse take precedence over ordinary confidentiality constraints. In general terms it is unwise to remove the girl from home because of the risk of parents closing ranks against her. In order to arrange further care for the girl and co-ordinate investigations, an urgent planning case conference should be called which will involve doctors, social services and police (CIBA Foundation 1984). A key worker should be appointed and the girl should not return home until it is safe for her to do so. Ideally this means that the alleged abuser should move out.

Not all cases will need to be handled by formal procedures; a girl may tell of abuse by a grandfather or uncle who lives some distance away, whereupon the parents must be brought in to decide how his access to their daughter can be stopped and whether charges should be brought.

The psychiatric treatment of sexually abused girls tends to follow the model pioneered by Giaretto (1981) and combines focussed family therapy in order to rehabilitate the abuser (Furniss et al 1984) with inclusion of the girl in a group for sexually abused teenagers (Herman & Schatzow 1984). It is important not to terminate treatment prematurely in the face of pseudo-mature coping behaviour on the part of the abused girl (Krener 1985). The family therapy component should involve the perpetrator but he need not live at home whilst it is in its initial stages. At what stage it is safe for the girl to be re-united with him and for him to return home is well discussed by Server & Janzen (1982) and the criteria are also appropriate objectives for family treatment:

1. Perpetrator acknowledges full responsibility for abuse
2. All family members and therapist consider child is safe
3. Abused girl has ability to seek help if abused again
4. Mother can protect girl from abuse
5. Mother does not blame girl for abuse
6. Marriage has improved and generational boundaries strengthened

7. Specific treatment for psychiatric pathology in girl and perpetrator, has been initiated.

Evaluation of the effectiveness of treatment along such lines is at an anecdotal level but such evidence as there is seems favourable in terms of relief of distress and restoration of more appropriate family and personal functioning in the short term.

REFERENCES

Ausubel D P, Montemayor R, Svajian P 1977 Theory and Problems of Adolescent Development. (2nd edn.) Grune and Stratton, New York

Baker A W, Duncan S P 1985 Child sexual abuse: A study of prevalence in Great Britain. Child Abuse and Neglect 9: 457–467

Bancroft J, Axworthy D, Ratcliffe S 1982 The personality and psychosexual development of boys with 47, XXY chromosome constitution. Journal of Child Psychology and Psychiatry 23: 169–180

Bentovim A 1987 The diagnosis of child sexual abuse. Bulletin of the Royal College of Psychiatrists 11: 295–299

Black D 1986 Schoolgirl mothers. British Medical Journal 293: 1047

Browne A, Finkelhor D 1986 Impact of child sexual abuse: a review of the research. Psychological Bulletin 99: 66–77

CIBA Foundation 1984 Sexual Abuse in the Family. Tavistock, London

De Jong A R, Hervada A R, Emmett G A 1983 Epidemiologic variations in childhood sexual abuse. Child Abuse and Neglect 7: 155–162

Feldman P, MacCulloch M 1980 Human Sexual Behaviour. Wiley, Chichester

Finkelhor D 1979 Sexually Victimised Children. Free Press, New York

Furniss T, Bingley-Miller L, Bentovim A 1984 Therapeutic approach to sexual abuse. Archives of Disease in Childhood 59: 865–870

Furstenburg F, Gordis L, Matz M 1969 Birth control knowledge and attitudes among unmarried pregnant adolescents. Journal of Marriage and the Family 6: 34–41

Gabrielson I, Klerman L, Currie J, Nyler N, Jekel J 1970 Suicide attempts in a population pregnant as teenagers. American Journal of Public Health and the Nation's Health 60: 2289–2301

Gagnon J, Simon W 1973 Sexual Conduct: The Social Sources of Human Sexuality. Aldine, Chicago

Giaretto G 1981 A comprehensive child sexual abuse treatment program. In: Mrazek P B, Kempe C H (eds) Sexually Abused Children and their Families. Pergamon, Oxford

Green J, Miller D 1985 Male homosexuality and sexual problems. British Journal of Hospital Medicine 32: 353–355

Green R, Roberts C, Williams K, Goodman M, Mixon A 1987 Specific cross-gender behaviour in boyhood and later homosexual orientation. British Journal of Psychiatry 151: 84–88

Herman J, Schatzow E 1984 Time-limited group therapy for women with a history of incest. International Journal of Group Psychotherapy 34: 605–616

Kinsey A G, Pomeroy W B, Martin C E 1948 Sexual Behavior in the Human Male. Saunders, Philadelphia

Klerman L, Jekel J 1973 School Age Mothers: Problems, Programmes and Policy. She String Press, Connecticut

Krener P 1985 After incest: secondary prevention? Journal of the American Academy of Child Psychiatry 24: 231–234

Meikle S, Peitchinis J A, Pearce K 1985 Teenage Sexuality. Taylor and Francis, London

Perez-Reyes M, Falk R 1973 Follow-up after therapeutic abortion in early adolescence. Archives of General Psychiatry 28: 120–126

Ratcliffe S, Bancroft J, Axworthy D, McLaren W 1982 Klinefelter's syndrome in adolescence. Archives of Disease in Childhood 57: 6–12

Russell J K 1983 School pregnancies — medical, social and educational considerations. British Journal of Hospital Medicine 29: 159–166

Schofield M 1968 The Sexual Behaviour of Young People. Penguin, Harmondsworth

Schofield M 1973 The Sexual Behaviour of Young Adults. Allen Lane, London

Server J H, Janzen C 1982 Contra-indications to reconstitution of sexually abusive families. Child Welfare 61: 279–288

Shaffer D, Pettigrew A, Wolkind S, Zajicek E 1978 Psychiatric aspects of pregnancy in schoolgirls: a review. Psychological Medicine 8: 119–130

Vener A M, Stewart C S 1974 Adolescent sexual behavior in Middle America revisited: 1970–1973. Journal of Marriage and the Family 36: 728–735

Walker, D The Times, 14 June 1984

Wild N J 1986 Sexual abuse of children in Leeds. British Medical Journal 292: 1113–1116

14

Schizophrenia

Whereas schizophrenia is rare among prepubertal children, its incidence increases throughout the teenage years. Although there are some differences in the clinical presentation according to developmental status, the condition, whether viewed as syndrome or disorder, is at root the same regardless of whether it is manifest in adolescence or young adult life. On account of this, the reader is directed to standard textbooks of psychiatry for accounts of aetiology, core psychopathology and neuropathology. Comment here will be selective and deal with issues most relevant to adolescence: the pathoplastic effect of age and developmental status, the importance of family relationships, and treatment approaches.

Presentation and psychopathology

All the classic forms of schizophrenia can be encountered in adolescence.

> Whilst on a school outing, 16-year-old Daniel became convinced that an assistant in a local shop was infatuated with him though the evidence that he advanced to support this assertion was nebulous, to say the least. Over the next few weeks he became convinced that he gave off an offensive odour and that other boys at school were commenting on this in secret code. He experienced sensations in his chest that he felt were imposed from outside and he came to believe that they were an indication that he had been selected for heart transplantation.
> Pandita, aged 15, was referred as a possible case of acute school refusal. She had shut herself in her bedroom from which her parents could not persuade her to emerge. At a domiciliary visit she was found

to be perplexed, alternately weeping and laughing for no clear reason. She was unable to talk coherently; her fragmented phrases failing to link together to yield an understandable theme. Whilst appearing generally self-absorbed, she would suddenly throw herself at her parents' feet in a gesture of appeal to them, yet then turn away and sing to herself before they could respond.

On holiday in London with her family, Shula, a mixed-race South African girl of 17, ceased to talk over a brief period of a few days. She began to pause in her walk and assume poses reminiscent of Balinese dancers. It was difficult to persuade her to continue walking and when she began to show disinterest in food admission to hospital was sought. On examination she was entirely remote and showed classical catatonic posturing, Mitmachen, and waxy flexibility of the limbs when these were placed in uncomfortable positions by the examining psychiatrist.

Although he had always been a somewhat retiring individual, prone to being bullied by his schoolmates, Darren had become remarkably uninterested in other people both at home and at school over a period of a year or so. He spent his sixteenth birthday shut in his bedroom but emerged in response to the pleas of his family without apparent misery or grumpiness. In fact, by their account, his mood was generally equable although he would make occasional fatuous remarks which could sometimes be insensitive. Most of his waking life was spent doing nothing except sitting in an armchair at home. It had long since been impossible to get him to carry out any schoolwork and he was a passenger in the classroom. Intelligence testing did not reveal a loss of cognitive skills, nor was he thought to be chronically depressed. Physical and neurophysiological investigations revealed nothing of note and a diagnosis of simple schizophrenia was made.

With respect to psychopathology one of the confusing elements is the common presence of affective symptoms. The first presentation of schizophrenia in late childhood is quite often preceded by a spell of depression (Eggers 1978) and clinical experience suggests that the same would seem to be true of first episodes occurring in young teenagers though this lacks systematic documentation. A self-depreciatory or grandiose aspect of delusions or ideas of reference is frequently accompanied by a depressed or expansive mood state respectively, consonant with the content of such beliefs. Anxiety or irritability are common and may be the focus of the initial complaint, whether by parents or adolescent.

The prominence of affective symptoms and the fact that phenomena such as ideas of self-reference or even catatonic signs can occur in bipolar affective disorder in adolescence (Hassanyeh & Davison 1980) mean that a precipitate diagnosis of either schizophrenia or affective disorder should be avoided when mental state examination reveals a mixed picture. Too rapid a commitment to a diagnosis of schizophrenia may mean that lithium is not considered and the chance of symptomatic relief or prophylaxis missed. Horowitz (1977) describes how this can happen.

The mode of onset and previous personality offer occasional clues. Zeitlin (1986) on the basis of a follow-up study suggests that acute onset is more typical of episodes of affective psychosis. Campbell (1952) noted a premorbid personality of anxious extraversion or cyclothymia among his cases of adolescent manic-depressive disorder. This may be set against the likelihood that self-absorption, lack of drive, and emotional unexpressiveness associates with schizophrenia in some instances. Most of the time, however, such descriptions of premorbid personality cannot be obtained to any discriminatory degree.

Considerable confusion can be caused by the presence of clear precipitating factors. These, and the presence of affective symptoms, often lead clinicians into discussions which use terms such as "psychogenic (or reactive) psychosis" with an implicit notion that this is a condition separate from schizophrenia. The dispute as to the usefulness of such an approach goes beyond adolescent psychiatry but it can be briefly noted that the implication of such a term is that the psychotic state can be expected to have a good prognosis and may well remit without the necessity for neuroleptic medication. This is not very different from saying that a clear precipitant and affective symptoms are indicators of a good prognosis for a schizophrenic episode (see review by Myers 1978). Rather similarly, an unusually sensitive previous personality in combination with an "understandable" precipitant and a mental state with affectively laden delusions of self-reference will be likely to generate a formulation along the lines of Kretschmer's (1966) *sensitive Beziehungswahn*. The practical relevance of such approaches is usually little different from making a diagnosis of schizophrenia with a good prognosis. Nosological "splitters" can generate a profusion of types of psychosis in adolescence but the implications of so doing are few, beyond the avoidance of an overt label of schizophrenia and a presumed sentence of protracted medication. Furthermore, the common difficulty of deciding whether a first instance of psychosis is fundamentally schizophrenic or affective, and the recognition that clear precipitation is a good indicator of outcome, might more logically lead to the use of a term "psychosis" with which to label such a first psychotic episode and to vary judgement on prognosis and the need for medication accordingly.

A rare group of adolescents will have a very long history of delusions and disturbed language, thought, mood and movement which reaches back into early childhood with no very clear onset (Cantor et al 1982). The distinction in nosology between "early-onset" and "late-onset" psychoses of childhood has been a useful device in differentiating autism from schizophrenia but has inhibited clinicians from recognising that schizophrenia can have an onset as early as the pre-school years. Unfortunately, such a picture has a poor long-term prognosis, consistent with the general finding that if schizophrenia occurs before puberty the outlook is gloomy (Eggers 1978, Kydd & Werry 1982, Warren 1965). Together with this there is, in my experience, a disappointing response in the short term to neuroleptic treatment.

The differentiation from common teenage concerns is not usually difficult. Certainly many adolescents display a sensitivity to how they are judged by others and may report fleeting ideas of self-reference or anxieties about bodily shape which are exaggerated; these may lead to a restriction of social activities. Hypochondriacal concerns which are connected with the physical maturation processes of puberty are common, as are speculations about cosmic principles, or idiosyncrasies of dress. The touchstone which differentiates such preoccupations from those more sinister and indicative of schizophrenia is how bizarre they are in the latter instance. Nevertheless, Steinberg (1985) makes the point that the converse is also true: that a morbid belief can underlie "what appear at first sight to be ordinary adolescent anxieties". Careful interviewing of the individual is clearly indicated in order to clarify whether this is so.

It is the parents who usually initiate medical contact in most instances of schizophrenia in school-age adolescents. Their complaints may include a number of elements of troublesome but normal teenage behaviour and it is obviously important to separate out what is morbid and what is not. However, common differences in attitudes or standards between parents and teenagers can provoke a family atmosphere replete with criticism and overinvolvement which may fulfil the criteria for high expressed emotion (Leff & Vaughn 1981) and promote relapse. The presence of such tensions offers an opportunity for useful family intervention which, although primarily focussed on issues which are not a function of the schizophrenic process, is likely to minimise the chance of relapse. The likelihood is that most schizo-phrenic youngsters will come from and return to living in the setting of their family and the perception and assessment of the reactions of their caretakers and siblings will require attention to a greater degree than is often the case with the schizophrenic adult.

Management

Virtually all adolescents in whom the diagnosis of schizophrenia is seriously entertained will require admission. The capacity of many adolescent units to respond to emergencies is notoriously limited and emergency admission may well need to be to an adult ward in the first instance. This is not as disastrous as often feared and is not contraindicated, since the first objective must be to offer the adolescent asylum in a place of healing wherein his or her mental state can be systematically assessed. The local resource for specialist adolescent psychiatry should be informed of the admission and the chance is that they will respond by offering a consultative liaison with the adult ward and arrange transfer to a suitable adolescent unit as soon as feasible.

Within an in-patient setting, full clinical description of the adolescent's mental state and a detailed history are the initial components of assessment. Although the parents and the patient will be the prime sorces of information, the family doctor and the relevant school doctor should be consulted. With parental permission a school report should be sought. It is usually wise to consider conducting a urine screen for amphetamines and to bear in mind the possibility of encephalitis (see Ainsworth 1987) which might require detailed neurological examination and investigation.

Not all young people with schizophrenia require psychotropic medication and a proportion will settle following admission with no more than conservative measures. If neuroleptics are necessary to control psychotic symptoms or to reduce excitation, then there is no evidence that adolescents differ from adults in their therapeutic response to various drugs and the choice of one specific neuroleptic should be made according to the individual psychiatrist's clinical judgement. There is a suspicion that young adolescents are more likely than adults to display extrapyramidal reactions (see e.g. Kydd & Werry 1982). One small point is that young teenagers tend not to heed warnings about photosensitivity and will sunbathe whilst taking chlorpromazine.

When a definite decision cannot be made as to whether the primary pathology is affective or schizophrenic it is appropriate to treat as for schizo-affective disorder with combined pharmacotherapy. At the same time it is essential to write very clear clinical notes describing mental state and separating observations from inferences. If there is a subsequent relapse, the clinical findings on the earlier presentation become crucial in formulation. It is supremely unhelpful to look at earlier records and find isolated statements such as "very confused and deluded" without any description of what clinical phenomena were present. Even a simple descriptive statement such as: "He has been sitting on the edge of his bed all morning smiling to himself but will not explain why" is preferable.

Whether the acutely psychotic adolescent should attend a Unit school is a decision that should be taken on common-sense grounds. There is little point in an acutely psychotic individual being forced into a classroom because attendance at school accords with the Unit routine. On the other hand, some diversionary activity during school hours may need to be provided. This may well be a nursing responsibility rather than a task for the occupational therapist.

Where possible, some attempt at helping the young person to make sense of the real world needs to be made. Lacking such an extensive and prolonged previous experience of the real world that adults with a first episode of schizophrenia will have, teenagers require the help of a counselling therapist to help them regain an appropriate perspective for their psychotic experience. There is advantage in adopting a clear model of mental illness rather than trying to be too clever in explanations. The intelligent psychiatrist can usually find a way of understanding mental content in schizophrenia; the professional task is to recognize abnormality in form. From the young person's point of view it may be a source of great relief to be told clearly and firmly that they do not smell and that others are not passing secret messages to one another. To enter into a discussion about subjective guilt without denying the delusion can be muddling for the patient.

Hopefully the acute symptoms will subside and a programme of rehabilitation into the Unit school and gradually into home life and local school can be put into operation. Parents will need advice and information; they need to be seen regularly. They may have been subjected to abuse or attack by their teenage child during the acute phase of the illness and are likely to feel bewildered and frightened. It is likely they will blame themselves for the development of their child's condition. Without proper attention to their needs it is only too easy for an atmosphere of criticism to develop within a Unit which may come to see itself (inappropriately) as a superior and more understanding alternative parent.

About 25% of adolescents with schizophrenia will make a complete recovery (see Weiner 1982). Among the remainder there will be those who relapse or who present a chronic, unimproved picture and for whom the question of long-term neuroleptics arises. This needs careful consideration since the younger the patient, the longer the duration of continuous treatment and the greater the risk of tardive dyskinesia. The need for depot preparations sometimes arises but compliance is rather less of an issue where the adolescent lives at home with parents who can supervise medication. On the other hand, this supervision may raise the hackles of a teenager who needs to exercise some sense of mastery and independence. Fine judgement is required.

There are advantages in seeing the young patient together with his or her parents and possibly with older siblings present. An opportunity can then be taken to create a shared family understanding of the problem and to correct any propensity for family members to adopt the unhelpful extremes of an overinvolved, overcritical manner, or an ingratiating, collusive stance towards the adolescent. The guidelines for this kind of approach derive from studies on expressed emotion and the success of interventions which aim to reduce this (Leff et al 1982, Falloon et al 1982). Straightforwardly, relatives should be helped to:

— avoid pandering to the adolescent's "sick" whims and beliefs whilst not falling into the trap of trying to argue him or her out of them
— stop being too inquisitive, protective or applying too much emotional pressure to the adolescent
— establish firm limits to, and expectations of, the adolescent's behaviour
— ensure the adolescent preserves sensible routines such as school or work attendance and maintains a sensible level of social involvement to avoid understimulation
— attend to sources of discord in family relationships and see that conflicts are brought to a resolution.

REFERENCES

Ainsworth P 1987 A case of 'lethal catatonia' in a 14-year-old girl. British Journal of Psychiatry 150: 110–112

Campbell J D 1952 Manic-depressive psychosis in children: a report of eighteen cases. Journal of Nervous and Mental Diseases 116: 424–439

Cantor S, Evans J, Pezzot-Pearce T 1982 Childhood schizophrenia: present but not accounted for. American Journal of Psychiatry 139: 758–762

Eggers C 1978 Course and prognosis of childhood schizophrenia. Journal of Autism and Childhood Schizophrenia 8: 21–36

Falloon I R H, Boyd J L, McGill C W, Razani J, Moss H B, Gilderman A M 1982 Family management in the prevention of exacerbation of schizophrenia: a controlled study. New England Journal of Medicine 306: 1437–1440

Hassanyeh F, Davison K 1980 Bipolar affective psychosis with onset before age 16 years. Report of 10 cases. British Journal of Psychiatry 137: 530–539

Horowitz H A 1977 Lithium and the treatment of adolescent manic-depressive illness. Diseases of the Nervous System 38: 480–483

Kretschmer E 1966 Der sensitive Beziehungswahn. 4th edn. Springer, Berlin

Kydd R R, Werry J S 1982 Schizophrenia in children under 16 years. Journal of Autism and Developmental Disorders 12: 343–357

Leff J P, Vaughn C E 1981 The role of maintenance therapy and relatives' expressed emotions in relapse of schizophrenia: a 2-year follow-up. British Medical Journal 139: 102–104

Leff J P, Kuipers L, Berkowitz R, Erberlein-Vries R, Sturgeon D 1982 A controlled trial of social intervention in the families of schizophrenic patients. British Journal of Psychiatry 141: 121–134

Myers D H 1978 Prognosis of schizophrenia. British Journal of Hospital Medicine 19: 516–523

Steinberg D 1985 Psychotic and other severe disorders in adolescence. In: Rutter M, Hersov L (eds) Child and Adolescent Psychiatry: Modern Approaches. 2nd edn. Blackwell Scientific, Oxford

Warren, W 1965 A study of adolescent psychiatric in-patients and the outcome six or more years later. II. The follow-up study. Journal of Child Psychology and Psychiatry 6: 141–160

Weiner I B 1982 Child and Adolescent Psychopathology. Wiley, Chichester

Zeitlin H 1986 The Natural History of Psychiatric Disorder in Children. Oxford University Press, Oxford

228

Gilles de la Tourette's syndrome

The common simple childhood tic is a recurrent, quick, sudden, purposeless, co-ordinated movement which recurs in the same place in the body, always taking essentially the same form. It can be suppressed by an exercise of will at the expense of mounting tension, increases with extremes of high or low arousal, and can be reproduced voluntarily on request. Such movements are more common in boys and affect about 10% of normal children aged between 5 and 10 years. They develop rapidly as an apparent habit and generally subside after a variable period of weeks or months in most cases. In a few instances they persist in the same basic form for more than a year and are termed chronic tics.

Common forms include blinks, screwing up the eyes, wrinkling the nose, shoulder-shrugging, flicks of arms or feet, sniffs, grunts or throat-clearing.

The coexistence of multiple motor tics and multiple vocal tics for more than one year indicates the presence of Gilles de la Tourette's syndrome. The initial diagnosis of this rare condition is usually made in early adolescence, though it will generally have begun in childhood with one or more motor tics indistinguishable from the common simple tics of childhood, the vocal tics tending to appear later, most commonly at around age 13.

In the minds of some clinicians, the vocal tics should be obscene or blasphemous (coprolalia) in order for the diagnosis to be made. However, only 5 out of Tourette's original 9 cases had coprolalia and most authorities in the field accept multiple vocal tics without demanding coprolalia as a requirement. This position is also taken by DSM-III. Using such criteria, about 60% of Tourette's syndrome cases will display coprolalia (Shapiro et al 1978). It is important to bear in mind that it can be suppressed voluntarily for brief periods and so may not be revealed at interview. Some youngsters are able to suppress their cursing until they can find a private place such as a lavatory wherein they can unburden themselves of their impulse. Others will convert the obscenity into a bark and then deny that they uttered anything scatological. Rarely, copropraxia (obscene gestures) may occur.

Other phonic tics include barking, hissing, sucking, whistling, grunting, coughing, throat clearing, snorting, fragmentary speech sounds, screaming, yelping, squeaking, clicking, moaning, unexpected emphasis on words, gasping, burping and lip-smacking.

About one-third of Shapiro et al's (1978) sample of 114 cases showed echolalia (repetition of the last word or words of a question directed to the patient) and another one-third demonstrated palilalia (the patient's repetition of his own last word or words in a phrase); rarely did both occur together.

Patients with Tourette's syndrome will also show other, more complex behaviours. Some are repetitive and compulsive: touching, pirouetting, posturing, slapping, clapping, squatting, stamping, skipping, sticking their tongue out. These can be carried out rapidly or at ordinary speed and do not always have the darting quality of tics. Although most rituals, like most tics, arise out of the blue in an inexplicable manner, patients often report how observing someone carry out an action results in them becoming captivated by a fascination with that action and experiencing a compulsion to repeat it themselves. In the short term this may manifest as echopraxia, seen in some Tourette's cases, but it is likely to persist long after the departure of the original observed person from the scene. In such a way a new action is added to the repertoire of the patient and may last for weeks or months. As a variant of this, actions such as throat-clearing in the course of an upper respiratory tract infection may acquire an inexplicable significance for the patient and persist after the infection has cleared as a tic. Some patients become fascinated by ideas or words that arise in conversation in a similar way and repeatedly return to them in reflection or talk; a kind of mental stereotopy.

This description of an inner urge to carry out an act is offered by some Tourette's patients (see e.g. Bliss 1980) as an explanation of their tics; they are seized by an accelerating, uncomfortable, tense mental sensation localised to a part of the body which they simultaneously recognize that they can discharge by a particular tic movement. On occasion they will repeat the tic in order to ward off a recurrence of the sensation or to get the movement "just right". It is clear that the distinction from obsessional phenomena is difficult, or, indeed, impossible. The impulse to carry out the tic or more complex manoeuvre may be resisted in the short term and viewed by the patient as an unwelcome intrusion. Unlike obsessional phenomena, though, such mental events are suppressed by haloperidol (Shapiro et al 1978). The consistency of such personal accounts is plausible, yet the absence of a pre-movement potential preceding tics in the EEGs of patients (Obeso et al 1981) is inconsistent with the idea that they are ordinary voluntary movements. The possibility remains that subcortical activity initiates both sensation and tic whilst the latter is potentially under the control of some voluntary inhibition.

Hyperkinesis and true obsessive-compulsive disorder are found more commonly than expected in association with Tourette's syndrome (Cohen et al 1985, Nee et al 1980). Some young people with the condition experience auditory hallucinations (Kerbeshian & Burd 1985).

The clinical course of the disorder is fluctuating and chronic with periodic waxing and waning of severity over weeks and months. This can breed illusions of the effectiveness of interventions or environmental change in the short term which are not borne out on follow-up. In the majority of instances, the condition persists indefinitely, though this is not at all inevitable and some cases will remit completely (Nee et al 1980). There is continuing change in the nature and pattern of the constituent tics and rituals; new ones appear and old ones fade away.

No very firm epidemiological data exist from which to draw prevalence estimates. Cohen et al (1985) and Schowalter (1980) both suggest a figure of around 5/10,000. Three times as many boys are affected as girls (Shapiro et al 1978).

Aetiology

Tourette's syndrome occurs in all the ethnic groups, cultures and social classes that have been surveyed. The evidence for a genetic component is accumulating (Comings et al 1984, Wilson et al 1978, Pauls et al 1981) and reflects the fact that chronic multiple motor tics and Tourette's syndrome aggregate together in families. As is often the case with conditions that are distributed unequally between the sexes, affected girls are more likely to have a strong family history; it is as if they require a larger genetic "dose" as reflected by the larger number of affected individuals in their relatives.

Just over one-half of all patients with Tourette's syndrome will show soft neurological signs and a broadly similar proportion will be found to have minor and non-specific EEG abnormalities, or performance scores signifiantly lower than verbal on the Wechsler intelligence scales (Shapiro et al 1978). None of this is good evidence for brain damage, though the condition has been reported to follow brain injury (Bleeker 1978).

Most recent interest has been devoted to neurotransmitter studies. The dramatic response to haloperidol and pimozide suggests that the condition results from a functional excess of brain dopamine. Some support for this suggestion is provided by the well-known tendency of stimulants, particularly pemoline, to provoke or exacerbate tics or, indeed, the full syndrome (Golden 1974, Lowe et al 1982). Direct assay of dopamine metabolites in cerebrospinal fluid have produced varying results, as have studies of the metabolites of serotonin, choline, and noradrenaline (Cohen et al 1979, 1985). The fact that clonidine is of therapeutic value suggests that an excess of noradrenaline is to blame. Clearly, the situation is still unresolved; conceivably several neurotransmitter systems are involved.

The association of Tourette's syndrome with non-specific emotional disturbance in older samples reflects, in part, the fact that these were drawn from psychiatric clinic populations. Nevertheless, specific associations exist. In childhood, hyperactivity and attentional problems are common accompaniments; Cohen et al (1985) estimate that 50–60% of childhood cases of the syndrome also fulfil the criteria for attention deficit disorder with hyperactivity. They also suggest a rate of 40% for associated obsessive-compulsive symptoms, though Nee et al (1980) found a higher rate of 68%. An association with sleep problems is also consistently reported (Mendelson et al 1980).

No contemporary authority on the condition supports a psychogenic hypothesis for the origin of Tourette's syndrome. Nevertheless, it is generally accepted that psychological factors influence the frequency and persistence of established tics so that anxiety, excitement or, conversely, boredom and fatigue will intensify them, and voluntary suppression, active concentration on a complex task or acting on stage will inhibit them (Fernando

1976). More particularly the personal significance of a tic or the amount of social attention it attracts may maintain it in a given individual. The sexual, scatological or aggressive content of many tics in Tourette's syndrome and the vigour with which they are discharged suggests strongly that what is awry in the condition is the normal process of inhibition of socially unacceptable behaviour. It thus becomes impossible to distinguish between a psychological and an organic model for the disorder. Further than this, it is necessary to account for the destructive impact of the condition upon the patient's personal development and the social repercussions of its embarrassing, offensive, handicapping symptomatology. Not unsurprisingly, secondary depressive moods, educational problems and sexual maladjustment may be manifest.

It has been suggested that motor tics are isolated components of the infant startle reaction which ordinarily appears at about 4 months (and is thus quite distinct from the Moro reflex), later to disappear. In response to a sudden, dramatic stimulus the baby screws up his face, hunches and flexes. The individual movements employed and the way in which they spread rostro-caudally, compare closely with tics (Corbett 1976, Moldofsky 1971).

Differential diagnosis

The differentiation of Tourette's syndrome from chronic multiple tics is probably of little practical value; in all probability the former is a more severe variant.

Some young people who present with classic features of Tourette's syndrome in their teens have been mistakenly diagnosed as having Sydenham's chorea in childhood. In fact the two conditions need not be confused: choreiform twitches are multiform and fragmentary and occur at unpredictable sites in the body.

Huntington's chorea, although often thought to be a possible cause of sudden involuntary movements, is more likely to present with extrapyramidal rigidity than chorea when it appears first in adolescence. Moreover, it will also be associated with progressive intellectual deterioration which is not a feature of Tourette's syndrome.

Dystonic syndromes such as dystonia musculorum deformans, spasmodic torticollis or oromandibular dystonia are unlikely to cause substantial diagnostic confusion. Wilson's disease may be associated with a variety of abnormal movements but can be excluded on the basis of inspection for a Kayser-Fleischer ring at the periphery of the iris and the performance of copper studies on blood and urine.

One possibility to be excluded in a teenager with a recent onset of tic-like jerks is covert amphetamine abuse, readily revealed by urinalysis.

Epilepsia partialis continua will result in repetitive myoclonus without impaired consciousness. The affected youngster may be heard to swear at the way in which his limb jerks uncontrollably but the absence of respite and the stereotyped nature of the movement mean that confusion is unlikely and, if necessary, resolvable by EEG and anticonvulsant trial.

Management

The guiding principles of treatment are to support normal psychosocial development and reduce suffering, not merely to abolish the tics. Indeed, it may not be appropriate to attempt total abolition of all tics if this requires vast doses of medication.

Given the manner in which the severity of the symptoms increases with anxiety, excitement or boredom, and decreases with involvement in skilled activities, it is obvious that the first task is to obtain a optimal social environment for the patient. To this end, parental counselling or even family therapy are crucial. The adolescent himself will need general advice and support to assist the establishment of personal equilibrium, as well as possible specific measures such as relaxation training or social skills tuition.

Because the condition fluctuates in intensity for endogenous as well as reactive reasons, early claims for the effectiveness of any intervention should be guarded. It is wise to rely on objective recording (counts or videotapes) of tics and rituals as well as global impressions though it is important to treat the patient and not the tic count.

Haloperidol has a more specific effect on the tics of Tourette's syndrome than just sedation. Quite low doses may well be effective, so that most adolescents may be managed on a daily dose of between 1 and 5 mg. Some adults will only experience benefit on much larger doses but the adverse effect of large doses of haloperidol on school performance and the risk of future tardive dyskinesia limit dosage in the young. Not all adolescents enjoy the drug: they may feel "zonked", "spaced out" or "zombified". A few develop anxiety reactions to school or social activities which remit on discontinuation of the drug (Mikkelsen et al 1981). Akathisia can be a problem with daily doses over about 3 mg and may require antiparkinsonian agents which in turn may mask emerging tardive dyskinesia and are thus inadvisable as a routine. It is sometimes said that persistent tardive dyskinesia does not occur as a treatment complication in Tourette's syndrome but Riddle et al (1987) have reported a case secondary to haloperidol taken continuously for 10 years at doses of between 1 and 7 mg/day. Weight gain and depressed or otherwise dysphoric mood are further reasons for older teenagers to discontinue halo-peridol on their own initiative, a not uncommon situation.

Pimozide at a daily dose of 1–10 mg/day is less sedative than haloperidol for equivalent tic blockade and is more acceptable to many patients (Ross & Moldofsky 1978).

Clonidine in an initial daily dose of 75 μg increasing gradually to 300 μg can succeed in cases where haloperidol is ineffective or poorly tolerated. The dose will often require to be increased over a period of months and there may be ultimate break-through of tics (Cohen et al 1980, Leckman et al 1985). Discontinuation can result in an exacerbation of symptoms. In the initial phase of treatment, the calming effect on the irritability which is often associated with the condition can be remarkable.

Whereas pharmacotherapy is without doubt the most effective single intervention, there is no reason not to combine it with behavioural measures, though none of these is dramatically effective when used alone (Turpin 1983). It seems likely that earlier reports failed to take into account the manner in which the condition waxes and wanes in severity. Some older teenagers improve temporarily when asked to monitor their own tics. Massed practice of a particular tic appears to be mainly of benefit as far as simple tics are concerned and, as Corbett & Turpin (1985) have pointed out, there have been many reported failures of massed practice in the treatment of Tourette's syndrome. Manipulation of response contingencies, by positive reinforcement of tic-free periods or withdrawal of social attention in response to tics, does not seem to have lasting effects.

Attention to the teenagers schooling is important since a substantial minority of patients experience educational difficulties. Bauer & Shea (1984), reviewing this area, make some specific suggestions as to how teachers may structure educational programmes and modify classroom procedures.

Depressive moods are not uncommon amongst Tourette's syndrome sufferers. Where the cause is not obvious and remediable, consider lowering the dose of haloperidol when this is prescribed. Avoid tricyclic antidepressants which worsen symptoms. If this is not recognised, there is a real risk of increasing the dose of antidepressant on the mistaken assumption that increasing tics represent increasing depression with the consequence that the tics are further exacerbated iatrogenically.

In all cases supportive and directive counselling of teenager and family is essential in order that the normal developmental hurdles may be overcome without failure or maladaptation. In essence this is the management of the condition for which the above interventions are the tools.

REFERENCES

Bauer A M, Shea T M 1984 Tourette syndrome: a review and educational implications. Journal of Autism and Developmental Disorders 14: 69–80
Bleeker H E 1978 Gilles de la Tourette's syndrome with direct evidence of organicity. Psychiatrica Clinica 11: 147–154
Bliss J 1980 Sensory experiences of Gilles de la Tourette syndrome. Archives of General Psychiatry 37: 1343–1347
Cohen D J, Shaywitz B A, Young J G et al 1979 Central biogenic amino metabolism in children with the syndrome of chronic multiple tics of Gilles de la Tourette: Norepinephrine, serotonin and dopamine. Journal of the American Academy of Child Psychiatry 18: 320–341
Cohen D J, Detlor J, Young J G, Shaywitz B A 1980 Clonidine ameliorates Gilles de la Tourette's syndrome. Archives of General Psychiatry 37: 1350–1357
Cohen D J, Leckman J F, Shaywitz B A 1985 The Tourette syndrome and other tics. In: Shaffer D, Ehrhardt A, Greenhill L (eds) The Clinical Guide to Child Psychiatry. Collier Macmillan, London
Comings D E, Comings B G, Devor E J, Cloninger C R 1984 Detection of a major gene for Gilles de la Tourette syndrome. American Journal of Human Genetics 36: 586–600
Corbett J A 1976 The nature of tics and Gilles de la Tourette's syndrome. In: Abuzzahab F, Anderson F (eds) Gilles de la Tourette's Syndrome. Vol. I. Mason, St. Paul, Minnesota
Corbett J A, Turpin G 1985 Tics and Tourette's syndrome. In: Rutter M, Hersov L (eds.) Child and Adolescent Psychiatry: Modern Approaches. 2nd · edn. Blackwell Scientific, Oxford
Fernando S J M 1976 Six cases of Gilles de la Tourette's syndrome. British Journal of Psychiatry 128: 436–441
Golden G 1974 Gilles de la Tourette syndrome following methylphenidate administration. Developmental Medicine and Child Neurology 16: 76–78

Kerbeshian J, Burd L 1985 Auditory hallucinosis and atypical tic disorder. Journal of Clinical Psychiatry 46: 398–399

Leckman J F, Detlor J, Harcherik D F, Ort S, Shaywitz B A Cohen D J 1985 Short and long-term treatment of Tourette's syndrome with clonidine. Neurology 35: 343–351

Lowe T L, Cohen D J, Detlor J, Kremenitzer M W, Shaywitz B A 1982 Stimulant medications precipitate Tourette's syndrome. Journal of the American Medical Association 247: 1729–1731

Mendelson W N, Caine E D, Goyer P, Elbert M, Gillin J C 1980 Sleep in Gilles de la Tourette's syndrome. Biological Psychiatry 15: 339–343

Mikkelsen, E J, Detlor J, Cohen D J 1981 School avoidance and social phobia triggered by haloperidol in patients with Tourette's disorder. American Journal of Psychiatry 138: 1572–1576

Moldofsky H 1971 A psychophysiological study of multiple tics. Archives of General Psychiatry 25: 79–87

Nee L E, Caine E D, Polinsky R J, Eldridge R, Ebert M H 1980 Gilles de la Tourette syndrome: clinical and family study of 50 cases. Annals of Neurology 7: 41–49

Obeso J A, Rothwell J C, Marsden C D 1981 Simple tics in Gilles de la Tourette's syndrome are not prefaced by a normal premovement EEG potential. Journal of Neurology, Neurosurgery and Psychiatry 44: 735–738

Pauls D L, Cohen D J, Heimbuch R, Detlor J, Kidd K K 1981 Familial pattern and transmission of Gilles de la Tourette syndrome and multiple tics. Archives of General Psychiatry 38: 1085–1090

Riddle M A, Hardin M T, Towbin K E, Leckman J F, Cohen D J 1987 Tardive dyskinesia following haloperidol treatment in Tourette's syndrome. Archives of General Psychiatry 44: 98–99

Ross M S, Moldofsky H 1978 A comparison of pimozide and haloperidol in the treatment of Gilles de la Tourette's syndrome, American Journal of Psychiatry 135: 585–587

Schowalter J E 1980 Tics. Pediatrics in Review 2: 55–57

Shapiro A K, Shapiro E S, Bruun R D, Gilles de la Tourette syndrome. Raven Press, New York

Turpin G 1983 The behavioural management of the tic disorders: a critical review. Advances in Behaviour Research and Therapy 5: 203–245

Wilson R S, Garron D C, Klawans H L 1978 Significance of genetic factors in Gilles de la Tourette syndrome: a review. Behavioral Genetics 8: 503–510

16

Disorders of sleep

Night-time sleep consists of an alternating cycle of rapid-eye-movement (REM) sleep with non-REM sleep (NREM). The latter can be categorised into four stages of increasing depth. REM sleep is a qualitatively distinct state from NREM and includes features such as binocularly synchronous rapid eye movements, suppressed muscle tone coupled with twitching movements, penile erection and rapid heart and respiratory rates; a state of high neurophysiological activity which is in contrast to the slowing of vegetative activity and inhibition of movement seen in the NREM state.

Vivid dreaming is confined to REM sleep but simple thoughts and images are recalled by individuals woken from NREM sleep.

On falling asleep, the NREM state progressively deepens through stages 1–4. There is then a rapid entry, 60–80 minutes after the onset of sleep, into REM state for a further 10 minutes or so. Thereafter the cycle repeats itself with re-entry into NREM followed by a further REM phase. The duration of the entire cycle in adolescents is about 70–100 min so that there are about 5 such cycles each night with the depth of NREM diminishing on each cycle. The first cycle may be prolonged by an increase of Stage 3/4 NREM following exercise or stress. REM sleep occupies about 20% of total sleep and each REM phase lasts 10–30 min, the duration progressively increasing with each cycle.

During adolescence there is a progressive increase in the relative amount of Stage 4 NREM sleep and a reduction in the total amount of sleep each night (Feinberg 1974, Karacan et al 1975, Williams et al 1972). At the same time there is a striking increase in the rate of daytime drowsiness and a preference for sleeping late in the mornings which is not typical of the prepubertal child. Some of this is obviously due to the late bedtimes preferred by adolescents and the chronic sleep deprivation resulting from the competing claims of school and work which is characteristic of contemporary life (Webb & Agnew 1975) but this is not the whole story since mid-afternoon drowsiness persists ever when total sleep time is held constant at 10 hours nightly (Carskadon 1981, cited by Anders 1981).

Poor sleep

Between 5 and 12% of teenagers surveyed in various studies regarded their sleep as poor or found it difficult to get off to sleep (Karacan et al 1976, McGhie & Russell 1962, Price et al 1978). It is readily apparent that such adolescents are distinguished by symptoms suggestive of depression and tension. In the study of 639 American high school pupils reported by Price et al (1978), those with insomnia (substantial difficulty falling asleep, waking for long periods during the night) were more likely to be female, to worry more, to have personal and family problems, possess poor self-esteem, and feel moody and dispirited. Such findings are comparable with studies on medical students (Johns et al 1971) and on other young adults (Kales et al 1976) and suggest that the poor sleep is secondary to psychological problems (particularly depression and anxiety) in many instances. A simple recourse to hypnotics would therefore miss the point.

Short sleep is not the same thing as insomnia and among the teenagers surveyed by Price et al (1978), there were 23 individuals who had 5 hours or less sleep a night; 12 of these had no reservations at all about the quality of their sleep. It is the complaint of insomnia which is clinically relevant. Given such a complaint it is necessary to explore the possibilities of the following:

— depressed mood: primary depression or secondary to loss etc.

— anxiety, whether primary or secondary to environmental stress

— licit or illicit medication with disruptive effects on sleep: nicotine, alcohol, coffee, tea, cola drinks and withdrawal of sedative agents are easily overlooked

— recent drastic dieting

— coexistent physical disorder such as uraemia or any condition causing pain

— sleep apnoea (see below) when coupled with daytime sleeping.

Management

If no underlying psychiatric condition or remediable environmental factor is evident, straightforward advice based on a combination of good sense (see Oswald 1984) and behavioural principles (France & Robson 1986) is a sensible recourse.

1. Minimal smoking, drinking and caffeine intake
2. Regular exercise
3. Routine bedtime and getting-up time
4. Regular evening meal with or without subsequent hot milky malted drink at bedtime
5. Avoid reading, watching TV and eating in bed unless clear that these assist getting to sleep
6. Systematic relaxation exercise once in bed
7. Avoid thoughts about getting enough sleep and worries about the day's events. Concentration on pleasant thoughts and images or on external noises: birds, traffic etc.
8. If no sleep after 10 minutes, get up and go to another room to read. Return to bed only when sleepy
9. Avoid sleeping during the day.

Waking during the night can be dealt with along similar lines:

1. Once fully awake, get up, avoid lying in bed fretting about not being able to sleep
2. Move to another room. Sit and read comfortably. Only return to bed when sleepy. Then as 6–9 above.
Prescription of hypnotics is to be undertaken sparingly, educating the patient as to the risks of withdrawal rebound, dependency and tolerance. Oswald (1984) has argued that very short-acting and long-acting benzodiazepines are less suitable than those with a medium elimination half-life such as lormetazepam or temazepam.

Parasomnias

These disturbances of sleep state tend to cluster within the same individual, to have a family history, and to be commoner in males. They include night-terrors, sleep-walking and sleep-talking. They are generally held to occur at the point at which stage 4 NREM shifts to REM during the first cycle of the night. The EEG during a parasomnia may be indistinguishable from a waking record and one mode of understanding the phenomena is to consider them as representing confused and dissociated activity resulting from very rapid arousal from very deep sleep. All are commoner in young children though may present in adolescence.

Night terrors are to be distinguished from nightmares, which are terrifying dreams, capable of subsequent recollection, and occurring during REM sleep. In a night terror the person sits up in bed or gets out of bed and wanders in an apparent state of terror with open eyes, extremely rapid pulse, sweating and breathing heavily. They may also appear hallucinated and be seen to fend of imagined threatening objects. It is almost impossible to rouse them or communicate with them in any detailed sense but if taken back to bed they usually settle back to normal sleep and have no memory of the episode in the morning. This latter fact may give rise to family rows, the teenager denying that he had a "bad dream" the previous night and disbelieving the account of his behaviour provided by his parents.

Sleep-walking bears an obvious resemblance with an abrupt onset, open eyes, an unsure walk and little response to questioning. As with night terrors, confusion and panic may cause sleep-walkers to injure themselves or, very rarely, others (Oswald & Evans 1985). Sleep-talking is likewise usually purposeless, mumbled, monosyllabic, and its content trivial. More co-ordinated, purposeful actions are rarely due to a parasomnia and should raise the possibility of hysteria, though this may be hard to diagnose or exclude without sleep laboratory studies.

Melanie was referred with a history of disturbed behaviour during the night starting shortly before her 18th birthday. She would suddenly run from her bed to other rooms in the house where she would be found to be inaccessible to attempts to communicate with her. At such times she appeared flushed, upset, frightened and incoherent. On one

241

occasion she had urinated in a wardrobe and on several others had injured herself by colliding with furniture.

After running semi-naked into the street she was seen urgently and a preliminary diagnosis of hysteria considered, though referred to a teaching hospital for confirmation. She was under some stress at school with a difficult course and under some parental pressure to succeed. Sleep laboratory studies showed her quasi-purposive behaviour to occur as she emerged from stage 4 NREM sleep at a remarkably abrupt rate with an "overshoot" into electrophysiological wakefulness before settling into sleep. The problem was abolished by a regular benzodiazepine but within a few months she developed nocturnal tonic-clonic seizures for which no cause has yet been identified.

Management

Sleep-talking does not reliably indicate psychological disturbance and should be treated by reassurance, unless external stressors can be identified as exacerbating influences which can be ameliorated. Stress is not a necessary pre-condition but may accentuate a predisposition. A similar principle applies to sleep-walking which is commonly (and erroneously) thought by parents to be provoked by disturbing dreams. Attention to the safety of the walker by locking doors and windows is necessary, there being no truth in the belief that sleep-walkers never injure themselves.

Night terrors should in the first instance be managed along the same lines. If persistent, they can usually be abolished by a medium-acting or long-acting benzodiazepine taken at bedtime in order to suppress Stage 4 sleep (Fisher et al 1972). Contrary to theoretical expectations, very short-acting agents such as triazolam are less useful since they may merely displace the night-terror to a later part of the night.

Hypersomnias

Drowsiness during the day is a normal experience, as discussed above. There are obvious common causes such as sleep deprivation and sedative drugs, and a few rare causes which tend to appear first in adolescence and are listed below.

Narcoleptic syndrome

The clinical diagnosis depends upon the demonstration of one or more of the narcoleptic tetrad:

1. Narcolepsy: sudden irresistible daytime sleep of a few minutes duration occurring several times a day and often provoked by particular activities

2. Cataplexy: a sudden loss of muscle tone lasting a few seconds affecting one or more muscle groups and resulting in partial slumping or even a fall. Classically, yet not constantly, such attacks are precipitated by strong emotion. They do not impair consciousness.

3. Sleep paralysis: inability to move whilst falling asleep or on waking but in either case whilst the subject is conscious and accompanied by panic

4. Hypnagogic hallucinations: vivid auditory or visual hallucinations at the point of falling asleep and possibly associated with sleep paralysis. Unlike those experienced by normal individuals, in the narcoleptic variety there is a powerful emotional accompaniment, usually fear.

The commonest presentation in adolescence is with narcolepsy alone. If cataplexy is also evident, the other features are likely to occur too (Parkes & Marsden 1974). Sleep EEG studies show immediate entry into REM state on falling asleep and subsequent sleep to be poorly organised. Indeed it is possible to understand the components of the syndrome as isolated aspects of REM state in particular.

The usual first treatment measure is to employ amphetamine in sufficient dose to counteract the sleep episodes. The risk of dependence appears small but there is the danger of amphetamine psychosis if large doses are used. Irritability and headache are commoner complaints and some individuals will do better on another stimulant such as methylphenidate. Cataplexy requires separate treatment and clomipramine is widely employed at a low dose, usually below 50 mg daily. Since the condition is lifelong, complications of management are likely.

Hypersomnia with sleep drunkenness

In this condition (Roth et al 1972), prolonged deep sleep at night extends well into the morning without spontaneous waking and the affected individual can be roused only with difficulty. A state of irritable disorientation, ataxia and drowsiness then follows. If not woken, he or she sleeps for sixteen hours or more, eventually waking spontaneously to clear consciousness. During waking hours the individual is prone to drowsiness but not the sudden spells typical of narcolepsy. Most cases are idiopathic and a family history is obtained in about one-third. A few instances follow encephalitis or head injury. The condition, which is static and shows no tendency to spontaneous remission, is ameliorated by stimulants on a symptomatic basis, one ruse being to give a dose of amphetamine when first rousing the patient, subsequently allowing him to sleep for a further half-hour from which he will wake spontaneously under the effect of the stimulant.

Kleine-Levin syndrome

This extremely rare condition of unknown cause (Critchley 1962, Orlosky 1982) affects males, typically with an onset during adolescence, producing recurrent episodes of hypersomnia accompanied by overeating, usually lasting several day, with intervening periods of normality which last for several weeks or months. During an episode, the teenager will sleep for 18 hours or more a day, though he can be roused with little difficulty. He will eat ravenously when food is placed in front of him and help himself to food from other people's plates though, if food is cleared from the house, will not complain excessively; it is as if the immediate availability of food is the trigger to gorging. Weight gain during an episode can be dramatic and produce abdominal stretch marks. Whilst asleep, he is typically troubled by morbid dreams and vivid fantasies with a cruel or sexual content. During waking periods, he is likely to be disorientated for time, masturbate excessively in a disinhibited way and wander restlessly around, mumbling rather than talking, and reacting irritably to intrusions. Following recovery there is little memory for events during a somnolent phase.

> David was seen at the age of 15 with a two-year history of episodes as described above. He knew when a somnolent phase was coming on; for a couple of days or so he would feel detached and unreal, finding it difficult to concentrate. No triggers for such episodes could be reliably identified though they recurred every three months or so. During one, he would sleep most of the day though he woke frequently and then wandered round the house, masturbating and

eating, and behaving in a generally surly, uncommunicative manner. He repeatedly checked on his mother's presence in the house, becoming anxious if she were not around. He would eat everything in the refrigerator, on one occasion devouring four gallons of ice cream in under an hour. Following recovery he could remember little, though he reported having experienced vivid hallucinatory episodes, not quite like dreams, such as visions of dogs running into barbed wire and decapitating themselves. When examined during a remission he was psychiatrically normal but, not surprisingly, had livid stretch marks around his umbilicus reflecting a rapid gain of weight, subsequently lost. His personality between episodes was impeccable and he was mature for his years. Methylphenidate had no effect either prophylactically or in terms of truncating an episode, but fenfluramine taken during a phase curtailed his eating and weight-gain as well as abolishing the morbid "dreams" which he had found distressing. At the time of writing, lithium appears to have prevented relapse.

There is no recognised treatment for the condition though, as above, a symptomatic approach may prove useful during acute episodes. The episodes become less frequent with age and commonly disappear during early adult life. Anecdotal reports suggest lithium may provide prophylaxis (Will et al 1988).

Sleep apnoea with diurnal drowsiness

Some adolescents have copious tonsillar and adenoidal tissue which obstructs their airway during sleep with resulting apnoeic spells of up to one minute in duration leading to disturbed nocturnal sleep and resulting daytime drowsiness. Dramatic snoring is an obvious clue. Intellectual functioning may be impaired and can lead to a mistaken diagnosis of mental handicap (Guilleminault et al 1976). Surgical management of upper airway obstruction can have a dramatic effect on both sleep and intellectual functioning. In severe cases, a permanent tracheostomy which can be blocked off during the day has been employed successfully (Anders 1981).

REFERENCES

Anders T F 1981 The development of sleep disturbances from infancy through adolescence. Advances in Behavioral Pediatrics 2: 171–190

Critchley M 1962 Periodic hypersomnia and megaphagia in adolescent males. Brain 85: 627–657

Feinberg I 1974 Changes in sleep cycle patterns with age. Journal of Psychiatric Research 10: 283–306

Fisher C, Kahn E, Edwards A, Davis D 1972 Effects of Valium on NREM night terrors. Psychophysiology 9: 91

245

France, R, Robson M 1986 Behaviour Therapy in Primary Care. Croom Helm, London

Guilleminault E, Eldridge F, Simmons B, Dement W 1976 Sleep apnea in eight children. Pediatrics 58: 23–30

Johns M W, Gay T J A, Goodyear M, Masterson J P 1971 Sleep habits of healthy young adults. British Journal of Preventive and Social Medicine 25: 236–241

Kales A, Caldwell A B, Preston T A, Healey S, Kales J D 1976 Personality patterns in insomnia. Archives of General Psychiatry 33: 1128–1134

Karacan I, Anch M, Thornby J, Okawa M, Williams R 1975 Longitudinal sleep patterns during pubertal growth. Four years follow-up. Pediatric Research 9: 842–846

Karacan I, Thornby J I, Anch M et al 1976 Prevalence of sleep disturbance in a primarily urban Florida county. Social Sciences and Medicine 10: 239–244

McGhie A, Russell S M 1962 The subjective assessment of normal sleep patterns. Journal of Mental Science 108: 642–654

Orlosky M 1982 The Kleine-Levin syndrome: a review. Psychosomatics 23: 609–621

Oswald I 1984 Insomnia. British Journal of Hospital Medicine 31: 219–224

Oswald I, Evans J 1985 On serious violence during sleep walking. British Journal of Psychiatry 147: 688–691

Parkes J D, Marsden C D 1974 Narcolepsy. British Journal of Hospital Medicine 12: 325–334

Price V A, Coates T J, Thoresen C E, Grinstead O A 1978 Prevalence and correlates of poor sleep among adolescents. American Journal of Diseases of Children 132: 583–586

Roth B, Nevsimalova S, Rechtschaffen A 1972 Hypersomnia with "sleep drunkenness". Archives of General Psychiatry 26: 456–462

Webb W D, Agnew H 1975 Are we chronically sleep deprived? Bulletin of the Psychonomic Society 6: 47–48

Will R G, Young J P R, Thomas D J 1988 Kleine-Levin syndrome: report of two cases by head trauma. British Journal of Psychiatry 152: 410–412

Williams R, Karacan I, Hursch C, Davis C 1972 Sleep patterns of pubertal males. Pediatric Research 6: 643–648

17

Interactions with physical conditions

The psychological and physical dimensions of personal functioning relate closely; any convention which separates mind and body simplifies matters, but at the expense of adequate clinical management. Relationships between the two may be construed in various ways as far as clinical phenomena are concerned.

A physical condition can give rise to psychological symptoms. The commonest of these are those related to acute pain and distress. Fear, despondency, passivity and regression are commonly encountered in acutely ill adolescents but there are also longer term issues of adaptation to chronic or damaging physical problems. These are discussed at greater length below.

Some physical conditions give rise directly to psychological phenomena: complex partial seizures are a case in point.

Kate, aged 14, had a repeated "day dream" which troubled her. She felt that someone was creeping up on her from behind, intending to strangle her. Whilst she was being interviewed, she said "It's happening" but was unable to explain further as she stared mutely into space. For several seconds she would not answer any questions and appeared to be unaware of her surroundings. Her hands drifted to her throat and then fell into her lap. She then shook her head as if to clear her thoughts, yawned and fell asleep. An EEG showed paroxysmal activity with a temporal lobe focus.

Alternatively, a physical condition may require medication which has psychological side effects.

An urgent call from the haematology ward for the duty psychiatrist led to a 15-year-old boy with haemophilia and on massive doses of steroids being admitted to the local adolescent unit on account of a schizophrenic-like psychosis which disappeared when his dose of steroids was carefully reduced.

247

In similar vein, the social restrictions placed upon ill adolescents may cause difficulties. Social isolation can result from unthinking (and often unnecessary) curtailment of activities such as swimming and disco dancing for those with seizure disorders.

Conditions which are considered primarily psychological can produce physical signs. The weight loss accompanying depression, or even anorexia nervosa, is an obvious example. Tetany secondary to hyperventilation accompanying acute anxiety is another. The topic of hysteria is considered below.

Sometimes the same phenomenon can be produced by either physical or psychological processes, even in the same individual. These may be objectively observable such as asthma, or symptomatic as in headache. The converse of this is when a condition of unknown aetiology such as Kleine-Levin syndrome (see Ch. 16) has clearly recognisable effects on both behaviour and the body.

As a further complication of the above mechanisms of effect, a number of younger teenagers will complain of physical symptoms rather than use psychological terms. They mention palpitations, neck pain, nausea, and a dry mouth with difficulty swallowing rather than say that they are anxious (though they agree that this is the case when it is put to them).

For such reasons, the psychiatrist needs to keep alive the knowledge and skills derived from his medical training in physical disorder. A number of distressed teenagers suffer more than they need because they, their caretakers and their doctors adopt an attitude which polarises mind and body, psychological causation of symptoms being considered only after the exclusion of even the rarest and most exotic physical causes, or physical conditions being overlooked by psychiatrists who will do no physical examinations. If a psychiatrist with several years of training in physical medicine cannot pursue a holistic approach combining mind and body, how can he expect physicians to do the same, bearing in mind the poverty of their psychiatric training?

Responses to acute serious illness or injury

The psychiatrist involved in hospital liaison work may be asked to advise when an ill or injured adolescent in hospital is found behaving oddly. Obviously a number of reasons suggest themselves: pre-existing psychiatric disorder, drug reactions, a confusional state secondary to infection or cerebral fat embolism from a fracture site. To such a catalogue should be added the vagaries of psychological adjustment to serious illness or injury. Dane Prugh (Prugh & Eckhardt 1980) has suggested that there is a recognisable sequence of phases in such adjustment: impact, recoil, and restitution.

Impact refers to the co-existence of realistic fears of death or disability with massive denial of the longer-term outlook. There may be fantastic ambitions: "when I get out of here I'm going to . . . . . ." which are probably helpful as a compensation for the helplessness enforced by acute illness or injury. At the same time, or instead, there is likely to be a marked regression with demands for nurturance, preoccupations with bodily needs and cravings for favourite foods and old toys. Psychological management throughout this stage amounts to warm support. Denial should not be challenged crudely and it is sensible to allow the adolescent his or her fantasies without going so far as to collude too actively with them. A special nurse can ensure continuity of care for both patient and parents. The latter will also need support in their own right and should not be confronted with a poor prognosis too harshly and too soon. If their hopes are dashed by cold pessimism, their own denial will be provoked to the extent that they shop around for alternative medical opinion and disrupt treatment.

A catastrophic reaction with marked withdrawal, refusal of food, mutism and loss of sphincter control may develop and raise questions of brain damage. Prugh & Eckhardt (1980) argue that this is a state of 'psychic shock' with a good prognosis. It may be seen in children as well as adolescents and usually responds to sympathetic nursing care. Attempts to 'break through' intrusively or rehabilitate forcibly are likely to be met with resistance and may foster entrenched regression. If this happens there is a risk of it being labelled by ward staff as malingering: if unchecked, this can lead to a vicious spiral of accusation or brusque imperatives to 'pull your socks up' which lead almost inevitably to further regression and withdrawal.

Recoil supervenes after several days or a few weeks when the seriousness of the situation is grasped realistically. There is less regression but a varying balance of guilt (often irrational) over the cause of the disorder, depression as a part of mourning the loss of health or bodily integrity; and irritability. This is a difficult stage for nursing staff and parents and is likely to last for several weeks.

Somehow, emotional acceptance of the person behind the behaviour has to be preserved. Staff and parents need to understand that this is a normal reaction which will pass, otherwise they will be tempted to react in a hostile manner themselves. Nevertheless they should be prepared to set limits upon demands and foster the development of independence: offering the patient choices of food or occupation and carefully allocating small tasks to him to encourage his returning capacity to help himself. This should not extend prematurely into a full rehabilitation schedule.

The parents will themselves progress from denial and numb disbelief to a stage where they question their own or each other's blame. They, too, will feel guilt and may be angry or despairing; they may need to mourn the loss of their expectations and ambitions for their child. There is no guarantee that they will progress through this phase in synchrony with the adolescent patient nor indeed with themselves. Marital rows may flare and they will need support as a couple, ideally always being seen together by any professional who provides information.

Restitution represents increasing acceptance and adaptation to any injury or convalescent weakness. According to qualities in the youngster's premorbid personality, there may be maladaptive coping such as overdependence and tearfulness on one hand or a blustering overcompensation on the other. Eventually an equilibrium is found within the family and social peer group.

Where required, a rehabilitation programme needs to involve parents as well as the patient. Hopefully they will move to a phase of rational acceptance of any lasting disability in their teenage child and begin to plan realistically. They too will need guidance if there are signs of overprotection or excessive reha bilitative zeal. Parents may develop an excessive identification with the needs of the child and sacrifice their own needs; this requires sensitive handling with a reminder that parents, too, have needs for privacy and satisfaction.

Specific physical conditions

Diabetes

Most adolescent psychiatry services see young diabetics with psychological problems associated with the management of diabetes itself. Whether there is an increase in the rate of formal psychiatric disorder apart from their adjustment difficulties is not clear from the literature: some studies find an increased rate of disorder (Sullivan 1978, Swift et al 1967), others not (Gath et al 1980, Hoare 1984, Simonds 1977, Starky 1963), a discrepancy which may relate to age of onset, later acquisition of diabetes being rather more likely to be associated with psychological problems (Rovet et al 1987).

Tattersall & Lowe (1981) point out how diabetes may interact with the adolescent developmental process itself (see Table 17.1). The physician in charge of a diabetic clinic and the liaison psychiatrist need to be aware of these specific issues, disentangle normal adolescent adjustment problems from the management of diabetes, and prevent the two becoming confused. This applies

Table 17.1 Adolescent development in diabetics (Tattersall & Lowe 1981)

Adolescent process	Diabetes-related difficulties
Accommodation to physical growth and maturation	Short stature Having an imperfect, flawed body
Sexual maturation	Delayed puberty Concerns about future pregnancy risks or impotence Invasion of personal privacy at repeated physical examinations
Independence and autonomy	Ordinary minor confrontations with parental authority become focussed upon control of diabetes Medical advice seen as authority to be confronted and questioned Use of hypoglycaemia or ketoacidosis as a manipulative threat Parental doubt as to youngster's ability to manage diabetes alone Experience of loss of control with hypoglycaemia
Identity	Chronic illness with risk of over-identification with sick role Self-consciousness at aberrant behaviour during hypoglycaemia Seeing older, disabled diabetics at adult clinic
Accommodation to peer group	Dietary restrictions may preclude prohibition of junk food, irregular snacks or alcohol Employment, licence and insurance difficulties.

to parents as well as the young diabetic. Normal parental concern over the safety of young teenagers out alone for long periods will naturally be heightened by the risk of hypoglycaemia or keto-acidosis; the risk of overprotection or even a lack of appropriate concern on the parents' part will need appraisal and guidance by the diabetologist. To these specific issues should be added the vagaries of the adaptation process described in the previous section: denial ("I don't want to be diabetic so I'm not") is a common inference drawn from the behaviour and posture of young adolescent diabetics seen in psychiatric clinics.

Psychiatric input may be valued at a consultative level to the clinic; it need not involve direct contact with the patient. Indeed this may cause risks of confused management. The psychological problems of most young diabetics can be managed by the clinic physician, especially if supported by specialist diabetic nurse, social worker and clinical psychologist. Referral to an adolescent psychiatrist is generally reserved for four main groups of diabetics.

1. Those with intercurrent serious psychiatric disorders (e.g. depression) requiring treatment in their own right.

2. Patients with adjustment problems specific to diabetes which do not resolve with sensible handling within the diabetic clinic, e.g. where issues of control within the family have become inextricably bound up with the management of diabetes and manipulation or deception of parents and doctors is rife.

3. Young diabetics who display vagaries of the normal adaptation process to chronic illness. Passage of responsibility for managing the diabetic from parents to the adolescent may provoke denial or over-identification with invalidity as typical maladaptive reactions. A strong reaction may coincide with the transfer of the young patient from a paediatric clinic to an adult diabetic clinic, the waiting room of which is populated by a number of diabetics with blindness or renal failure or who have had amputations. There may also be a change in medical attitude from indulgence of the individual child (free diet and one injection a day) to a tighter and more impersonal control of blood sugar level.

4. Brittle diabetics, often adolescent girls, whose blood sugar level varies abruptly and in an exaggerated manner leading to unstable control. This may derive from biochemical responses to emotion (Minuchin et al 1978), poor dietary control by parents (Loughlin & Mosenthal 1944), excessive insulin dosage (Rosen-

bloom & Giardano 1977) or manipulation of diet or insulin by the patient (Rosen & Lidz 1949). Tattersall (1985) offers a concise and lucid review which emphasises the risk of factitious illness in apparent insulin resistance.

It follows from consideration of the above reasons for referral that close parental involvement is inevitable. In many cases this will be in the form of family therapy, considering family functioning as a whole (see Newbrough et al 1985). Empirical justification for this is provided by the studies of Minuchin and his colleagues (1978) who were able to demonstrate improved biochemical stability as well as positive changes in psychological and interpersonal functioning in a group of families containing a young diabetic. It needs emphasising that their therapeutic input was intensive and prolonged.

Epilepsy

A seizure disorder may arise anew during adolescence, though more commonly it will be a continuing problem which developed during childhood and has persisted. Life will be easier for the physician in the latter instance as habits of medication and awareness of the dangers of seizures will already have been established and be that more resistant (though by no means totally so) to denial or maladaptive extremes of parental concern. Life for the parents will, however, be more difficult with the danger that "the interminable nature of the strain" of chronic epilepsy may have exhausted their capacity to cope (Taylor 1985).

Epilepsy which is newly diagnosed in adolescence presents problems for the teenager who must adapt to the idea that he has a condition which is invisible, may not become overt even when medication is overlooked for a few days, and yet arouses fear and antagonism in others. Many teenagers who develop epilepsy seem unable to relinquish a notion of their own invulnerability, listen to medical explanations or advice without seeming to hear, and shrug off any suggestion of future problems with employment, alcohol or relationships.

Specific issues which arise in association with epilepsy and cause psychological difficulty for the adolescent centre upon trust, truthfulness and alarm.

Trust. Seizures do not necessarily occur when medication is missed. The adolescent has to trust the authority of his doctor as to whether it is important to continue anticonvulsant treatment. If the seizures are nocturnal only he must trust his parents' report that he has had one. Should the doctor abide by the rule that anticonvulsants should not be discontinued during puberty, but that this should await physical maturity (Tanner grade 5), then the adolescent must trust medical advice on that topic even though he may have had no seizures for four years. It has to be admitted that the rules for eligibility for a driving licence offer considerable support to physicians urging compliance with medication. He must ask his friends, parents and teachers to trust him to take his tablets and not to put himself at risk. In addition he must trust them to accept him if he tells them of his disorder.

Truthfulness arises within the peer group first of all, as implied above. Most teenagers with epilepsy welcome some guidance sooner or later as to how much to tell their friends, particularly those of the opposite sex. The issue may arise because a thrice daily medication regime means tablets must be taken at school. Alternatively, it may need confronting if alcohol, drugs, pillion rides or midnight swims are on the social agenda. Or it may occur most dramatically following a seizure in public or the discovery by friends of a medical identity bracelet. Whilst it is difficult to establish rules for disclosure, variations on the "need to know" principle on one hand and the foolishness of covering up something that is obvious to all concerned on the other are crude guidelines. It is a little more difficult with employers. A teenager who has been free of seizures for three years, is not exceptionally hot-headed, and is not applying for a job wherein a seizure would be dangerous should not, I suggest, be pressurised into offering disclosure of his controlled condition.

Alarm may apply to the adolescent's own reactions or to those around him. On learning of the diagnosis, many patients fear for their intelligence, sanity and social acceptability. The first two fears can be met with reassurance but anxieties about how others will respond will receive regular reinforcement. Teenagers with epilepsy may be unreasonably prohibited from participating in plays, outings or sport at school, from going out to discotheques by parents (though there is no great risk from stroboscopic lights: Berney et al 1981), from employment or from representing others at formal functions "in case he lets us down". At a finer grain, the squeamish anxiety of friends can quickly turn to rejection or revulsion. Fears of loss of control belong both to the patient and his associates, particularly in sexual matters. An alert teenager can sometimes take advantage of this. "I can't let you do it, you might have a fit in the middle" one adolescent boy was told by his girlfriend. "I only have fits when I'm tense and frustrated" was his answer. She did let him and he didn't have a fit.

In practice there are few restrictions that are necessary and hardly any that can be enforced. Swimming alone, cycling on busy roads and rock climbing are unwise, as is working with machinery such as lathes or balers which would be lethal if a fit resulted in collapsing forward. Most teenagers are going to experiment with alcohol or other intoxicants. I suspect that solvents and marijuana are both comparatively neutral as ictogenic agents though amphetamines and barbiturates are indeed dangerous. It is wise for the physician not to be excessively censorious; usually the adolescent has had a basinful of remonstration from his parents. He may welcome the opportunity to talk things over in a more neutral setting and jointly to reflect on any risks he might take with the support of a knowledgeable adult. Too many restrictions provoke the dangers of helpless invalidity or blustering bravado.

In comparison with diabetes, epilepsy seems more prone to foster dependency (Hoare 1984) and is well known to be associated with a higher rate of formal psychiatric disorder, the reasons for which are various (Shaffer 1985). Care should be taken that there is no iatrogenic contribution: unnecessary restrictions are dealt with above, medication should not be allowed to burgeon, the patient and not the blood anticonvulsant level must be treated, disfiguring agents such as phenytoin are to be avoided if possible and so forth.

One condition to be particularly aware of is non-convulsive status, an uninterrupted sequence of absence or complex partial seizures (Stores 1986). It may present with fright, apparent psychosis or dementia, a vacant expression, near-mute withdrawal; lack of self-care and loss of much spontaneous activity being key signs. An EEG reveals 3 Hz spike and wave activity which can readily be terminated with intravenous diazepam.

Myalgic encephalomyelitis and other post-viral syndromes

Although depression can follow influenza, this is not likely to be a common association (Paykel 1984, Sinahan & Hillary 1981).

Nevertheless, most out-patient psychiatric services will see a number of adolescents and young adults who present with a number of debilitating symptoms, physical and psychological, after an illness of apparent viral origin: most typically, infectious mononucleosis, an upper respiratory tract infection or hepatitis.

The best described complex of complaints is that entitled myalgic encephalomyelitis, Royal Free disease, Iceland disease, Otago mystery disease or epidemic neuromyasthenia; labels which reflect the fact that it is often described as occurring in epidemics within an institution. Although regarded as a manifestation of epidemic hysteria in the earlier psychiatric literature (McEvedy & Beard 1970), this view was criticised as inadequate at the time by some of the physicians involved (Acheson 1970, Compston et al 1970) and is no longer accepted as a complete explanation (British Medical Journal 1978), a number of physical correlates having been described, though the final position is still far from clear (Dawson 1987). Certainly some cases within a closed community affected by myalgic encephalomyelitis may be individuals who are introspective and hypochondriacal or who are hyperventilating with apprehension, but such mechanisms cannot account for most cases which conform to a reasonably consistent clinical picture and can present sporadically.

Following a 'flu-like illness or pharyngitis with lymphadenopathy, the teenager fails to make a satisfactory recovery. Some cases will have shown evidence of abnormal lymphocytes in a blood film or have had a positive monospot test for infectious mononucleosis but most will not. The most obvious feature is persisting subjective weakness and fatiguability, a lowered tolerance for exercise and concentration and a general malaise. This can be utterly at variance with previous personality. In addition to this core feature there may be:

— pain, particularly in the neck or head, which is constant and yet not associated with observable local pathology

— hyperacusis such that loud noise is painful and moderate noise (as in a classroom) distressing

— scalp tenderness which makes combing hair painful

— blurred vision and intermittent diplopia

— irritability and a propensity to tearfulness, with an increase in clinging behaviour directed towards attachment figures.

Less frequent complaints include night sweats, micturition difficulties, paraesthesiae and fainting, possibly secondary to functional hypoglycaemia. Behan & Behan (1980) and Ramsay (1978) provide good descriptive accounts. Routine investigations are normal and the temptation to plump for a psychological aetiology usually proves irresistible to the doctor, much to the irritation of the patient.

Abnormal pathology is not absolutely constant, though various small series have shown abnormally raised IgM immunoglobulins and lactic dehydrogenase levels in many cases. Less frequently, eosinophil counts are raised, electromyograms are abnormal and serological tests (anti-nuclear factor, smooth muscle antibody etc.) are positive (Behan & Behan 1980, Winbow 1986). Viral studies can show recent Coxsackie B virus infection (Calder et al 1987) though this is inconstant (see Dawson 1987).

Early attempts to mobilise the youngster are usually counter-productive, eliciting distress and ultimately a withdrawal to bed, a response which confirms the unwary in their belief that the aetiology is psychological. It seems only sensible to acknowledge openly that the affected individual is ill and that their assumption of the sick role is appropriate. Indeed it has been suggested that the duration of subsequent residual disability is minimised by bed rest in the acute phase (Ramsay 1981) but hard evidence is lacking. Pain may respond to a non-steroidal anti-inflammatory drug in some instances. Antidepressants, although commonly given, are frequently useless. Gradual and sympathetic rehabilitation with support to girl and family is indicated though may be prolonged.

> Jill developed a sore throat, headache and aching limbs shortly before her fourteenth birthday. She was clearly ill with a pyrexia, which cleared up but left her with severe neck pain and an inability to concentrate or undertake more than the briefest physical activity. Her parents found her to be irritable, weepy and clingy. At first she was thought to be depressed although she was still able to enjoy things and preserved an optimistic view of the future. Antidepressants were of no avail. She found attending school a trial but asked for work to be sent home. She did not appear to be a classic case of school refusal since her symptoms continued throughout weekends. Her parents were alarmed when a passing aeroplane caused her to fall to the ground crying and holding her hands over her ears. On review of her history it was thought likely that she had a post-viral syndrome and a referral to an infectious diseases specialist resulted in the demonstration of high IgM and Coxsackie B titres and a high anti-nuclear factor. She was gradually reintroduced into school over a period of

two terms but it was just over a year before her neck pain abated and she began to feel well again.

Infectious mononucleosis is notorious for producing a spectrum of neurological and psychological sequelae. It may also present with perceptual distortions such as depersonalisation, micropsia, hyperacusis and tinnitus. Copperman (1977) described three cases, two teenagers and a child, who saw objects around them increasing and decreasing in size alternately, an "Alice in Wonderland syndrome". There may be a clinical picture resembling that of myalgic encephalomyelitis but sometimes with more depressive colouring and suicidal ideation (Cadie et al 1976, Hendler & Leahy 1978). Although some authorities suggest that monoamine oxidase inhibitors are useful in such circumstances, the more usual finding is that they are not, and continuing support for teenager and family is the best that can be offered, allowing the condition to heal in its own time and minimising any secondary handicap.

An organic basis for such enduring changes in mood and energy is strongly suggested by the findings of abnormal T cell function (Hamblin et al 1983) in patients with anergia and mood lability following infectious mononucleosis, and excessive intracellular acidosis on exercise in a man with excessive fatiguability and asthenia after chickenpox (Arnold et al 1984).

Hysteria

The term "hysteria" is no more satisfactory in adolescent psychiatry than in general adult psychiatry. If the misleading term "hysterical personality" is set aside, the word is usually employed when an incapacity or a disturbance of function of an organ normally under conscious control cannot be shown to have a physical cause. There are well-known traps in such an approach: hysterical alteration of function can co-exist with physical pathology, and an inability to demonstrate a physical cause does not mean the aetiology is psychogenic, nor that a physical process will not reveal itself rather later in the course of the condition.

It is conventional to distinguish between conversion and dissociation in the discussion of psychological mechanisms in hysteria. Both notions presume a concept of mental energy which sits awkwardly with more contemporary ideas of interpersonal processes and, since it has no particular bearing on management, the distinction is not further pursued.

In a series of scholarly articles, Taylor (e.g. 1979, 1986) argues that hysteria is not best construed as a physical or mental illness but as an enactment of sickness, a claim to illness laid by an individual in an intolerable predicament from which other lines of escape are blocked. A notion and model of a particular sickness is required and the experience of the adolescent and his or her allies (which can include the medical profession) will provide this. Varying degrees of conscious awareness and social skill mean that the borders of the condition blur into Munchausen's syndrome, malingering and other forms of factitious illness.

One advantage of such conceptualisation is that it emphasises the extent to which the propagation of the condition is a consensual phenomenon; the support of allies who will pursue an explanation of the symptoms in terms of physical illness: parents, nurses and doctors. "Like magic", writes Taylor (1986), "it has no real properties beyond belief." As such, mass hysteria (see below) as a consensual phenomenon is seen to have links with conversion syndromes, the stuff of which forms the usual grounds for diagnosing hysteria. A further advantage is the fact that having a physical disorder (such as epilepsy) does not debar the adolescent in an impossible predicament from presenting symptoms and signs that conform to his or her idea of sickness and what doctors might expect to find. Indeed, such a personal experience of illness provides a template for a model of sickness which can then be enacted. Marsden (1986) makes the point that patients commonly have a "desire to convince or help the doctor to determine the real cause of their problems. Their anxiety leads to elaboration or exaggeration of their real deficit."

Such an approach rests implicitly on the framework of concepts such as sick role (wherein a person gains exemption from normal social responsibilities by agreeing to co-operate with a physician in a process of getting well) and illness behaviour, which includes all the personal reactions, psychological and social, displayed by someone who experiences the symptoms of illness. Illness behaviour may be abnormal in the sense that it is maladaptive or persists inappropriately after medical advice and information. In the broadest sense of the term, abnormal illness behaviour includes hysteria, hypochondriasis, malingering, denial of disease and so on. A useful discussion of terms in this field is provided by Mayou (1984). Understanding such descriptions of the relationship between an adolescent and his doctor enables hysteria to be seen as a non-verbal communication about help-lessness and plight, sanctuary from which is achieved by becoming ill, usually physically (Chodoff 1974, Hersov 1985).

The clinical presentation of hysteria will vary according to the type of service within which a case presents. Pseudoseizures are familiar to epileptologists, stiff joints to orthopaedic surgeons and so on. The types of problem experienced by a given psychiatric service will depend upon its liaison links, though disturbances of voice, eye, ear and limb functions feature in most psychiatric departments. Amnesic syndromes and fugues are not at all common among adolescents, though trances may be seen, usually as short-lived emergencies in accident and emergency depart-ments. It is commonly said that hysteria is proportionally commoner among recently immigrant families whose teenagers may possess more direct or indirect knowledge of physical illness than established British families with less experience of crippling physical disorder in the young. Assuming that such an increased prevalence can be confirmed by systematic study, it may also arise from a putative increase in the number of adjustment prob-lems to which first- or second-generation immigrant families seem prone, particularly in the different expectations of teenage behav-iour that parents and school peer group may hold.

> Aisha, at 16, was the eldest girl of an Indian family who had moved to Britain eight years previously. Her parents arranged a marriage for her, according to their custom, but she found this impossible to accept, having thrown in her lot with a group of white girls at school and adopted their slang, standards and expectations. Pressure from her parents mounted and she developed a tight spasm of her adductor thigh muscles which prevented her from walking (and, indeed, from future marital sexual intercourse). An elderly relative, living nearby, was wheelchair-bound.
>
> Following a series of family interviews, Aisha's parents dropped their demands that she marry the man of their choice. She accepted rehabilitative physiotherapy and was walking normally after a month. Two years later she showed no evidence of physical disease.

A further anecdotal impression is that Freud was right and that sexual abuse is common in the aetiology of predicaments from which adoption of the sick role is the only perceived escape for the adolescent girl abused within her family.

The principles of management are well established (Bebbington & Hill 1985, Brooksbank 1984, Dubowitz & Hersov 1976):

— early consultation between physical specialist and psychiatrist

— avoid unhelpful polarisation of aetiology into organic and psychological

— ensure an adequate psychiatric assessment is performed

— stop unnecessary physical investigations

— active physical rehabilitation directed at the symptom

— provide the patient (and family) with an honourable exit from the sick role; avoid confrontations which produce loss of face for the patient.

Goodyer (1981) points out that an approach which links individual and family system approaches is logical even though evidence from systematic study is lacking. It would be foolish to disagree with this since both the adolescent's personal view of his symptom and the family's perception of it must be explored. Granting sick role status and privileges hinges upon parental reaction and a model of sickness may exist within the wider family. To take an exclusively family-centred approach would rob the psychiatrist of the opportunity to explore the adolescent's own private perspective as well as the responsibility to undertake a physical examination of his patient. Given that a number of children exist with physical symptoms which are initially regarded as psychogenic but can subsequently be shown to relate to neurological disorder (Caplan 1970, Rivinus et al 1975), it seems at least likely that the same would be true for adolescents, as it is for adults (Slater 1965). The posture to be struck is not a total eschewal of physical involvement but a rejection of the drive for even more physical investigation in an attempt to assuage the family's anxiety. To repeat what has already been said in this chapter: there is no point in psychiatrists bemoaning the lack of a holistic approach to disorder among their physically-orientated medical colleagues if they do not themselves operate across the mind-body divide and display themselves to their patients as doctors of both mind and body. Such a stance conveys by example the futility of a mind-body split in understanding the individual patient's symptom.

Some cases of hysteria with an acute onset will respond readily to an out-patient approach but the chronic case will usually be admitted. A prolonged sojourn on a general medical ward is probably not helpful as the accusation of malingering is often made by nursing staff who have serious physical disorders to cope with. The process of punitive rejection can follow rapidly with the adolescent accentuating his claim to sickness to counteract such dismissal of his plight. For such reasons, a psychiatric ward is preferred, though this may be unacceptable to parents (who fear stigma and the possibility that undetected physical disorder will be overlooked) and unacceptable to the adolescent (who may see it as defeat). A united front needs to be presented by all the adolescent's medical advisors; even in the face of admitted diagnostic uncertainty they must all insist that psychiatric admission is advisable. This is not always easy to achieve.

Mass hysteria

A rapid spread of symptoms such as fainting, overbreathing, tetany, nausea, itching, shaking or complaints of abdominal pain throughout a closed community of adolescents, particularly girls, is a phenomenon well documented historically and in the scientific literature. Those outbreaks which have been investigated medically demonstrate that affected girls usually have no physical basis for their symptoms beyond the contribution of respiratory alkalosis secondary to hyperventilation (Levine et al 1974); the effects of suggestion and a general state of high emotional tension within an "in group" are obvious. The relevance of the symptoms to preoccupations within the group is a further prerequisite (Kerckhoff et al 1965). Typically an episode starts with the development of symptoms in a few individuals with some importance or influence over others and spreads rapidly though unevenly (Benaim et al 1973, Levine 1977). A physical disorder in one or a few girls may trigger an infectious reaction of emotional imitation which girls are likely to say is beyond their control (Benaim et al 1973, Moss & McEvedy 1966). Those who succumb are more likely to have high N scores on the Eysenck Personality Inventory (Moss & McEvedy 1966) and can amount to about one-third of the group. If uncontained, an outbreak can persist for months (Mohr & Bond 1982).

The management of such an outbreak is well established (British Medical Journal 1979, Forrester 1979). The preoccupations or fears affecting the group as a whole (such as anxiety about poisoning, black magic or an outbreak of true infection) should be met by firm reassurance addressed to the group as a whole. Medical management needs to be centred on one clinic or a defined network of doctors who are in close communication with each other. A positive diagnosis of an emotional basis for symptoms in each individual case should be made early and the temptation to investigate all cases physically must be resisted. Affected individuals should be isolated from the rest. Rarely it may be necessary to close a school to limit contagion. Individuals with positions of prestige or influence within the peer group who are seen as lead figures in the outbreak may need individual psychiatric attention in their own right but most affected girls can be managed by simple reassurance.

REFERENCES

Acheson E D 1970 Epidemic malaise (letter). British Medical Journal i: 363

Arnold D L, Bore P J, Radda G K, Styles P, Taylor D J 1984 Excessive intracellular acidosis of skeletal muscle on exercise in a patient with post-viral exhaustion/fatigue syndrome. Lancet i: 1367–1369

Bebbington P, Hill P, 1985 A Manual of Practical Psychiatry. Blackwell, Oxford

Behan P, Behan W 1980 Epidemic myalgic encephalomyelitis. In: Rose F C (ed) Clinical Neuroepidemiology. Pitman, London

Benaim S, Horder J, Anderson J 1973 Hysterical epidemic in a classroom. Psychological Medicine 3: 366–373

Berney T P, Osselton J W, Kolvin I, Day M J 1981 Effect of discotheque environment on epileptic children. British Medical Journal 282: 180–182

British Medical Journal 1978 Leader: Epidemic myalgic encephalomyelitis. British Medical Journal i: 1436

British Medical Journal 1979 Leader: Epidemic hysteria. British Medical Journal ii: 408–409

Brooksbank D 1984 Management of conversion reaction in five adolescent girls. Journal of Adolescence 7: 359–376

Cadie M, Nye F J, Storey P 1976 Anxiety and depression after infectious mononucleosis. British Journal of Psychiatry 128: 559–561

Calder B D, Warnock P J, McCartney R A, Bell E J 1987 Coxsackie B viruses and the post-viral syndrome: a prospective study in general practice. Journal of the Royal College of General Practitioners 37: 11–14

Caplan H L 1970 Hysterical "conversion" symptoms in childhood. Unpublished M.Phil. dissertation, University of London

Chodoff P 1974 The diagnosis of hysteria, an overview. American Journal of Psychiatry 131: 1073–1078

Compston N, Dimsdale H, Ramsay A M, Richardson A T 1970 Epidemic malaise (letter) British Medical Journal i: 362–363

Copperman S M 1977 "Alice in Wonderland" syndrome as a presenting symptom of infectious mononucleosis in children. Clinical Pediatrics 16: 143–146

Dawson J 1987 Royal Free disease: perplexity continues. British Medical Journal 294: 327–328

Dubowitz V, Hersov L 1976 Management of children with non-organic (hysterical) disorders of motor function. Developmental Medicine and Child Neurology 18: 358–368

Forrester R M 1979 Epidemic hysteria — divide and conquer. British Medical Journal ii: 669

Gath A, Smith M A, Baum J D 1980 Emotional, behavioural and educational disorders in diabetic children. Archives of Disease in Childhood 55: 371–375

Goodyer I 1981 Hysterical conversion reactions in childhood. Journal of Child Psychology and Psychiatry 22: 179–188

Hamblin T J, Hussain J, Akbar A N, Tang Y C, Smith J L, Jones D B 1983 Immunological reason for chronic ill health after infectious mononucleosis. British Medical Journal 287: 85–88

Hendler N, Leahy W 1978 Psychiatric and neurologic sequelae of infectious mononucleosis. American Journal of Psychiatry 135: 842–844

Hersov L 1985 Emotional disorders. In: Rutter M, Hersov, L (eds) Child and Adolescent Psychiatry: Modern Approaches. 2nd edn. Blackwell Scientific, Oxford

Hoare P 1984 Does illness foster dependency? Developmental Medicine and Child Neurology 26: 20–24

Kerckhoff A C, Back K W, Miller N 1965 Sociometric patterns in hysterical contagion. Sociometry 28: 2–15

Levine R J 1977 Epidemic faintness and syncope in a school marching band. Journal of the American Medical Association 238: 2373–2376

Levine R J, Sexton D J, Romm F J, Wood B T, Kaiser J 1974 Outbreak of psychosomatic illness at a rural elementary school. Lancet ii: 1500–1503

Loughlin W C, Mosenthal H O (1944) Study of the personalities of children with diabetes. American Journal of Diseases of Children 68: 13–15

McEvedy C P, Beard A W 1970 Royal Free epidemic of 1955: a reconsideration. British Medical Journal i: 7–11

Marsden C D 1986 Hysteria — a neurologist's view. Psychological Medicine 16: 277–288

Mayou R 1984 Sick role, illness behaviour and coping. British Journal of Psychiatry 144: 320–322

Minuchin S, Rosman B L, Baker L 1978 Psychosomatic Families: Anorexia Nervosa and Diabetes in Context. Harvard University Press, Cambridge, Mass

Mohr P D, Bond M J 1982 A chronic epidemic of hysterical blackouts in a comprehensive school. British Medical Journal 284: 961–962

Moss P D, McEvedy C P 1966 An epidemic of overbreathing among schoolgirls. British Medical Journal ii: 1295–1300

Newbrough J R, Simkins C G, Maurer H 1985 A family development approach to studying factors in the management and control of childhood diabetes. Diabetes Care 8: 83–92

Paykel E 1984 How frequent is postinfluenzal depression? British Medical Journal 289: 1061

Prugh D G, Eckhardt L O 1980 Stages and phases in the response of children and adolescents to illness or injury. Advances in Behavioral Pediatrics 1: 181–194

Ramsay A M 1978 Epidemic neuromyasthenia, 1955–1978. Postgraduate Medical Journal 54: 718–721

Ramsay M 1981 Myalgic encephalomyelitis. Stanford le Hope: Myalgic Encephalomyelitis Association

Rivinus T M, Jamison D L, Graham P J 1975 Childhood organic neurological disease presenting as psychiatric disorder. Archives of Disease in Childhood 50: 115–119

Rosen H, Lidz T 1949 Emotional factors in the precipitation of recurrent diabetic acidosis. Psychosomatic Medicine 11: 211–215

Rosenbloom J, Giardano B 1977 Chronic overtreatment with insulin in children and adolescents. American Journal of Diseases in Children 131: 881–885

Rovet J, Ehrlich R, Hoppe M 1987 Behaviour problems in children with diabetes as a function of sex and age of onset of disease. Journal of Child Psychology and Psychiatry 28: 477–491

Shaffer D 1985 Brain Damage. In: Rutter M, Hersov L (eds) Child and Adolescent Psychiatry: Modern Approaches. 2nd Ed. Blackwell Scientific, Oxford

Simonds J F 1977 Psychiatric status of diabetic youth matched with a control group. Diabetes 26: 921–925

Sinahan K, Hillary I 1981 Post-influenzal depression. British Journal of Psychiatry 138: 131–133

Slater E 1965 Diagnosis of hysteria. British Medical Journal i: 1395–1399

Starky G 1963 Family background and state of mental health in a group of diabetic schoolchildren. Acta Paediatrica 52: 377–390

Stores G 1986 Psychological aspects of nonconvulsive status epilepticus in children. Journal of Child Psychology and Psychiatry 27: 575–582

Sullivan B J 1978 Self-esteem and depression in adolescent diabetic girls. Diabetic Care 1: 18–22

Swift C F, Seidman F, Stein H 1967 Adjustment problems in juvenile diabetics. Psychosomatic Medicine 29: 555–571

Tattersall R 1985 Brittle diabetes. British Medical Journal 291: 555–556

Tattersall R, Lowe J 1981 Diabetes and adolescence. Diabetologia 20: 517–523

Taylor D 1979 The components of sickness: diseases, illness and predicaments. Lancet ii: 1008–1010

Taylor D C 1985 Psychological aspects of chronic sickness. In: Rutter M, Hersov L (eds) Child and Adolescent Psychiatry: Modern Approaches, 2nd Ed. Blackwell Scientific, Oxford

Taylor D 1986 Hysteria, play-acting and courage. British Journal of Psychiatry 149: 37–41

Winbow A 1986 Myalgic encephalomyelitis presenting as psychiatric illness. British Journal of Clinical and Social Psychiatry 4: 29–31

18

Developmental disability

Mental handicap

As with individuals of normal intelligence, adolescence for the mentally handicapped represents a developmental phase within which the rate of physical growth accelerates, sexual maturation proceeds apace, social expectations increase and horizons widen beyond the family and school. Such issues complicate the personal and family lives of adolescent mentally-handicapped individuals and can give rise to clinical problems or complicate the provision of education.

Schooling

It is now accepted that a large number of moderately and severely mentally handicapped teenagers will remain in full-time education until the age of 19, nearly always at schools for children with moderate or severe learning difficulties (MLD and SLD schools). Some will progress to tertiary education at a local college of further education at or before that age. Adolescence thus occurs within the years of daily school attendance and teachers share with parents the teaching of skills appropriate for adulthood. The emphasis within the curriculum during the final years of schooling is likely to be on training in life skills such as self-care, use of public transport, handling money and so forth, according to level of ability. Since such achievements are learned and practised at both home and school, the partnership between teachers and parents in assisting the development of such skills needs to be close. It is likely that the school will have a detailed picture of the adolescent in question because of the small size and high staff/pupil ratio of SLD schools. It follows that clinical involvement with any severely mentally-handicapped teenager should lead to liaison with his school provided that his parents agree. Contact with school is desirable in the assessment and treatment of schoolchildren of any level of intellectual ability but there is reason to think that it is of especial value in the instance of mental handicap.

Physical growth

It is a common experience in clinical practice that a mentally-handicapped child who is somewhat disobedient or aggressive can be managed at home or at school until he enters the pubertal growth spurt. The behaviour itself may then not alter, but the increasing size of the youngster makes it more threatening. The parents' complaint that he is now unmanageable needs evaluation. It is likely that what they are saying is realistic; that their old methods of containing unacceptable behaviour are no longer feasible. Alternative approaches will need to be considered such as accelerator operant programmes to build up prosocial behaviours or to reinforce competing, prosocial behaviours or other, less formal, ways of encouraging activities that are incompatible with the unacceptable behaviour. The use of a "time-out" procedure which involves the parent removing their attention rather than the child being removed from the room may be required to extinguish some behaviours. Very occasionally, medication such as haloperidol or propanolol is indicated to curb aggressive outbursts that are not functionally linked to environmental factors which can be changed but, as at all ages, this must not be a way of keeping a handicapped individual in an inappropriate environment.

Although parents are usually right in what they say about their own children, their statement that their pubertal child has become unmanageable may indicate that their adjustment to the fact that he is handicapped is arrested at the bargaining stage (see Bicknell 1983) in the sense that they have implicitly agreed to look after their child whilst he is young, physically appealing and physically manageable. As he loses such characteristics with the onset of adolescence, the parents feel that it is now the turn of the health service or social services to take over his care.

Another variant of the same theme is the use by parents of an indulgent, infantilising stance in their approach to the handicap which can yield a "spoilt brat" in childhood whose increased stature and strength at puberty enables him to tyrannise the household. In such instances a focus on handling skills may miss the point that it is the parents (or grandparents) who need counselling in a more psychotherapeutic mode in order to counteract a chronic issue in family dynamics.

For some families, the handicapped teenager's understandable wish for freedom and independence gives rise to parental fears that he will be exploited and infantilisation appears as a new issue, not having been evident previously. Clashes over the choice of clothes for girls, or the use of public lavatories for boys may have, at root, apprehensions about sexual exploitation by adults.

Sexual maturation

The commonest sexual issue arising in clinical work with male mentally handicapped adolescents is a failure to observe social propriety while masturbating. This may reflect the fact that no privacy is available for the young person. In very general terms it pays to teach where masturbation is acceptable rather than attempting to stop it. Although the practice is obviously innocent, there is a slight risk of it dominating waking life at the expense of other activities which may benefit development. There is also the problem of sanctioning behaviour which would diminish public acceptability in wider society.

Crude sexual overtures to others can be problematic, particularly if these take the form of genital exposure or attempting to fondle someone else. Mere prohibition is insufficient and must be coupled with tuition in what is appropriate in the way of social overtures. It is possible to mistake ordinary physical affection or attachment behaviour for a sexual approach. Given the fact that most severely-handicapped adolescents will be attending school, their supervision is usually adequate to guard against the risk of unwanted pregnancy.

Social expectations

As Russell (1985) points out:

> It is vital for mentally handicapped young people to be helped to enter life as an adult citizen free of those aspects of appearance and behaviour which mark them out as different from other members of the community.

Such a stance follows from the contemporary professional assumption that the mentally handicapped have a right to life in the general social community and merit such assistance as makes this possible. The rejecting attitudes of others are themselves a handicap to such integration, so that promoting social acceptance is pragmatic management. To this end, training in self-grooming, social skills, posture and decorous behaviour have a purpose, namely to lessen the likelihood of social rejection, not merely to manipulate cosmetically the handicapped individual in order to spare the embarrassment of others.

Teaching the right setting for sexual activity has been mentioned. Careless dress or toilet behaviour may provoke similar responses from the public. One problem that arises with remarkable frequency is the difficulty within the family home in persuading a young mentally handicapped teenager to close the lavatory door. Excited shouting, hand-flapping or other forms of boisterous behaviour can offend; the British public like their handicapped (and, indeed their non-handicapped) teenagers to be reserved in public, even though such activity may well have been sanctioned in childhood. Self-injury by biting or hitting is particularly unacceptable and leads to marked social avoidance. The assessment and management of such behaviour is difficult at any age (Corbett 1975, Corbett & Campbell 1980) and if not tackled before adolescence may have become ingrained as a reaction which is by now chronic and doubly difficult to treat.

The issues of civic participation and employment are unresolved. Use of the vote, appropriate independence in financial affairs (own bank account), taking risks in sport and entering into legal contracts will all need positive consideration for the individual in question. Given the current level of unemployment, it seems likely that some moderately handicapped individuals who might previously have been able to seek paid work will be permanently unemployed and never become financially independent. Sheltered workshops and segregated work settings may offer suitable alternative experience of work for such individuals and promote work skills, even though the principle of normalisation might seem thus to be violated.

Wider horizons

With the development of hostels and specially constructed housing, an increasingly large proportion of mentally handicapped teenagers can look forward to the possibility of life outside both hospital and their family of origin. This is reflected in the fact that much of their secondary education is devoted to independence training. They may therefore be expected to participate in a wider social field than would have been the case had they remained at home with their parents. The philosophy of normalisation (Flynn & Nitsch 1980) assumes that it is the right of mentally handicapped people to have access to the same range of services as the non-handicapped population. As a consequence, communication skills are crucial. It is alarming, therefore, to note that two studies of mentally handicapped teenagers record that only one-third or less could make themselves understood to others and only a minority could tell the time, handle money or use a telephone (Mittler & Preddy 1981, Cheseldine & Jeffree 1982). Their plight is accentuated by the dearth of specialist services devoted to the needs of mentally handicapped adults compared with those for children; the contrast is dramatic: health visitors pull out, paediatric follow-up is discontinued, school social workers remain attached to schools. By the late teens, the only services provided in many districts are the general practitioner and the social education centre (previously known as the adult training centre or ATC). The allocation of a social worker is by no means automatic and may well go by default. The police are reluctant to get involved with petty crime, and opportunities for the probation service to become constructively involved are lost.

Left to their own devices mentally handicapped adolescents may flounder socially and react idiosyncratically. Bicknell (1980) points out how behaviour disorders such as withdrawal, negativism or aggressive outbursts can be understood as communications of distress, particularly when a mentally handicapped person finds himself in an inappropriate, unsympathetic or uncomprehending environment. The risk is that inadequate formulation of the problem can lead to superficial attempts to control such behaviour by medication (Taylor & Bicknell 1986).

Even when formal social education can no longer be provided by the school, good social education centres can provide social skills training or promote experiences and arrangements which allow a chance to achieve or excel, such as the Duke of Edinburgh's award sheme.

The family

Mentally handicapped teenagers quite often have adolescent siblings who may react variously as they themselves achieve sufficient maturity to be able to make choices about their own lives. Whilst there are no grounds for thinking that they will automatically react adversely (see Mittler & Mittler 1983) there is some evidence from studies of the siblings of younger handicapped children to suggest that older sisters may be disproportionately at risk (Gath 1978) so that the picture is by no means clear. At the risk of creating superficial generalisations it may be ventured that a few siblings will throw themselves into activities concerned with handicap generally or the welfare of their mentally handicapped sibling in particular. On occasion this may reflect their guilt at being unscathed themselves, a phenomenon parallel to the "survivor guilt" noted in some of those who lost relatives in the holocaust in Nazi Germany. This is not always a satisfactory explanation and the possibility of ordinary and appropriate altruism should be allowed for. Others find that it is embarrassing to bring their friends home and deal with this either by removing themselves from family life or, conversely, by cutting themselves off from ordinary social friendships and staying in. Both extremes raise the question as to whether such siblings need counselling themselves in order to preserve their own psychosocial development.

For the parents the major issue is likely to be "letting go" of their handicapped teenager. In order for him to achieve a measure of independence it will be necessary for them to allow others to participate in his social education and care. Respite care may be refused because of a fear that no-one else will be sensitive to his needs, and a few parents find themselves in an impossible position, having exhausted themselves by continuous caretaking yet refusing to trust any other person to look after their youngster. Haunted by fears of what should happen when they die, they may talk of suicide and "taking him with me", a signal of personal distress which should be taken very seriously.

> Richard had always been severely mentally handicapped and was difficult to look after because of his boisterous behaviour, particularly at night. His mother was a small lady who had experienced an unsatisfactory childhood herself and was prone to bouts of anxious helplessness during which she would shoplift with increasing abandon until caught. Now he was 16, Richard was too big for his mother to handle and she had agreed to respite care. Whilst away on a group holiday with other handicapped teenagers he had a fit which, although harmless, confirmed to his mother that only she could look after him properly. As a single parent, she found this exhausting. In despair she tried to sedate her son with a motley collection of tablets and then attempted to suffocate him with a cushion. He fought her off, breaking her fingers in the process, so that she called an ambulance and was taken to a hospital casualty department where the full story emerged.

The whole matter may give rise to marital dispute if one parent has adjusted to the fact of handicap at a different pace to the other. One may be prepared to "let go" while the other persists in ministering to every need. This discrepancy tends to polarise as an issue about caring with one partner becoming "overinvolved" as they see the other "pulling out". Actual divorce is not obviously commoner in families containing a young mentally handicapped child (see e.g. Davis & Mackay 1973) but clinical experience suggests that it is sometimes postponed until the youngster has completed schooling, at which point one partner may abruptly leave or have an extra-marital affair. The understandable bitterness that follows can prejudice the development and independence of the handicapped teenager who may find himself at the centre of custody and access disputes which are bewildering and frightening for him.

Families shrink with time. Other children leave home and grandparents die. For the parents, such changes may result in an increasing burden of care with fewer pairs of hands available. Conversely, there may be less criticism or carping; not all leavings are a loss. The older teenager who is mentally handicapped may settle into a cosier style of life with ageing parents. There are attendant risks: infantilisation, incest, and non-accidental injury can all occur in response to changes in the parents and their relationship. The social world of the teenager after school is likely to be that of their middle-aged or elderly parents rather than that of teenagers generally. Loneliness becomes a serious problem. As other siblings marry and have babies, the social isolation of the handicapped teenager can breed jealousy. Such feelings may not be expressed in the absence of a confidante outside the family and be overlooked. Rather similarly, grief following a bereavement can easily go unobserved.

Autism

The diagnostic term "infantile autism" is somewhat unfortunate since autism is a lifelong condition, best regarded as a selective handicap affecting language development, the ability to extract patterns of meaning from experience so as to predict the future, the capacity to generalise learning from one situation to another, and the ability to engage in ordinary reciprocal social interactions and form deep personal relationships.

Textbooks describe a clinical picture as presented in middle childhood, usually in a child of near-normal intelligence. The presentation of autism in the child with substantial intellectual retardation is less well described and recognised. Nor is how the autistic child presents in adolescence and in adult life usually considered, though there are important changes in the clinical picture (Hill 1986).

For most clinicians, the central feature of autism is the indifference to other people. Autistic children are classically remote and impersonal in their social behaviour; they do not afford people the normal, central position in their personal universe, make no eye contact with them, cannot play reciprocally, form no friendships and do not display selective attachments to their parents. The autistic adolescent may have acquired some skills and some understanding of other people so that such a description no longer obtains in detail.

For instance, a number will now use eye contact, albeit rather clumsily: standing too close for comfort with a fish-like stare. Similarly, the withdrawal from people which can be seen in some younger autistic children may be replaced by approaches to others and attempts to initiate social encounters (Mesibov 1983).

Paradoxically, this may cause new problems since the capacity of autistic adolescents to understand facial expressions and non-verbal social cues is likely to remain very poor (Hobson 1986) and the person with whom they are talking may overestimate their communicative capacity. Since autistic people characteristically lack metacommunicative skills it is unlikely that they will interrupt to say that they do not understand. Instead they may impulsively break off a conversation in which they find themselves out of their depth, or persist with ritualistic, sterile questioning on a favoured topic. The consequence is that non-autistic people misinterpret their motives in doing so and regard them as rude and tiresome.

Their lack of empathic judgement and their difficulty with the pragmatic aspects of language (the ability to use and comprehend language by reference to its social context) means that autistic adolescents appear brusque and insensitive, embarrassing their caretakers in shops and restaurants. The end result may be that other people come to avoid them or that their parents are less inclined to take them out: their social isolation persists for rather different reasons.

Although full affectional bonds do not develop, clinging behaviour and homesickness can be seen in some autistic adolescents. This may be misunderstood because of the way in which it has been delayed and displaced from early childhood. The characteristic difficulty in anticipating the future and tolerating imposed change leads to repetitive questioning about, for instance, weekend visits for those in boarding schools.

Tantrums precipitated by uncertainty and change in routines become less easy to handle because the erstwhile small child is now a large teenager. Some impulsive, aggressive outbursts are learned devices for manipulating the situation and require appropriate firmness and consistency on the part of parents and teachers. Rarer and more difficult to control are the attacks on others which are apparently intended to produce observable distress in the victim which a few autistic teenagers find fascinating. Once again, such attacks represent a social overture rather than a withdrawal from people.

The ritualistic aspect of autism often reaches a peak in late childhood and may wane a little during adolescence (Rutter 1970). A very few teenagers will develop a true obsessional disorder with an obvious compulsive quality, subtly different from the resistance to imposed change and ritualism of the classical autistic picture.

It is well recognised that autistic children may develop seizures for the first time in adolescence (Deykin & MacMahon 1979). For the most part, these are infrequent, occurring every six months or so, and can be managed by simple precautionary measures rather than anticonvulsants.

Some individuals with autism show a deterioration in behaviour and academic skills, even intellectual capacity, in adolescence. The behavioural changes include the development of self-injurious behaviour, unpredictable tantrums, the appearance of new mannerisms, and an increase in uncooperative behaviour. In a report of five such cases, Gillberg & Schaumann (1981) estimated that about one-third of autistic children would show such deterioration. However they did not distinguish clearly between behavioural and cognitive deterioration and only one of their cases showed definite intellectual decline. Whilst a worsening of aggressive and self-injurious behaviour in early adolescence is not very unusual and may be associated with a temporary fall in academic achievement, loss of intellectual capacity is rare. In the author's experience of over 100 autistic teenagers under continuous review for several years, far fewer than one-third have shown a dramatic worsening at puberty and only one girl has displayed a definite and permanent loss of language and performance skills on formal testing, possibly due to a lack of motivation, previously not a problem. She simultaneously developed other curious behaviour including giggling, appearing suddenly distracted, and exceptional hesitancy at walking through doorways, signs suggestive of schizophrenia, a condition which can supervene in autistic as well as non-autistic individuals.

Depression is a more common phenomenon in the autistic teenager, particularly the brighter or more socially active individual who becomes aware of his or her handicap (Wing 1983). The less intelligent or communicative may develop mood swings with accompanying behavioural changes. Paradoxical though it may seem, some autistic teenagers can experience loneliness and pine for friendship. On occasion, it appears that their first attachment forms towards an age peer.

Philip, a boy of 16 with classical autism diagnosed in childhood by an international authority and educated at a boarding school for autistic children, began to follow a male classmate around the school. When away from him, he would become upset and ask the staff repeatedly what his friend, Alan, was doing. In the playground he followed Alan closely and would sometimes hold on to his coat from behind. Alan was remarkably uninterested in all this though he would sometimes try to shake Philip off, with the result that Philip would hover even closer. Neither spoke to each other or shared any activity. There was

275

absolutely no evidence of sexual arousal on Philip's part. When Philip fell ill with chicken-pox and was isolated in the boarding department, he cried and moaned for Alan, wanting to see him and asking about him. He would accept little reassurance and became withdrawn, mute, refused food, curled up in a ball and looked the picture of misery until he was allowed a visit from Alan.

Awareness of their limitations in making friends seems to be at the core of some depressive states in autistic adolescents who are verbal enough to state their preoccupations. In Rutter's (1970) words, their lack of friends is "the result of a lack of social skill, not of social interest". How to deal with such depressive reactions is more difficult. Simple counselling seems the best approach but it is outstandingly difficult and many psychiatrists have early recourse to antidepressants though there is very little, if any, evidence that they are effective. Prophylactically, there seem to be advantages in intensive social skills training but the gains in skills are small using existing techniques.

Hyperactivity, a common problem in childhood, tends to calm down in adolescence (Ando & Yoshimura 1979) and is sometimes replaced by a dramatic and pervasive underactivity resulting in an inert individual, reluctant to stir from a preferred position and angry when required to do so. Such immobility can superficially mimic depression, particularly when there is an associated reluctance to perform classwork or move to a lavatory to urinate. There is no specific treatment and the resulting management problem can be serious if the family or the class all have to march at the pace of the slowest or else leave him behind.

The development of sexual interest can present management problems, particularly with boys. They usually discover masturbation for themselves though their technique is commonly less than deft. Having no social inhibitions, they will indulge anywhere and can easily spend most of the day masturbating, at the expense of their education and wider life experience. It is highly unlikely that their sexual behaviour will develop into overtures to others, though if they continue to masturbate in public, this may be mistaken for exhibitionism. The most straightforward tactic is to insist that they only masturbate in their bedroom and can only have a limited amount of time there. Whilst most autistic adolescents are "comfortably celibate" (Dewey & Everard 1974), the occasional adventurous and capable autistic adolescent boy discovers that sweets or other treats can be obtained by prostituting himself, but this is rare.

The risk to attractive autistic girls from unscrupulous men is rather greater.

For those autistic teenagers who show a partial abatement of the more severe social withdrawal and disinterest in people, who have good language ability and have become less ritual-bound, the clinical picture can develop into that of a rather solitary individual with grammatically stilted but adequate speech and a preoccupation with a narrow range of rather sterile topics of interest such as bus routes, within which there is a curious emphasis on trivial detail and little interest in sharing the interest with others. Often rather scruffy in appearance, insensitive to the feelings of other people and betraying a one-sidedness in conversation, such an individual may easily be described as an instance of Asperger's syndrome (Asperger 1944, Wing 1981, and see Ch. 7). Whether there is value in distinguishing between Asperger's syndrome with and without normal early speech milestones is currently debated without clear advantages for either stance emerging. Although Asperger originally stressed the significance of normal early speech, the term is in wide use as a synonym for "mild" autism in adolescent and adult life and as such includes individuals with aberrant and delayed early speech. At present it is therefore rather a rag-bag term, a behavioural syndrome with no consistent developmental course and no specific aetiology.

Irrespective of labels, social adaptation can improve very substantially indeed with time and effort as illustrated by the case of Jessy Park (Park 1967, 1983). The way in which this is promoted is arduous and does not hinge upon any particular treatment approach in isolation. Behavioural programmes based in the home or school are useful, as is structured education with an emphasis upon language development and communication (including sign language). Psychoanalytic psychotherapy can waste time better spent at school and is of no direct benefit. Medication can alleviate some secondary behavioural and emotional problems but there is no good evidence that it affects the core disorder (Rutter 1985). Given sensible management and education, the rate and probably the final level of development depend upon the level of intelligence. Since most autistic adolescents are of limited intellect, their prognosis is poor and many of the issues raised in the section on mental handicap (q.v.) will apply to them and their families too.

Physical disability

As with children, rates of psychiatric disorder among physically handicapped adolescents are elevated. Most epidemiological studies in this area have grouped children and adolescents together, mentioning no differences in point prevalence of psychiatric disorder between the two developmental stages (see e.g. Breslau 1985, Seidel et al 1975). There are only a few studies specifically of adolescents with conditions such as cerebral palsy or spina bifida.

Dorner (1975, 1976) studied a group of 63 adolescents with spina bifida, finding a high rate of depressive feelings (two-thirds had definite and recurring misery) and an absence of conduct problems. Broad confirmation of this pattern is provided by McAndrew's (1978) study of Australian adolescents with spina bifida; depression and low self-esteem being very common. In a detailed and controlled study of adolescents with spina bifida and cerebral palsy, Anderson & Clarke (1982) found about half (52%) of their sample to have psychological problems compared with 15% of controls. Nearly three-quarters of the psychological problems were neurotic with a marked lack of self-confidence, extreme self-consciousness, social anxieties, excessive worrying and frequent feelings of misery. Irritability, tantrums and aggressive behaviour were found in most of the remaining quarter but in half of these, such symptoms were thought to arise from anxious insecurity and poor self-esteem.

It is important to note that cerebral palsy always associates with brain dysfunction and spina bifida often does so. Rates for psychiatric disorder as high as these would not be expected in conditions which are not associated with brain dysfunction (Seidel et al 1975). Indeed, a number of recent studies of young cystic fibrosis sufferers (see Breslau 1985) have not shown marked differences from controls in this respect.

In the studies by Minde (1978) and Anderson & Clarke (1982), many of the features repeatedly shown to be associated with psychiatric disorder in the non-handicapped were confirmed as relevant to the severely physically handicapped: maternal mental ill-health, poor family relationships, low intelligence in the individual adolescent and so on. Factors specific to the disability, or nearly so, also emerged. Social isolation, extreme parental attitudes of denial of disability or gross pessimism and despair, the presence of a urinary appliance and the presence of epilepsy were all important whereas the presence of a speech problem curiously was not. A simplified conclusion from the results of these studies would be that encouragement of the teenager's independence and the provision of a full social life are protective factors.

Indeed, Minde's (1978) study indicated that a friendship with a non-handicapped individual was negatively associated with psychological deviance. This is not a matter for the simple prescription of environmental manipulation since moving a teenager to normal, mainstream schooling was not associated with improvement in psychiatric adjustment. Almost certainly, detailed consideration of the teenager's social activities needs to be undertaken, particularly as it is in the early teens that a physically handicapped adolescent is likely to experience his siblings' rejection, perhaps because they may have themselves experienced some relative privation of parental attention during childhood because of the burden of care presented by the handicapped child.

To this might be added, as a preventive measure as well as a humane courtesy, the provision for the adolescent of information about his disability. Many of the young adults with a variety of handicaps in the survey by Brimblecombe et al (1986), said they had not enough information about their disability and did not know to whom to turn for medical advice: in the previous year less than half had seen a specialist and only a quarter had seen their general practitioner. Sexual counselling and advice about basic health problems were identified as unmet needs by about one-quarter of the sample in each instance. This parallels the observation by some of Minde's (1978) parents: doctors lose interest as the child becomes an adolescent and the pace of improvement slackens.

REFERENCES

Anderson E M, Clarke L 1982 Disability in Adolescence. Methuen, London
Ando H, Yoshimura I 1979 Effects of age on communication skill levels and prevalence of maladaptive behaviours in autistic and mentally retarded children. Journal of Autism and Developmental Disorders 9: 83–93
Asperger H 1944. Die "autistischen Psychopathen". Archiv für Psychiatrie und Nervenkrankheiten 117: 76–136
Bicknell D J 1980 Treatment and Management of Behaviour Disturbance in the Mentally Handicapped Person. Sandoz Products Ltd, Feltham, Middx
Bicknell D J 1983 The psychopathology of handicap. British Journal of Medical Psychology 56: 167–178

Breslau N 1985 Psychiatric disorder in children with physical disabilities. Journal of the American Academy of Child Psychiatry 24: 87–94

Brimblecombe F, Kuh D, Lawrence C, Smith R 1986 Role of general practitioners in the care of disabled young adults. British Medical Journal 293: 859–860

Cheseldine S E, Jeffree D M 1982 Mentally handicapped adolescents: a survey of abilities. Special Education, Forward Trends 9: 19–22

Corbett J A 1975 Aversion for the treatment of self-injurious behaviour. Journal of Mental Deficiency Research 19: 79–95

Corbett J A, Campbell H J 1980 Causes of severe self-injurious behaviour. In: Mittler P, de Jong J M (eds) New Frontiers in Mental Retardation, Vol. 2. University Park Press, Baltimore

Davis M, Mackay D 1973 Mentally subnormal children and their families. Lancet ii: 974–975

Dewey M A, Everard M P 1974 The near normal autistic adolescent. Journal of Autism and Childhood Schizophrenia 4: 348–356

Deykin E, MacMahon B 1979 The incidence of seizures among children with autistic symptoms. American Journal of Psychiatry 136: 1310–1312

Dorner E 1975 The relationship of physical handicap to stress in families with an adolescent with spina bifida. Developmental Medicine and Child Neurology 17: 765–776

Dorner S 1976 Adolescents with spina bifida — how they see their situation. Archives of Disease in Childhood 51: 439–444

Flynn R, Nitsch K 1980 Normalisation, Social Integration and Community Services. University Park Press, Baltimore

Gath A 1978 Down's Syndrome and the Family: The Early Years. Academic Press, London

Gillberg C, Schaumann H 1981 Infantile autism and puberty. Journal of Autism and Developmental Disorders 11: 365–372

Hill P 1986 Identifying the autistic child. Maternal and Child Health 11: 386–389

Hobson R P 1986 The autistic child's appraisal of expressions of emotion: a further study. Journal of Child Psychology and Psychiatry 27: 671–680

McAndrew I 1978 Adolescents and young people with spina bifida. Ability Press, Melbourne

Mesibov G 1983 Current issues in autism and adolescence. In: Schopler E, Mesibov G (eds) Autism in Adolescents and Adults. Plenum Press, New York

Minde K K 1978 Coping style of 34 adolescents with cerebral palsy. American Journal of Psychiatry 135: 1344–1349

Mittler P, Mittler H (eds) 1983 Parents, Professionals and Mentally Handicapped People — Approaches to Partnership. Croom Helm, London

Mittler P, Preddy D 1981 Mentally handicapped pupils and school leavers: a survey in North West England. In Cooper B (ed) Assessing the Handicaps and Needs of Mentally Handicapped Children. Academic Press, London

Park C C 1967 The Siege. Harcourt, Brace and World, New York

Park C C 1983 Growing out of autism. In: Schopler E, Mesibov G (eds) Autism in Adolescents and Adults. Plenum Press, New York

Russell O 1985 Mental Handicap. Churchill Livingstone, Edinburgh

Rutter M 1970 Autistic children: infancy to adulthood. Seminars in Psychiatry 2: 435–450

Rutter M 1985 The treatment of autistic children. Journal of Child Psychology and Psychiatry 26: 193–214

Seidel U P, Chadwick O F D, Rutter M 1975 Psychological disorders in crippled children. Developmental Medicine and Child Neurology 17: 563–573

Taylor E, Bicknell J 1986 The psychiatry of mental handicap. In: Hill P, Murray R, Thorley A (eds) Essentials of Postgraduate Psychiatry, 2nd Edn. Grune and Stratton, London

Wing L 1981 Asperger's syndrome: a clinical account. Psychological Medicine 11: 115–130

Wing L 1983 Social and interpersonal needs. In: Schopler E, Mesibov G (eds) Autism in Adolescents and Adults. Plenum Press, New York

19

School-related problems

Schools

The British education system comprises two main types of school: state, which are free and provided by the local education authority, and independent or private which require fees. Independent schools include "public" schools for 13–18-year-olds, and a small number of special schools for children and adolescents with learning difficulties. Most adolescents attend state secondary schools, usually comprehensive schools which serve a locality and do not select children on the grounds of ability (though they may not take those who have special educational needs because of, for example, seriously limited intellect). In a few areas, children are directed at the age of 11 or 13 either into grammar or high schools, or into secondary modern schools, the former two taking the brightest children and offering a more academic curriculum.

At about the age of 16, most children take the General Certificate of Secondary Education (GCSE) in various subjects and a minority will take "A level" examinations in a few subjects at about age 18. In some areas, A level courses are taught at sixth-form colleges which allow teaching resources to be rationalised. Good grades at A level make it possible to apply for a place at university.

Other forms of higher education (after the age of 16) include colleges of further education and polytechnics which offer a number of courses, academic and vocational.

Schoolchildren thought to require special education are assessed and a statement of their special educational needs is drawn up according to the procedures specified in the Education

Act (1981). A psychiatric contribution to this statement may be requested, though confidentiality concerns mean that parental permission must be obtained by the psychiatrist before it goes to the education authority. According to the educational needs specified in the statement, special educational provision may be provided in the child's present school or at a special school. Among the latter are schools for children with severe and moderate learning difficulties (the old ESN(S) and ESN(M) schools), schools for emotionally and behaviourally disordered (maladjusted) children and schools for autistic children. Any of these may be boarding schools.

At the end of compulsory schooling, a teenager has a number of options such as further education, youth training programmes (under various names), employment, or indeed unemployment. The amount of consideration given to planning for this varies enormously; for some teenagers and their parents it forms a substantial preoccupation. Schools offer careers guidance to their pupils but this is sometimes perfunctory and requires supplementation by sources outside the educational system.

Educational underachievement

Academic achievement at school depends upon an interplay between the adolescent's cognitive capacities (intelligence, ability to concentrate, memory etc.), the amount and quality of the teaching he receives, the opportunities for learning within and outside school, and his motivation. Clearly it can be undermined by a number of factors. The concept of underachievement suggests that a standard has been set for an individual's work which is not being met. In the clinical assessment of educational underachievement, the first task is to determine how expectations of performance have arisen. The usual sources are the standard of past work and measured intelligence (IQ for the purposes of this discussion).

The issue of IQ is important. A number of intelligence tests are validated against academic performance so it is not surprising that IQ and academic achievement correlate well. Nevertheless, such correlation is not perfect and because of this it is incorrect to pro-rate an expected standard of classwork by straightforward extrapolation from known IQ. For instance, an IQ of 120 does not mean that a pupil should achieve 20% above average.

Because of the less-than-perfect correlation between IQ and academic achievement, the expectation will be that he should achieve a level of work somewhere between average and 20% above; the exact level depending upon the skill in question. A discussion of how this sort of thinking can be applied to reading by the use of a regression equation is provided by Yule et al (1974).

The assessment of academic achievement is best carried out by a psychologist, most commonly an educational psychologist. It is obvious that the expectations of teachers and parents will need to be ascertained. The adolescent's actual level of achievement in all class subjects requires inspection. Further evaluation nearly always involves standardised tests of achievement and intelligence.

Assuming that such procedures do demonstrate reasonable expectations on the part of teachers and parents and that a discrepancy is apparent between ability as reflected by intelligence testing and performance on standardised tests of academic achievement, then a series of possibilities arise. These may be grouped into those that are long-standing and have endured throughout the pupil's educational career, and those that have an onset.

The first group includes problems that should have been identified during primary school:

— unsuspected low intelligence, perhaps masked by nice manners and a sociable demeanour.

— deafness or poor visual acuity

— unsupportive or anti-educational family

— unrecognised, chronically poor attendance at school

— specific learning difficulties such as those affecting reading ("dyslexia"), arithmetic or spelling

— hyperactivity associated with attentional difficulties

However, some individuals who find their lack of achievement an embarrassment will have learned to avoid public failure by resorting to diversionary tactics whenever they are asked to do something in class which is beyond them. Their misbehaviour becomes the focus of concern and their academic shortcomings are overlooked in the excitement. This can continue until (or beyond) transfer to secondary school at the age of 11. Remediation at this stage is difficult, because their self-esteem is now compromised so that they are unwilling to risk failure, their preferred stance being non-co-operation and a stubborn refusal to attempt the classroom tasks set. They can be wary of praise since it sets standards they fear cannot be maintained. Tragically, such individuals will find secondary schooling even more demanding yet the remedial resources are scarcer than at a primary school level.

When the onset of underachievement (relative to ability), resulting in a drop in the standard of work, is clear, causes may include:

— a bad relationship with a particular teacher

— boredom (but beware the use of the self-description of "bored" in depression)

— preoccupation secondary to e.g. parental divorce, bullying etc.

— depression

— tiredness (too little sleep, sedative medication for e.g. hay fever)

— unsuspected truancy

— drug abuse

— epilepsy with subclinical seizures

— rebellion against parental ambition or a "swot" label

— sexual abuse

— dementia (rare but important)

— schizophrenia.

It is wise to interview the adolescent individually since a number of the above causes are not easily admitted in an interview which includes parents. Some of these conditions can be treated directly, though in others the psychiatric contribution may be formulation followed by advice or consultation to parents or, with their permission, the school.

Mobbing

The distinction between bullying by one or a few individuals and mobbing wherein a victim is taunted, laughed at derisively, or frozen out of social activities by a large group of his peers is an old one but the term "mobbing" for the latter (by analogy with the behaviour of birds) has come into use comparatively recently (Orton 1975, Pikas 1975).

The victim of such group persecution usually has some oddity of speech, stature or origin that marks him out as different. He is often accused of betraying accepted standards in some way by being bad at games, a member of an ethnic or religious minority, or atypically sensitive and artistic. Alternatively he has a florid yet ineffectual temper or a propensity to dissolve into tears. It is usually easy to see how a quality of vulnerability which other boys (and it seems more prevalent among boys) feel uneasy about in themselves is projected upon a convenient scapegoat for attack. Any attempt by the victim to defend himself is highly likely to intensify the attacks. Some victims accept the situation in despair and may try to play up to their assigned role by inviting derision. This is done with little subtlety and it is at this point that the problem may first come to the attention of staff who will conclude, not unsurprisingly, that "he asks for it". In my experience, many victims are friendless and lack the social skills necessary to forge friendships. Not uncommonly they are obese or have a history of developmental clumsiness with consequent poor self-esteem.

A group of mobbing boys appear to exult in a shared sense of identity and sadistic purpose. If taxed individually, they tend to confess some remorse or sympathy for the victim yet this does not appear to deter them from future group offensives. Ordinarily, the school is unaware of the practice and mobbing is denied by both perpetrators and victim; the latter only too aware that complaints to staff will result in fiercer persecution.

Such behaviour is not confined to the human race, nor to adolescents. Lynching, for instance, is carried out by adults whereas the evocative episode in William Golding's *Lord of the Flies* in which Piggy is chased nearly to his death involved younger children. The persecution of ineffectual teachers by their pupils in class is a similar phenomenon involving different generations. There remains an abiding impression, though, that mobbing is most typically a feature of hierarchically-organised boys' secondary schools, particularly boarding schools.

Although it is easy to say that prevention is better than cure, the problem is hard for a school to detect and harder still to anticipate. From a psychiatric viewpoint, the problem is most likely to come to light when a victim takes an overdose or loses control in school as a result of mobbing.

> Stuart was referred as an emergency after he had threatened to throw a petrol bomb at a group of 14-year-olds in his class who were teasing and provoking him daily, snatching his books and hiding his games kit. A small boy with an explosive temper but no good as a fighter, he had a stammer and a past history of developmental dyspraxia. He had no friends and was an only child, used to adult company.

Pikas (1975) has suggested some guidelines for schools based on Swedish experience. In essence these boil down to being non-punitive to mobbers and tackling them individually about the mobbing. The victim will need considerable support and advice as to how to reduce any provocation he offers. Psychiatric management should extend this by providing supportive counselling and social skills training for the victim. Anger management techniques and video feedback probably add a little to this as a second line of treatment but many cases will be helped sufficiently by more routine measures. It is obvious that the school authorities should be kept well aware of the extent of the problem (which they often deny is real) but should be dissuaded from stern lectures in assembly which can exacerbate the problem alarmingly.

School refusal

School attendance is obligatory until the age of sixteen. Technically, a 16-year-old will not be entitled to leave school until the end of the Easter or Summer term, depending upon when his birthday is. In practice, a blind eye is often turned and it is unlikely that an education authority would take action against a teenager who did not attend after his sixteenth birthday.

The reasons for failure to attend school

Non-attendance at school during term-time may occur for various reasons. Physical illness is the commonest of these but truancy

287

becomes increasingly prevalent during the years of secondary schooling so that about 25% of London fifth-year pupils (15- and 16-year-olds) truant intermittently (Gray et al 1980). A small number of teenagers are withheld from school by their parents and a few (perhaps 1% of all young teenagers: Berg 1980) will find attendance at school impossible on account of emotional upset, especially anxiety or fear. Such anxiety or fear is associated with attending school but is not necessarily of school itself so that the term "school phobia" is not strictly correct. Because of this the term "school refusal" is preferred even though the word "refusal" carries unintended connotations of truancy.

"Truancy" is absence from school which is pursued covertly by a child who is aware that his non-attendance is illegal. The parents do not know where their child is when not at school. There is commonly an association with other antisocial behaviour and low academic attainment. The usual view of truancy as a form of delinquency can underestimate the extent to which school is seen as unwelcoming or irrelevant by the older school-age child.

It is important to recognise that these reasons for non-attendance may co-exist in any one individual. Anxiety related to school attendance can present as somatic symptoms such as tension headache, palpitations, diarrhoea or nausea secondary to hyperventilation. The absence of such symptoms at week-ends and during school holidays is an important clue since anxiety as such may be denied by an adolescent who feels demeaned if he admits to it. A few truants may become apprehensive about returning to school, fearing punishment, academic failure or the loss of a position in the peer group. Such apprehension can escalate to handicapping proportions in an unassertive escapist whose truanting is based more on a wish to evade the social and academic challenges of school than on the positive pursuit of pleasurable activities.

Truancy which results in solitary wandering or a return home after both parents have left for work seems often to be associated with emotional symptomatology and may require management along similar lines to school refusal. It may also arise out of adverse factors in the school such as bullying or perceived harshness on the part of staff members:

> Dawn began to absent herself from school without her parents' knowledge and would wander alone around the local cemetery. She was in her third year at secondary school and diabetic. Lately her diabetes

had been poorly controlled and she had polyuria secondary to an osmotic diuresis. Her teachers were curiously unaware that her frequent requests to go to the lavatory during lessons were connected with her diabetes and had assumed that she was seeking attention. In consequence she had not been allowed to excuse herself from a lesson on several occasions and had wet herself twice in the classroom. This was seen as further evidence of attention-seeking behaviour and she was told off. Her solution to the dilemma was to avoid the risk of further humiliation by solitary truancy.

Whereas some teenagers will be withheld from school by their parents for uncomplicated reasons such as a wish for help with a new baby or to give father a hand with a heavy job, in some instances staying at home is sanctioned because a parent is agoraphobic, alcoholic or depressed. The youngster perceives their parent's need for help or company and stays at home out of loyalty. The parent may, indeed, protest feebly that their child should be at school but give way too early for any insistence on school attendance to be effective. The situation is essentially that of withholding, yet psychiatric involvement will be indicated with the parent as identified patient in order to relieve the parentified child.

The clinical picture of school refusal

School refusal in adolescence may be part of a chronic pattern of uneven attendance with protracted convalescences, and numerous days off sick with little definite to show in the way of identifiable physical pathology. This may have gone unremarked, especially if there is a chronic condition requiring frequent hospitalisation or otherwise leading to absences from school which are medically justified but which mask intermittent neurotic refusal. On investigation, abnormalities or deficiencies of personality are evident, commonly overlapping with a common core of high dependency (Berg 1980). Clinical experience suggests the following:

— chronic timidity in the face of novelty with a well-established tendency to withdraw from challenge

— an inability to face challenges without precise, detailed knowledge of their nature

— a persisting emotional immaturity resulting from the fact

289

that the normal separation anxiety of toddlerhood has never been resolved by the development of adequately secure affectional bonds with attachment figures. This may present as a neurotic fear that a parent will not survive without the adolescent's presence but the end result is the same: he does not feel secure unless close to his parent, a situation precluded by school attendance.

— a lack of confidence in peer relationships and a difficulty in forging durable friendships

— a precarious self-esteem coupled with a tendency to panic when this is threatened by academic or social failure, which breed panic rather than disillusionment

— demanding, manipulative, yet dependent; characteristic of the "spoilt brat".

For such a personality, a minor setback at school or difficulty at home can trigger a spell of non-attendance.

However, the onset of school refusal in an adolescent previously able to cope with the demand of school attendance suggests a different underlying psychopathology:

— depression. This should always be considered as a likely cause of school refusal arising anew in adolescence (Kolvin et al 1984). It may have separation anxiety with clinging or a morbid concern for a parent's safety as a symptom. This is to be distinguished from a long-standing emotional insecurity (as mentioned above) by the fact that it has an onset and is at variance with previous personality.

— realistic fear of some aspect of school such as bullying

— social anxieties arising out of the adolescent developmental process, such as embarrassment at delayed puberty revealed in showers after games. Some social fears may be morbid and akin to social phobia (fear of being seen eating or of eye contact with others) or may have a dysmorphophobic nature.

— fears of travelling, crowding in assembly, or queueing for lunch which are homologous with adult agoraphobia

— rarely, the development of conditions such as schizophrenia or obsessive-compulsive disorder.

The typical presentation is well described in textbooks of child psychiatry since school refusal is most likely to present in late childhood. At the time of having to leave for school, affected teenagers become tearful, protesting unconvincingly that they feel unwell, or alternatively becoming withdrawn, even mute. As parental pressure mounts they may react irritably or appeasingly with promises to go to school the next day. They may dash for their bedroom or the lavatory in order to hide. The sheer size of teenagers usually makes it impossible to drag them forcefully to school so the running home from school which may be seen in the younger child who has been firmly taken to school is less frequent. Although they may declare a wish to return to school there is usually a reason why tomorrow is better than today. In a number of households they sullenly refuse to get out of bed on schoolday mornings and their truculent manner leads the behaviour to be seen merely as defiant rather than as a crude cover for feelings of vulnerability.

Assessment

Contact with the school and with the education welfare service is essential in order to obtain details of past attendance, current academic and social functioning, and the attitude of school staff to the child.

Most school refusers are of normal intelligence but if there has been a long history of patchy attendance, achievement may also be uneven. A very few school refusers have specific learning disabilities such as the spelling difficulties which represent the later stage of specific reading retardation. Such errors are often inconsistent and may be falsely attributed to laziness, thus eliciting harsh criticism from secondary school teachers unaware of the previous history of reading difficulty. Contact with the educational psychologist is thus important if there is any suspicion of a learning disability, though this is rarely the case.

It is always wise to conduct separate interviews with parents and their teenager in addition to seeing them together. Often it is only when seen alone that a school refuser will reveal details of depressive symptoms or specific fears about school or home. There may be value in quantifying self-esteem or depressive mood by the use of self-administered questionnaires in order to assess progress and time re-entry to school.

Management

The treatment of school refusal involves two components: a return to school, and the treatment of the underlying psychiatric condition. In most instances the two will interweave and it is wise to plan this in any case. Otherwise the risk is that a successful return to school is seen by the family as an indication to discontinue treatment and the underlying problem is not adequately dealt with. Contemporary opinion is that the return to school should be as soon as possible; postponing this to allow for treatment of an underlying condition first is likely to provide time for anticipatory fears of school to incubate and intensify the avoidance. Depression is a partial exception to this general rule and in such circumstances it is humane to treat the affective disorder first, though a return to school need not await complete restitution of mood, concentration and self-confidence.

A prompt return to full-time school on an agreed date with parents, teachers and teenager all well prepared to provide firm support is occasionally successful with a young teenager whose attendance has only recently collapsed and who has a good previous personality and record of attendance. It is most likely to succeed in cases where events at school have triggered non-attendance and these have subsequently been seen to be dealt with so that they will not recur.

The more usual story is that the adolescent in question has a long history of marginal adjustment and patchy attendance with particular difficulties after holidays and illnesses. In such circumstances a graded return is indicated; the re-entry is taken at a pace which the adolescent and his family can manage. Initially some form of contact with the school is established: a visit from a favoured teacher for instance. Arrangements are made for some schoolwork to be done at home and preliminary trips to the vicinity of the school are planned. These are graded according to difficulty and accomplished whilst accompanied by a supportive adult. Often it is appropriate for this to be the adolescent's father or failing this, an education welfare officer (education social worker). A first visit to the school might well be undertaken whilst other children are safely in class, and consist of a visit to the head-teacher or the staff room to return some completed work. A longer visit can include working alone in the library or a single period with a sympathetic teacher. The duration of time spent in school can be extended gradually over a period of weeks with an ultimate goal of full-time attendance.

Whilst this is being carried out the parents are provided with support and are encouraged to take over the responsibility for maintaining attendance. A graded approach enables them to regain control of the situation at a pace that they can tolerate. The overall principle is for them to manage matters on a step-by-step basis, neither jumping in too rashly with extreme demands which will fail, nor allowing progress to stagnate. The pace is set by negotiation between the adolescent and his parents and the therapist. One of the principal tasks of the latter is to ensure adequate liaison with the school, particularly as the teachers involved will not often have had any experience of children with school refusal. It is usually necessary for the adolescent to rehearse the reason he will give enquiring schoolmates for his absence and similar thought should be given as to how he will respond to other eventualities like class detentions. A full account of this approach is given by Yule et al (1980).

Some adolescents will benefit from simultaneous training in social skills or relaxation techniques in order to enhance their ability to cope with re-entry. Most clinicians find medication to be of very little value with adolescents except where depression is evident, a view confirmed by Berney et al (1981), in spite of claims that imipramine is an effective addition to ordinary attempts to return a group of somewhat younger children to school (Gittelman-Klein & Klein 1971), presumably because it can block separation panic.

The question of whether a change of school would solve the problem is often raised. Unless there are grounds for thinking that the present school is unsuitable, a change is nearly always unwise. An unfamiliar curriculum, new rules, and a strange peer group present a confusing situation which is more destructive than the apparent advantage of a "clean start" can offset. Serious bullying by staff or other pupils is a possible exception to this general rule though it is remarkable how many individuals elicit bullying in virtually any school they may attend.

A similar issue is the advisability of home tuition, a facility provided on a part-time basis by the local education authority. A useful rule of thumb is to avoid this if it is to be delivered in the adolescent's home since this can lull everyone into a sense of something being done whereas the fact of the matter is that he remains isolated from his peers and his academic education is minimal. Attendance at a home tuition centre away from home itself has no such disadvantages and can be a useful stage in a graded return programme.

Failure of a graded return is an indication for admission to an adolescent unit. This allows education to continue whilst therapeutic attention is given to underlying problems, particularly personality deficits. The subject is well discussed by Berg & Fielding (1978) and Hersov (1985).

The other component of treatment is directed towards the underlying psychological problem and this is probably the most significant psychiatric contribution (Baker & Wills, 1979). By and large this is self-explanatory. When agoraphobic or social fears are evident, for example, these can be treated on their own merits. Obviously the business of returning to school involves a partial exposure to the feared stimuli in such instances and this needs to be managed within an overall programme. The treatment of personality immaturity or deviance will need protracted therapy on group, family or individual lines according to individual formulation. Cognitive methods can help the individuals with poor self-esteem improve their concept of themselves. Whatever the underlying psychiatric pathology (whether framed in individual or family terms) it is crucial to press for its treatment since this seems to be the most important element in long-term outcome (Valles & Oddy 1984). Unfortunately many cases drop out of treatment once a return to school has been achieved. It follows that it is sensible to agree with the family at the outset that both the inability to attend school and the reasons for this need treating.

Prognosis

Most school refusers can be managed on an out-patient basis and, within that setting, most will achieve a return to school. Not infrequently they drop out of treatment at that point. Only a small proportion will require admission to hospital and they will be the more severe cases. Most follow-up studies of adolescent school refusers have been carried out on those who have been in-patients and would ordinarily be expected to convey a gloomier view of adult outcome than would apply to school refusers in general. It seems as though those who have required hospital admission will continue to be handicapped by persisting emotional symptoms in adulthood, one-third will experience minor symptoms and a final third will be asymptomatic (see e.g. Berg et al 1976, Berg & Jackson 1985, Warren 1965). Only a minority of those with persisting symptomatology will be found to have agoraphobia on follow-up.

REFERENCES

Baker H, Wills U 1979 School phobic children at work. British Journal of Psychiatry 135: 561–564

Berg I 1980 School refusal in early adolescence. In: Hersov L, Berg I (eds) Out of School. Wiley, Chichester

Berg I, Fielding D 1978 An evaluation of hospital inpatient treatment in adolescent school phobia. British Journal of Psychiatry 131: 500–505

Berg I, Jackson A 1985 Teenage school refusers grow up. British Journal of Psychiatry 147: 366–370

Berg I, Butler A, Hall G 1976 The outcome of adolescent school phobia. British Journal of Psychiatry 128: 80–85

Berney T, Kolvin I, Bhate S R et al 1981 School phobia: a therapeutic trial with clomipramine and short-term outcome. British Journal of Psychiatry 138: 110–118

Gittelman-Klein R, Klein D F 1971 Controlled imipramine treatment of schoolphobia. Archives of General Psychiatry 25: 204–207

Gray G, Smith A, Rutter M 1980 School attendance and the first year of employment. In: Hersov L, Berg I (eds) Out of School. Wiley, Chichester

Hersov L 1985 School refusal. In: Rutter M, Hersov L (eds) Child and Adolescent Psychiatry: Modern Approaches. 2nd edn. Blackwell Scientific, Oxford

Kolvin I, Berney T P, Bhate S R 1984 Classification and diagnosis of depression in school phobia. British Journal of Psychiatry 145: 347–357

Orton W T 1975 Mobbing. Health and Social Services Journal, p. 2027

Pikas A 1975 The treatment of mobbing in schools — principles for and the results of an anti-mobbing group. Scandinavian Journal of Educational Research 19: 1

Valles E, Oddy M 1984 The influence of a return to school on the long-term adjustment of school refusers. Journal of Adolescence 7: 35–44

Warren W 1965 A study of adolescent psychiatric in-patients and the outcome six or more years later. 2. The follow-up study. Journal of Child and Adolescent Psychiatry 6: 141–160

Yule W, Hersov L, Treseder J 1980 Behavioural treatments of school refusal. In: Hersov L, Berg I (eds) Out of School. Wiley, Chichester

Yule W, Rutter M, Berger M, Thompson J 1974 Over- and underachievement in reading: distribution in the general population. British Journal of Educational Psychology 44: 1–12

20

Substance abuse

The abuse of substances for the purpose of altering one's state of mind or in order to conform socially is widespread amongst human societies. Although tobacco abuse is not uncommon amongst young adolescents, with an overall prevalence rate of about 10–15% among teenage schoolchildren and a peak prevalence of about 25% among 16-year-old boys (Bewley et al 1980, Rawbone & Guz 1982) and has obvious health risks, it is almost never perceived as a symptom which merits medical referral. The same might be said about moderate use of alcohol by teenagers under 18. The usual substances which excite psychiatric referral are drugs, solvents, and alcohol in large quantities. Solvent (or volatile substance) abuse and heavy drinking are treated in separate sections of this chapter.

Young people who abuse drugs are not especially likely to be teenagers. More usually they are young adults, but the age spectrum for certain types of drug abuse extends downward into the teens. For most teenagers, their contact with drugs is likely to be exploratory; they will take them out of curiosity. The opportunity to do so is nearly always provided by the generosity of an acquaintance, not the incitement of a "pusher". Indeed, the latter character is largely fictional as far as the adolescent drug scene is concerned. In the UK, the illicit drug most often used by adolescents is cannabis, followed in order of prevalence by stimulants and heroin. Although a few older teenagers will abuse substances such as LSD, barbiturates and cocaine, their clinical management is much more the province of the adult psychiatrist with specialist interests in dependency and addiction and the reader is referred elsewhere, particularly to the companion volume in this series (Raistrick & Davidson 1985), for information on these drugs and their abuse.

Cannabis

The grey-green leaves (marijuana, grass) or the brown, solid resin (hashish) obtained from the flowering heads of the plant *Cannabis sativa* can be smoked when mixed with tobacco in a roll-your-own cigarette (joint). A dozy euphoria results with heightened perception of music, humour and (for some) sex. A number of rituals surround the preparation and smoking of joints, which is essentially a social activity among a few friends. In common with most illicit drugs, various slang terms are used to describe the substance and its use: these change quite rapidly and it is unwise for the naive professional to try and emulate street terminology; the risk of being out of date and thus betraying one's social distance is large. At the time of writing, the generic term "dope" has been widely used for some years in South London to refer to all types of cannabis.

Cannabis is easily available and not very expensive though the risk of buying poor-quality samples is high. It can be grown with a little effort in Southern England but the potency of such a crop is low. Most teenagers who wish to use cannabis regularly will know a friend of a friend who can obtain a small quantity; the supply lines are typically long and erratic. The risk of dependency is low and physical addiction not a problem. Occasional social use is not uncommon among older teenagers and although there are no very reliable prevalence figures, an estimate that about 10% of British school-age adolescents have tried it seems plausible (Kosviner 1976), though rates of about 20–30% for the same age group would apply in the USA (Fishburne et al 1980, Johnston 1985). The rates will be highest in inner urban areas, among those with Caribbean roots, and among students (Wiener 1970, Plant 1975a).

The clinical relevance of cannabis is minimal. In a few susceptible individuals it can precipitate a psychotic episode, the form of which varies with schizophreniform, delusional, manic and confusional states all recorded (see e.g. Carney et al 1984), though the likelihood of this happening to an adolescent is very small. A few first-time users will panic and may present in casualty as an emergency. Some individuals can take too much too quickly on top of too much alcohol with the result that they appear confused and barely able to move. They, too, may be brought to casualty but the intoxication soon passes and they fall asleep with no subsequent ill-effects.

Stimulants and other pills

A number of stimulants such as dexamphetamine sulphate, methylphenidate, and appetite suppressants such as diethylpropion may be taken recreationally by older adolescents, sometimes in large quantities together with alcohol and quite often with other drugs such as benzhexol. Sedatives such as barbiturates and benzodiazepines may be used to "come down" after a week-end spent taking stimulants. The term "speed" which used to refer strictly to intravenous methylamphetamine is now often used to cover all stimulants taken by whatever route.

Among teenagers in a particular locality, the use of stimulants comes and goes according to availability and fashion. There is a trend towards their use mainly by the rowdy element as a component of the "hard stuff" expressed by football hooligans; they are not generally popular within the black community. A group may take them to enhance a party or a rock concert. Indiscriminate and excessive use is a commoner issue than dependence though a mild depressive downswing after a bout is not uncommon. Occasionally this is intense and carries a suicidal risk (Connell 1968) though this is rare among adolescents. Likewise the paranoid state well described by Connell (1958) is rare in florid form in this age group.

Although the signs of amphetamine abuse are easy to recognise (dilated pupils, tachycardia, restlessness and tremor), they may well not be present and urine examination is indicated when suspicion is aroused. A positive result indicates use but not necessarily dependence (Strang & Connell 1985).

Heroin

In the last few years, the abuse of heroin by inhaling the smoke of heroin heated on silver foil (chasing the dragon) has become widespread in certain areas. Some users will try other routes of administration, particularly sniffing (snorting), but injection is less common among adolescent, as opposed to adult, users. Recently, street heroin has become cheaper so that young abusers will be less likely to abuse codeine or dipipanone though these are popular alternative opioids with adult abusers.

Heroin itself (scag, smack, and numerous other terms) is a white or brown powder, extremely bitter to the taste and often

Table 20.1 Physical signs of opiate intoxication

Small pupils
Drowsiness (nodding), leading to unconsciousness
Slowing of mental processes
Slowing of pulse and respiration
Generalised pruritus
Delayed urination and ejaculation
Constipation

wrapped in paper torn from glossy magazines. Unlike cocaine it does not numb the tongue on tasting.

The signs of intoxication and withdrawal are well described elsewhere (e.g. Raistrick & Davidson 1985) and are only tabulated here (see Tables 20.1 and 20.2). Strong evidence that a teenager is abusing heroin may be gathered from these clinical pictures, or from the discovery of equipment such as tinfoil (kitchen foil or chewing gum wrapper) with dark tracks on one side and blackening on the other, straws or tubes of tinfoil, a dessert spoon blackened underneath, pledgets of cotton wool (for filtering dissolved heroin as it is drawn up into the syringe) and, rarely, needles and syringes. Unexplained blood stains on clothing or on an item such as a tie which can be used as a tourniquet are suspicious.

There may be behavioural changes. Associating with known heroin users is a powerful indicator. Telephone calls late at night from people who leave no message, long absences from home

Table 20.2 Signs of opiate withdrawal

Apprehension leading to panic
Racing thoughts
Yawning
Lacrimation
Runny nose
Sweating
Shivering
Dilated pupils
Gooseflesh
Anorexia
Aching back and legs, stabbing stomach pains
Restlessness coupled with subjective exhaustion
Sudden clonic jerks
Increase in pulse and respiratory rate
Vomiting
Diarrhoea
Frequency of micturition
Easily triggered orgasm or spontaneous ejaculation

with excuses that cannot be verified, going out at odd hours, excessive sleepiness, and an irritable, self-centred manner may all have an innocent explanation when taken individually but as a cluster are suspect.

In order to sustain a habit of half a gram a day, money to the extent of well over £200 a week will be required. This in turn leads to selling possessions, theft from home (possibly made to look like a burglary), dealing in heroin, or street crime.

Heroin users tend to see themselves as somewhat different to those who abuse cannabis or pills such as stimulants. The urgency of heroin withdrawal is of a totally different order to any other withdrawal syndrome, alcohol included. It does not follow that in the first place, all heroin users are more inadequate or disturbed than other drug abusers. Indeed, various statements by ex-addicts make the point that it is fairly easy to drift into heroin abuse by way of social introductions which lead to frequent use, rapidly followed by physical dependence (see, e.g. Field 1985). Abuse can arise out of chance, boredom and carelessness. Although heroin abuse is, at first sight, more serious a phenomenon than other forms of drug abuse and quite often associated with individual vulnerabilities, it is not helpful to postulate a primary psychiatric disorder (as opposed to psychological vulnerability) as causal in all cases of heroin abuse: "the concept that every addict is by definition a person of flawed character is not only mistaken but a potential hindrance to recovery" (Edwards 1986). It may be true that given the opportunity to try heroin, only those with substantial inhibitions will refuse a first offer: robust psychological health or strong moral principles may be protective but their absence does not ordinarily indicate psychiatric disorder. Many drift into heroin abuse and addiction for lack of any substantial alternative motivation and because for many, taking heroin is pleasurable. The idea that dependence may eventually supervene is met by omnipotent denial until it is too late.

Concepts of drug abuse

The distinction between psychoactive drug use and abuse hinges upon social convention and will thus vary between cultures and from one time in history to another. Some drugs are sanctioned in Western society, either for recreational use (alcohol) or for medical purposes, others proscribed. Those that are allowed are usually controlled in some way, particularly by age limits or licence to dispense. Alcohol is legally used as a social drug by adults and many young teenagers will ape this usage. They may also extend the repertoire of drugs used sociably and a large number of teenagers will come into contact with illicit drugs through groups of acquaintances and at parties. In such settings, group pressure to conform or share an exploratory experience is likely to be strengthened by the disinhibiting effect of alcohol use. The first contact with a drug is usually experimental, may not progress further, and reflects the combination of individual curiosity and the interests of the peer group (Glynn 1981). To this may be added the difficulty adolescents have with learning to moderate their own risk-taking behaviour. Alcohol and tobacco are usually the first drugs taken, with volatile substances and/or cannabis following in some instances. Which drug is used seems to depend upon peer group familiarity and subculture: cannabis among black teenagers; alcohol, stimulants and solvents among whites. There is a well-recognised tendency for those teenagers who are active delinquents also to use drugs such as tobacco and alcohol; most regular illicit drug abusers are similarly likely to be delinquent, both features often reflecting a common causal field involving personality and social background (Johnston et al 1978).

If exposure to drugs is a phenomenon largely dictated by the peer group, what elements indicate repetition of the experience? Availability and advertising seem the simplest answers for alcohol and tobacco. Widespread use among like-minded friends seems to be the case with cannabis. Although virtually all heroin users have used cannabis, few cannabis users go on to heroin (Kandel & Yamaguchi 1985). Progression to other drugs from cannabis is poorly understood. Introduction by an acquaintance certainly applies to many, though why they should persist thereafter and become regular users is not always clear. Sometimes it is simply because the experience was enjoyable or alleviated some distress. It does not appear that progression beyond cannabis to the regular use of "harder" drugs depends upon peer pressure alone, but factors such as depressive feelings, lack of closeness between parents and their children and parental drug use come into play (Kandel & Yamaguchi 1985). This suggests that various factors predispose to repetition and that no single model will explain why certain teenagers will go on to use a drug regularly and become

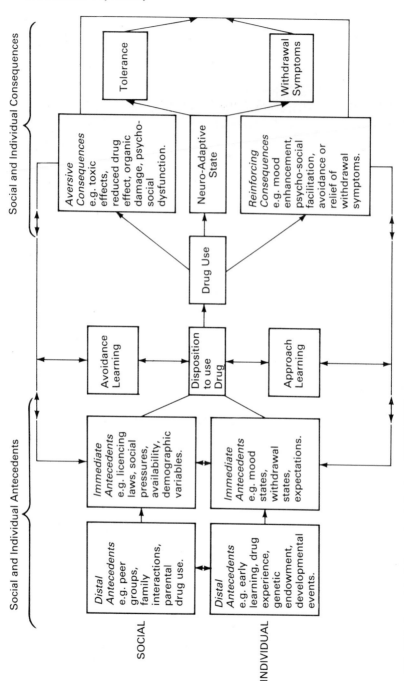

Fig. 20.1 A model of drug-using behaviour (WHO 1981)

physically dependent where this is a possible consequence. Whilst it seems at first sight likely that there is, for many, "a require-ment of adverse personal characteristics in addition to cannabis use for the move to heroin" (Raistrick & Davidson 1985), the importance of context may be overlooked in favour of such individual personality factors. There is evidence that coarse social variables such as unemployment (Peck & Plant 1986) and war service (as in Vietnam) increase general drug misuse among those involved. Ultimately, a multifactorial model such as that proposed by the World Health Organisation (WHO 1981) and illustrated in Figure 20.1 inevitably becomes adopted in order to accommodate the various elements implicated in aetiology.

Such models are necessarily depicted in broad brush-strokes. One idea that can thus be overlooked but which is of particular relevance to adolescence is the concept of deviancy amplification. Plant (1981) suggests that the attempts by society to control illicit use of drugs promote a reactive counterculture among drug misusers. On the basis of his study in Cheltenham (Plant 1975a) he proposed that use of particular drugs provides a ticket of entry to various cliques; conversely that abuse of a drug became a condition of acceptance to such groups. The way in which this mechanism interacts with common adolescent concerns about personal identity is clear. As a drug taker and a member of a drug-taking circle with its own argot, counter-authoritarian atti-tudes, shared thrills and secrecy, an adolescent can adopt and enjoy an image liable to be glamourised as wickedly exciting and tragic by the mass media; a young person who lacks solid identi-fication with any other group may superficially resolve uncer-tainties about what sort of person he is.

Clinical management

The psychiatrist faced with a teenager who is regularly abusing drugs to an appreciable degree will probably refer him to a specialist in drug dependency. Certainly the treatment of opioid dependence should always be implemented by a clinic with substantial experience in the clinical management of individuals whose life has become dominated by the issue of procurement.

At the other end of a spectrum of severity, the adolescent of reasonably sound personality who is using cannabis or pills socially with a group of friends will neither welcome nor benefit from any psychiatric intervention.

The general adolescent psychiatrist will probably want to manage those cases of soft drug abuse wherein it appears that drugs are being abused to alleviate dysphoria, personality difficulties and family relationship problems, since these, if primary, may prove amenable to standard psychiatric interventions. Most adolescent units will be wary of admitting drug abusers for fear of contagion spreading the practice to other patients; admission to a drug dependence unit is preferable for those cases which require detoxification. The concern shared by most parents is that such an admission will result in their child learning more about drugs and identifying with a drug culture. Whereas these are reasonable concerns, by the time detoxification is required identification has nearly always occurred. Out-patient management on eclectic lines (see Raistrick & Davidson 1985) employing family interviews, supportive individual counselling and an encouragement of close parental supervision, with attempts to structure free time and the choice of companions, is thus the mainstay of most attempts at treatment. If the primary issue is control and supervision, younger adolescents (16 and under) may be received into local authority care but the risk of contagion still applies and the local social services department may be unwilling to risk drug-taking spreading through one of their residential children's homes.

The importance of voluntary agencies and projects cannot be underestimated and no account of management principles can afford to neglect them. The Standing Conference on Drug Abuse (1–4 Hatton Place, London EC1N 8ND, tel 01-430 2341) provides a comprehensive information service on such services.

Alcohol

It is generally assumed that heavy drinking among adolescents is increasing. Certainly there has been a remarkable increase in the number of British teenagers convicted for offences directly related to drunkenness (Royal College of Psychiatrists 1979). Similarly, various American surveys demonstrate a steady increase in the proportion of teenagers who drink regularly (Fishburne et al 1980). In Kandel & Yamaguchi's (1985) study, 20% of American children had used alcohol by the age of 10 and after the age of 15 a steep rise in the initiation rate ensured that virtually all (95%) had tried it by the age of 18. The peak use of alcohol in the same study cohort was between the ages of 18 and 20, at which time half of the (representative) sample were drinking at least four days a week and a quarter were drinking daily. Half of the drinkers were drinking an average of five drinks on a drinking day. These rates of drinking fell quite rapidly thereafter for the cohort as a whole. For the population as a whole, heavy drinking is a common phenomenon of late adolescence.

Physical dependence upon alcohol is rare in adolescence (Vingelis & Smart 1981). Problems associated with teenage drinking are those associated with intoxication or its sequelae. Academic achievement at school can obviously be impaired by drinking strong lager in the lunch break or by a hangover. Social rejection by exasperated peers can follow repeated drunkenness which results in passing out or vomiting. Disinhibited behaviour may lead to brushes with authority or the law. Drunken driving causes accidents in which people are killed.

The emotional consequences of such mishaps can themselves lead to increasing drinking (sometimes secretly) in order to manage painful emotions arising from failure, rejection and culpability. The psychiatrist is most likely to be involved at this stage, may fall into the trap of offering treatment without enquiring closely about alcohol use, and find himself counselling a mildly intoxicated individual; a less than profitable activity.

Some adolescents will turn to alcohol in order to anaesthetise dysphoria arising from events or moods originally unconnected with alcohol, but the same caveat applies: asking about alcohol intake is a necessary activity in assessment. It is important to bear in mind that many heavy drinkers in this age group will also abuse other drugs (Wechsler 1976) and these should be specifically enquired about.

In line with this observation that teenagers will drink to obliterate psychic pain, the term "affect tolerance" has been coined by Krystal & Raskin (1970). The assertion is that a number of teenage heavy drinkers lack the capacity to bear unpleasant feelings and accordingly use alcohol. As a corollary, it is suggested that helping such adolescents to acknowledge and express their feelings is appropriate therapy. Whereas this is common sense, the question arises as to how much heavy drinking can be thus explained. In one study, only 5% of teenage abusers of alcohol were thought to suffer an affective disturbance (Smart 1976).

Many teenage heavy drinkers are delinquent (Blacker et al 1965) or express antisocial attitudes: alcohol use for them is often the reverse, the creation of excitement as a relief from boredom. Certainly some will use group drinking as a forum to exhibit drinking prowess in order to compensate for doubts about their own competence and to drown fears of dependency (MacKay 1963) but to assume that individual or group counselling on a voluntary basis will engage them is optimistic; they do not see their drinking as a problem and certainly not as a psychiatric one. This is frequently reinforced by the fact that substantial numbers of teenage heavy drinkers have a parent who is also abusing alcohol (MacKay 1963). For those teenagers who consider that they have a drinking problem, there are grounds for thinking that their response to treatment along the lines advocated for adults is about as good as for adults (Unger 1978).

The long-term outlook for teenage heavy drinkers is not necessarily poor. In line with the generally decreasing alcohol intake by age in the general population after the early twenties, the absolute numbers of heavy drinkers also falls. Fillmore (1974) in a follow-up of American college students aged 16–25 found that only half the problem drinkers identified whilst at college had a drink problem twenty years later.

Volatile substance abuse

The practice of inhaling volatile substances for fun is virtually confined to teenagers as far as the United Kingdom is concerned. Using inhalants to produce intoxication is centuries old but sniffing hydrocarbons is a recent phenomenon, presumably related to their ready availability in contemporary society. Although the first reports of glue sniffing by adolescents in the United States stem from the early 1960s (e.g. Glaser & Massengale 1962) it was not until about 1970 that the first British cases were recognised (Watson 1982).

The prevalence of the problem is hard to define precisely since its extent appears to fluctuate with fashion. Clinicians recognise that in one year a given housing estate may contain a number of individuals who are abusing solvents, yet the following year the practice has all but died out. Most cases have been reported from urban areas, and have been reported to be particularly associated with social deprivation and a family history of alcohol abuse (Oliver & Watson 1977). In a Glasgow study, Ramsey (1982) found a point prevalence of 9.8% for 13–15-year-old boys. Nevertheless, more privileged areas also experience the problem. An unpublished study of the same age group in three Surrey schools (Morgan 1984, personal communication) found a rate for present and past use of 7.9% for boys and 4.2% for girls. The general consensus is that most abusers are aged between 13 and 15, and that boys outnumber girls. Only a minority will be referred to treatment agencies; the majority of these will only abuse volatile substances and not involve themselves with other drugs (see Gay et al 1982).

Materials and methods

The wide range of substances used (see Table 20.3) indicates the inadequacy of the common terms "glue sniffing" and "solvent abuse", even though adhesives and solvents are still the most commonly abused substances. Glue is smeared around the inside of a polythene bag or crisp packet which is then held to the nose and mouth whilst being squeezed with the other hand, a practice known as "bagging". Fluid solvents or petrol are sniffed from the can or poured onto a rag which may also be placed inside a bag. A disposable cigarette lighter with its flint removed provides an easily concealed source of intoxication for use during lessons or at concerts. Aerosols are squirted straight into the mouth during inhalation.

Table 20.3 Volatile substances commonly abused

Glues, adhesives, plastic cement
Rubber solution
Typing eraser (Tipp-Ex etc.)
Lighter fuel
Paint thinner
Acrylic paint
Nail polish and remover
Dry-cleaning fluid
Petrol
Amyl nitrite
Aerosols: hair lacquer, oven cleaner, Damp Start, de-icer, cellulose paint, fire
         extinguisher, stain remover, lighter refill

Effects

All such methods allow a concentrated dose of volatile substance to be presented to the vast surface area of the lungs from which absorption is rapid. Given the high lipid solubility of solvents, intoxication is rapid. The initial response is that of mild central nervous system excitation, followed by a depressive effect, in other words a pattern corresponding to alcohol intoxication. Subjective symptoms include euphoria, disinhibition, dizziness and blurred vision. With higher doses, a few youngsters will experience visual or auditory hallucinations in the context of a delirious state. Dysarthria, ataxia, irritability, and impaired judgement are obvious in the early stages and will progress to drowsiness or coma with higher doses. Pain in the chest or abdomen, bronchospasm or vomiting may occur (Sourindrhin 1985) and convulsions, even status epilepticus, have been reported (Alister et al 1981).

The picture of acute intoxication may be complicated by the concurrent use of alcohol or illicit drugs which may potentiate the above effects (Skuse & Burrell 1982).

An erythematous rash around the mouth may be seen in heavy users of bags. Apparently reversible impairment of renal function, with diminished creatinine clearance, haematuria and proteinuria, is seen in some abusers and this can be combined with hepatic damage (O'Brien et al 1971). Eosinophilia or even aplastic anaemia can occur (Powars 1965). A wide range of neurological damage has been reported but Ron (1986), in a scholarly review, considered that faulty methodology reduces the confidence that can be placed in most studies. A subacute cerebellar syndrome persisting for weeks or months and associated with structural cerebellar changes in a minority of heavy abusers of toluene is accepted, as is the likelihood of a very few toluene abusers developing optic atrophy or sensorineural deafness. The difficulty of differentiating functional effects due to the persistence for days of volatile substances in the brain from true long-term effects makes further conclusions hazardous as far as teenagers are concerned, though there is some suspicion that older users of toluene may be at risk for cerebral atrophy, intellectual and memory deficits. Older reports of peripheral neuropathy in solvent abusers probably reflect poisoning by *n*-hexane (no longer widely used) rather than toluene.

There is evidence to suggest that volatile hydrocarbons can

cause cardiac arrhythmias as an acute complication, and a strong suspicion that chronic abuse can produce a dilated cardiomyopathy in the longer term (Boon 1987).

Mortality

Between 1971 and 1983, there were 282 deaths from volatile substance abuse in the United Kingdom. During this period a rising rate resulted in 80 deaths in 1983, virtually all male and mostly under the age of 20 (Anderson et al 1985). There was a proportional increase in Social Class V and in the armed forces, though all social classes were affected and the overall association with social class was not strong. For those under 18, the rate among those in local authority care was increased tenfold over expectation. Such deaths accounted for 2% of all male deaths in the 10–19 age group. In most cases the victim had been sniffing alone and in 8% of cases for which inquest data were available, there was evidence of accompanying auto-erotic behaviour: bondage or self-strangulation. The actual causes of death included asphyxiation (plastic bag over the head, hanging), inhalation of vomit, drowning, head injuries or, most commonly, direct toxic effect. Only a few cases were due to poisoning by halogenated halocarbons; most followed toluene intoxication (data from Anderson et al 1985). It seems likely that some deaths resulted from ventricular fibrillation or myocardial infarction secondary to coronary artery spasm (Boon 1987).

Most abusers will escape serious morbidity or death. Sourindhrin (1985), referring to his own work, commented that "the lack of morbidity and mortality in a group of 300 glue sniffers seen at a Glasgow clinic is reassuring".

Course

Most sniffers have their first experience when introduced to the practice as a member of a group of youngsters. They may well be bored and thus curious. The vast majority will only indulge on a very few occasions, nearly always in company. Davies et al (1985) estimate that about 10% will go on to become chronic abusers. The remainder abandon the practice.

A clinical impression is that local fashion dictates the extent and duration of the practice. A given school, children's home or housing estate may house one or more groups of adolescents who share recreational activities. Such groups may go through a phase of sniffing moderately regularly for a few weeks and then progress to another activity.

Whether there is causal continuity between obtaining intoxication by inhaling volatile substances and developing a habit of harder drug use is unclear. Davies et al (1985) describe four individuals who progressed to abuse opiates. All had been chronic abusers of solvents for between 3 and 6 years and had pre-existing personal psychopathology. Interestingly, in each case inhalation of heroin fumes preceded the use of injection (though, of course, this practise is not uncommon). There is no means of predicting which solvent abusers will progress to hard drug use or alcohol dependence.

Psychological issues

The typical social abuser of volatile substances who sniffs only with others is unlikely to be particularly disturbed. There is a clinical impression that most such youngsters resemble the large number of teenagers who engage in mildly antisocial behaviour and petty delinquency. They tend to be somewhat undersupervised and possess anti-authoritarian attitudes but do not exhibit a higher rate of psychiatric disorder than non-sniffing delinquent controls (Lockhart & Lennox 1983). Put another way, very few solvent abusers need psychiatric referral (8 out of 134 in Sourindhrin and Baird's (1984) study).

Skuse and Burrell (1982) examined chronic, sporadic and occasional abusers referred to a child psychiatry department and found no differences in rate or type of psychiatric disorder between them. This does not mean that overall rates of disorder in the general population are the same in each group since their sample was drawn from referrals to a psychiatric clinic. It does suggest that heavy abuse does not cause psychiatric disorder.

The abiding impression from clinical practice and from a number of descriptive accounts is that solitary chronic abusers are likely to have experienced disruption or disorganisation of family life as a result of parental alcoholism, discord, divorce or death (Masterton & Sclare 1978). Although not necessarily psychiatrically disordered, such individuals seem to sniff in order to escape feelings of despair, inadequacy, emptiness and misery and the effect of environmental stress.

It appears that the death rate is higher among solitary abusers, partly because they are more likely to use unsafe methods such as putting their heads completely inside large polythene sniffing bags. They may also inhale greater quantities or place themselves at higher risk of cardiac dysrhythmias by simultaneous auto-erotic activities such as self-strangulation and masturbation (Anderson et al 1985).

Detection

Social association with other volatile substance abusers is suspicious; the practice is contagious, especially among the bored and disaffected. Being found in a locale favoured by sniffers is equally suspect. Such places are likely to be littered with bags containing dried glue, milk bottles or empty containers for cleaning solvents. Such debris can be found in the teenager's bedroom or in the household dustbin.

The signs of acute intoxication resemble drunkenness. Giggling, shouting, unsteadiness, dysarthria, difficulty concentrating on a conversation, and drowsiness are common but there may also be evidence of hallucinations.

Spillage of glue on clothing may be seen. Less obvious are the light patches on clothes where solvents such as cleaning fluids have been spilt. The smell of solvents on the breath can be very strong. "Glue sniffer's rash" around mouth and nose indicates heavy abuse.

Levels of toluene can be measured in breath and blood. Of more practical use is the presence of its metabolites benzoic acid and hippuric acid in the urine. Both are present in non-abusers but a urine hippurate/creatinine ratio greater than 1 indicates recent exposure to toluene (Ramsey & Flanagan 1982).

Most volatile substances are cheap or easy to steal so that only those with heavy habits (e.g. 2–3 pints of glue a day) will need to spend much money.

Management

Most youngsters who sniff in groups will abandon the practice sooner rather than later without having damaged themselves.

They do not require psychiatric referral — which is not to say that volatile substance abuse is not a social problem which needs to be taken seriously. Community intervention to educate children, parents, teachers and retailers is a multidisciplinary enterprise involving social, medical and police services as well as voluntary agencies.

It is the chronic and especially the solitary abuser who will benefit from systematic psychiatric appraisal. This advisedly includes both separate and joint interviews with the adolescent and his parents as well as consultation with his teachers. Particular attention should be paid to self-esteem, mood stability, coping strategies for stress, sources of pleasure, social skills, the intensity of attachments, parental alcohol abuse, and the extent of parental support and supervision.

Physical investigations (plasma urea and electrolytes, liver function tests, full blood count, urinalysis) are usually negative but their performance may bring home to the youngster that he is possibly damaging his body.

Where individual or family pathology is revealed by the above, it will obviously require treatment on its merits. The extent of continuing abuse should provide an indicator of success, if there is a genuine functional link between identified pathology and abuse.

Individual or group counselling, social skills training, advising parents, and the provision of alternative recreational opportunities are interventions that are often best carried out by knowledgeable professionals who are not psychiatrists (see O'Connor 1984). The efforts of youth workers or intermediate treatment programmes can supplement and often replace psychiatric endeavour. The most specific help that the medical profession can provide is likely to be in health education. This can take the form of advising the youngster how to sniff safely: in company, in a safe place, avoiding aerosols, dry-cleaning fluid or bags over the head, not simultaneously smoking or drinking alcohol, and the use of the coma position in first aid. If such information is given without histrionics and without an authoritarian, patronising manner it has a chance of being listened to and may take some of the anti-authoritarian sting out of the practice. There is little point in delivering a moralistic lecture which has all been heard before. The art is to make it clear that, whilst not supporting the abuse of solvents, one is still the teenager's doctor and concerned that they look after their own health.

REFERENCES

Alister C, Lush M, Oliver J S, Watson J M 1981 Status epilepticus caused by solvent abuse. British Medical Journal 283: 1156

Anderson H R, Macnair R S, Ramsey J D 1985 Deaths from abuse of volatile substances: a national epidemiological study. British Medical Journal 290: 304–307

Bewley B R, Johnson M R D, Bland J M, Murray M 1980 Trends in children's smoking. Community Medicine 2: 186–189

Blacker E, Demone H, Freeman H 1965 Drinking behavior of delinquent boys. Quarterly Journal of Studies in Alcohol 26: 223–237

Boon N A 1987 Solvent abuse and the heart. British Medical Journal 294: 722

Carney M W P, Bacelle L, Robinson B 1984 Psychosis after cannabis abuse. British Medical Journal 288: 1047

Connell P 1958 Amphetamine Psychosis (Maudsley Monograph No. 5) Chapman and Hall, London

Connell P 1968 The use and abuse of amphetamines. Practitioner 200: 234–243

Davies B, Thorley A, O'Connor D 1985 Progression of addiction careers in young adult solvent misusers. British Medical Journal 290: 109–110

Edwards G 1986 Drugs: no simple answer. The Times, 15.7.86.

Field T 1985 Escaping the Dragon. Unwin, London

Fillmore K M 1974 Drinking and problem drinking in early adulthood and middle-age: an exploratory 12-year follow-up study. Quarterly Journal of Studies in Alcohol 35: 819–840

Fishburne P, Abelson H, Cisin I 1980 National Survey on Drug Abuse: Main Findings: 1979. National Institute on Drug Abuse, Rockville, Md.

Gay M, Meller R, Stanley S 1982 Drug abuse monitoring: A survey of solvent abuse in the County of Avon. Human Toxicology 1: 257–263

Glaser H H, Massengale O N 1962 Glue sniffing in children. Journal of the American Medical Association 181: 300–303

Glynn T J 1981 From family to peer: a review of transitions of influence among drug-using youth. Journal of Youth and Adolescence 10: 363–383

Johnston L D 1985 The etiology and prevention of substance use: what can we learn from recent historical changes? In: Jones C L, Battjes R J (eds) Etiology of Drug Abuse: Implications for Prevention (NIDA Research Monograph 56) National Institute on Drug Abuse, Rockville, Md.

Johnston L D, O'Malley P M, Eveland L K 1978 Drugs and delinquency. A search for causal connections. In: Kandel D B (ed) Longitudinal Research on Drug Use. Empirical Findings and Methodological Issues. Hemisphere, Washington D.C.

Kandel D B, Yamaguchi K 1985 Developmental patterns of the use of legal, illegal, and medically prescribed psychotropic drugs from adolescence to young adulthood. In: Jones C L, Battjes R J (eds) Etiology of Drug Abuse: Implications for Prevention, (NIDA Research Monograph 56) National Institute on Drug Abuse, Rockville, Md.

Kosviner A 1976 Social science and cannabis use. In: Graham J (ed) Cannabis and Health. Academic Press, London

Krystal S, Raskin A 1970 Drug Dependence: Aspects of Ego Functions. Wayne State University Press, Detroit

Lockhart W H, Lennox M 1983 The extent of solvent abuse in a regional secure unit sample. Journal of Adolescence 6: 43–45

MacKay J R 1963 Problem drinking among juvenile delinquents. Crime and Delinquency 9: 29–38

Masterton G, Sclare A B 1978 Solvent abuse. Health Bulletin 36: 305–309

O'Brien E T, Yeoman W B, Horby J A E 1971 Hepatorenal damage from toluene in a "glue-sniffer". British Medical Journal ii: 29–30

O'Connor D J 1984 Glue sniffing and the abuse of solvents by school children. Maladjustment and Therapeutic Education 2: 2–13

Oliver J S, Watson J M 1977 Abuse of solvents "for kicks" — a review of 50 cases. Lancet i: 84–86

Peck D F, Plant M 1986 Unemployment and illegal drug use: concordant evidence from a prospective study and national trends. British Medical Journal 293: 929–932

Plant M A 1975a Drug takers in an English town. Tavistock, London

Plant M A 1975b Drug takers in an English town: factors associated with the use of injected drugs. British Journal of Criminology 15: 181–186

Plant M A 1981 Drugs in perspective. Hodder and Stoughton, London

Powars D 1965 Aplastic anaemia secondary to glue sniffing. New England Journal of Medicine 273: 700–702

Raistrick D, Davidson R 1985 Alcoholism and Drug Addiction. Churchill Livingstone, Edinburgh

Ramsey A W 1982 Solvent abuse: an educational perspective. Human Toxicology 1: 265–270

Ramsey J D, Flanagan R J 1982 The role of the laboratory in the investigation of solvent abuse. Human Toxicology 1: 299–311

Rawbone R G, Guz A 1982 Cigarette smoking among secondary schoolchildren 1975–79. Archives of Disease in Childhood, 57: 352–358

Ron M A 1986 Volatile substance abuse: a review of possible long-term neurological, intellectual and psychiatric sequelae. British Journal of Psychiatry 148: 235–246

Royal College of Psychiatrists 1979 Alcohol and Alcoholism. Tavistock, London

Skuse D, Burrell S 1982 A review of solvent abuses and their management by a child psychiatric outpatient service. Human Toxicology 7: 321–329

Smart R G 1976 The New Drinkers: Teenage Use and Abuse of Alcohol. Addiction Research Foundation, Toronto

Sourindhrin I 1985 Solvent misuse (leader) British Medical Journal 290: 94–95

Sourindhrin I, Baird J A 1984 Management of solvent misuse. A Glasgow community approach. British Journal of Addiction 79: 227–232

Strang J, Connell P 1985 Clinical aspects of drug and alcohol abuse. In: Rutter M, Hersov L (Eds.) Child and Adolescent Psychiatry: Modern Perspectives. 2nd edn. Blackwell Scientific, Oxford

Unger R 1978 The treatment of adolescent alcoholism. Social Casework 59: 27–35

Vingelis E, Smart R G 1981 Physical dependence on alcohol in youth. In: Israel Y et al (eds) Research Advances in Alcohol and Drug Problems. Vol. 6. Plenum, New York

Watson J 1982 Solvent abuse: presentation and clinical diagnosis. Human Toxicology 1: 249–256

Wechsler H 1976 Alcohol intoxification and drug use among teenagers. Journal of Studies in Alcohol 37: 1672–1677

WHO Memorandum 1981 Bulletin of the World Health Organization, 59: 225–242

Wiener R S P 1970 Drugs and Schoolchildren. Longman, London

21
Treatment interventions.
I. provisions

Many adolescents with psychiatric disorder are never seen by a psychiatrist. Adolescence is, in terms of physical medicine, a comparatively healthy phase, with the consequence that adolescents do not commonly see doctors and are therefore not very used to seeking medical opinion from a general practitioner who might refer them to a psychiatrist. Those who are seen by psychiatric services usually present a fairly chronic picture, referral having been delayed for a number of reasons, including a false hope that the psychological difficulties will go away if ignored. The fear of stigma — which itself creates stigma — leads families (and their medical advisors) to postpone psychiatric consultation until the problem is so ingrained that the treatment problem which confronts the psychiatrist is comparable to that of a general surgeon referred a case of terminal malignant cachexia; medical skills which might have been relevant had the referral been earlier are now irrelevant or can only be rehearsed by an exploratory laparotomy.

Within psychiatric services, it is as out-patients that most adolescents will be seen. The current organisation of services cuts uneasily across the teenage period with child (or "child and adolescent") psychiatry taking responsibility for those up to the age of 16 or, in some areas, up to the time of leaving school, adult services taking over thereafter. This tends to mean that the 16–18-year-olds get a raw deal. The Health Advisory Service (1986) document *Bridges over Troubled Waters* suggests that local adult and child psychiatric services need jointly to establish a service for older adolescents to overcome such difficulties. Most psychiatrists have experienced the problem of the two specialities squabbling unhelpfully over who should take on the case of a 16-year-old. Not that there are no real difficulties in this area — adolescents do not readily warm to the idea of being seen in a department for children — but it is often the family-orientated child psychiatrists with their links with the education service and their readiness to take a developmental perspective who have relevant skills to offer. Adult wards and clinics do not necessarily offer the best ambience for the more immature individuals in their mid-teens, but the ethos of general adult psychiatry is more orientated towards in-patient treatment and adult psychiatric wards are geared to acute admission in a way that many adolescent units are not, and in an emergency involving a psychotic adolescent this may prove helpful.

Many regions have a specialist adolescent psychiatric service but this tends to be centred upon an adolescent in-patient unit (called an adolescent unit for short) and will thus see the most severe cases. It is obvious that, for disordered adolescents generally, the psychiatric services are patchy and lack a clear identity. As a result, the knowledge base of adolescent psychiatry is poorly developed and the physical and manpower resources for adolescent patients are scanty (Health Advisory Service 1986). The psychiatrist working with an adolescent clientele will need to be familiar with a network of services and agencies within the health service, the education service, social services and the voluntary sector, most of which he will have no control over. Given the amount of diversity, only a sketch of what might be locally available is mentioned here.

General out-patient and community services

Younger disturbed adolescents will be seen in child guidance clinics, hospital departments of child and adolescent psychiatry or by child or adolescent psychiatrists working in association with local social services or in special schools. Those a little older will be seen in adult psychiatry clinics, psychotherapy departments, clinics for drug dependence or eating disorders, and by forensic or mental-handicap psychiatrists. The district clinical psychology service will see some teenagers, though not often within a specific psychological service for adolescents as a client group. A certain amount of treatment (mainly counselling) may be carried out by student health services, school medical officers and psychologically-minded paediatricians.

Outside the health service, a large number of disturbed adolescents will be managed within schools (including schools for emotionally and behaviourally disturbed children), by social services, and by voluntary agencies.

Adolescent units

Most health service regions have one or more adolescent units for those adolescent psychiatric patients who need residential assessment or treatment. As a rough generalisation they tend to be neglected by the managing authorities, are poorly equipped with dilapidated premises and a chronic shortage of nursing staff, which limits their ability to admit disturbing young patients. Some have been notoriously selective in the cases they will accept and the types of treatment they offer. The best (of which there are an appreciable number) contain highly skilled staff and have a school attached, offer a range of treatments, a prompt service to potential referrers, and link with out-patient services on- and off-site. Because young people need space, adolescent units are often sited in the grounds of large mental hospitals even though this limits their accessibility in both psychological and geographical terms. Waiting lists for admission are common and admissions tend to be for months rather than days.

Admitting a teenager to a psychiatric hospital away from his or her family for a lengthy period is a major step and it is appropriate that some hurdles are placed to impede unnecessary or precipitate admission. Furthermore, the reason for admission is frequently a suitable issue around which therapeutic work may be organised if the aim is to return the patient to his original family and school (Bruggen et al 1973). Nevertheless, the test of a good unit is the promptness with which it can respond to a genuine emergency, not at all an easy managerial task. Some acutely psychotic teenagers who need admission to hospital have to be admitted first to a general adult ward and transferred to an adolescent unit after a few days when a bed becomes available. The success of such a procedure depends upon the readiness of the adolescent unit staff to liaise with the adult ward.

Three groups of disturbed teenagers are notoriously difficult to find in-patient resources for. The behaviourally-disturbed autistic and mentally-handicapped adolescents are not usually welcomed by the average adolescent unit and are also barred from mental handicap hospitals by rigid policies about not admitting "children". Aggressive "acting-out", conduct-disordered teenagers (especially offenders) of normal intelligence are likewise shunned because of their disruptive impact and excessive demands on sparse nursing time. Drug abusers, particularly those using hard drugs, are generally excluded because of the risk of contagion. The reasons why such disturbed teenagers are not admitted are understandable in each instance but alternative facilities are usually lacking.

A frequent misunderstanding about adolescent units is to confuse their residential and therapeutic purposes. They are in-patient units in which adolescents with psychiatric disorder live so that they may receive more intensive psychiatric assessment and treatment than would be possible if they were living at home. They also provide a measure of supervision and protection for the individual patient on the principle of asylum as well as, in some instances, protecting the community from a dangerous, disturbed adolescent. The pivot of these functions is the principle that a young person having a psychiatric disorder is the primary problem. Adolescents whose first need is someone to look after them or look over them should be catered for by social services. Those who, without being primarily psychiatrically disordered, are excessively naughty, unruly or malevolent and from whom society needs a measure of protection which cannot be provided by their parents, are likely to need custodial care rather than health service treatment. Although slanted toward the consideration of psychiatric in-patient units for children, the chapter by Hersov and Bentovim (1985) provides a clear and concise statement about the purposes of admission to hospital and the way in which this needs to be seen as a component of a total treatment plan.

Clinical practice within an adolescent unit is a specialised topic with an obvious need for interdisciplinary collaboration. Steinberg (1986) has edited a useful guide, focussing on the practice in one particular unit run on eclectic lines.

A common problem in adolescent unit work is finding an adequate living setting or school for the adolescent who cannot or should not return home. Many teenagers stay in adolescent units past the optimal time for treatment because they need to transfer to a residential school or hostel but no place is available or the paperwork involved is cumbersome and protracted. A large number of adolescents who need in-patient treatment will also have special educational needs but these take a notoriously long time for education authorities to arrange for and the number of boarding schools who are prepared to take a new pupil at the age of 15 is severely limited.

Day units

Many adolescent units will have a number of patients attending daily, particularly as part of the rehabilitation process. A recent development has been to create specialist day units which can serve a more local area than a more expensive and remote in-patient unit. The Health Advisory Service report (1986) envisaged a practice of seeing day-patients in so-called resource centres which would provide a local centre of expertise and knowledge. It seems likely that this arrangement will be developed in a number of districts. Experience suggests that this approach to children, which allows continuing contact with their families, need not be confined to the treatment of moderately severe disorder but can be applied to severe conditions for which in-patient treatment would ordinarily be considered (Linnihan 1977).

Walk-in clinics

There is a respectable tradition of offering exceptionally accessible advisory or counselling services for teenagers who are likely to be shy of the more statutory services and procedures. Many of the successful walk-in or drop-in clinics in the UK have been managed by voluntary agencies (often with support funding from social services departments) and it is not obvious that the health service can successfully usurp this pattern without frightening off the clients who currently use such a service. Perhaps understandably, the focus for concern in walk-in clinics tends to be the individual adolescent, in contrast to the family orientation common in health service practice (Laufer 1980).

Resources provided by social services departments

Quite apart from the provision of field-workers for individual adolescents and their families, and the children's homes maintained by residential social workers, there exists a range of other services for disturbed teenagers:

— Intermediate Treatment (Ch. 8, p. 110)

— adoption and fostering services, particularly including specialist fostering as an alternative to residential care

— community homes with education on the premises

— resource centres and reception centres for families and teenagers in acute crises of care and support

— sheltered accomodation and hostels

— remand homes and other facilities for offenders and those at risk

— day assessment centres for those with possible special care needs

— information about voluntary services.

It is impossible to overestimate the contribution of social service departments to the psychological welfare of numerous adolescents. The pattern of provisions will obviously vary from one local authority to another, so that some departments will have, for example, a specialist family therapy team or run a centre for the young unemployed. Local knowledge becomes essential and, in theory, can be made available through the social workers attached to departments of psychiatry, since they are employed by social services departments. There is a well-established practice of child and adolescent psychiatrists providing consultation services to the social services department with special reference to the way in which disturbed young people can continue to be helped by local provisions.

Resources provided by education departments

The concept of special educational needs enshrined in the 1981 Education Act has revolutionised the way in which the schooling of disturbed children and teenagers can be provided. Whereas previously a distinction was made between ordinary and special schools, this structure is being replaced by an attempt to provide special facilities on an individual basis within mainstream schooling as far as possible. Undoubtedly a need for schools for the emotionally and behaviourally disturbed (maladjusted), those with learning difficulties (including the mentally handicapped), the delicate, the autistic, and those with hearing and visual difficulties will persist in the medium term, yet the general trend is to move their expertise into ordinary schools and address it towards individual children with special educational needs who will thus remain integrated into the ordinary peer group and community. Exactly how this is achieved will depend upon the local education authority in terms of strategy and finance, and the schools psychological service in terms of the individual. Educational psychologists thus become central to the process of determining special educational needs and how they may be met. Psychiatrists are likely to be involved in the process of supplying evidence to the full assessment procedure which assists this.

One impact of contemporary educational thought about curriculum development has been to provide some momentum for the development of pastoral care services within schools. The school counsellor movement prominent in the 1970s (Jones 1984) seems to have abated somewhat, the provision of support, advice and counselling being increasingly seen as one of the general duties of all teachers. Nevertheless, many secondary schools will have a number of teachers with posts of responsibility in the area of pastoral care, a system quite often administered by a deputy headteacher.

Outside the school itself, the education welfare service, although historically preoccupied with non-attenders and informing parents about welfare rights, has in many areas moved towards a more therapeutic position with the development of casework skills, so that educational welfare officers (EWOs) or educational social workers may prove valuable allies for psychiatrists. An EWO is commonly the professional who refers an adolescent with a school-related problem to a child guidance clinic.

Most education authorities will have established a number of units in or adjacent to schools to accommodate adolescents with difficult behaviour or educational needs that can be met without full-time provision. Discontent about "sin-bins" has led to a more cautious use of their deployment but home tuition services, including centres separate from schools for groups of pupils unable to attend full-time school, are in the ascendant, being commended, for instance, by the Health Advisory Service report (1986).

The voluntary sector

Some voluntary organisations relevant to disturbed teenagers are national in scale and well recognised: the Richmond Fellowship, schools and communities run by the Rudolf Steiner and Camphill Village organisations, schools and hostels belonging to the National Autistic Society, the Family Welfare Association, Family Service Units, and Alateen, to name but a few. They are outnumbered by the local groups and enterprises which complement the statutory services in any particular district but can be relatively invisible to the clinician. An important recommendation of *Bridges Over Troubled Waters* (Health Advisory Service 1986) is the establishment in each district of a directory of resources for disturbed adolescents covering the work of all agencies, statutory and voluntary.

Other resources

The clinical medical officers and the specialists in community medicine who have a designated responsibility for child health are part of the health service though before 1974 they were employed by the local education authority as school medical officers. The Court report (DHSS 1976) envisaged an integration of their role with that of general practitioners (which was eventually opposed by the medical profession) and a screening task for pupils who would, at the age of 13, have the chance of at least one confidential interview with a doctor. Although school doctors in state schools are not permitted to prescribe medication, they can have a useful counselling role and make referrals to psychiatric departments.

Community psychiatric nurses most commonly see themselves as clinically involved with adult psychiatric patients though there are a small number specifically involved with children and adolescents. It seems likely that this practice will increase.

The probation service is active in providing support, counselling and hostel provision for older adolescent offenders and may administer local projects such as groups for exhibitionists or social skills training.

Churches have a long tradition of involvement with teenagers in emotional difficulties and may have powerful authority in individual cases where marital work with parents or bereavement counselling with an adolescent is required.

REFERENCES

Bruggen P, Byng-Hall J, Pitt-Aikens T 1973 The reason for admission as a focus of work in an adolescent unit. British Journal of Psychiatry 122: 319–329
DHSS 1976 Fit for the Future. Cmnd 6684. HMSO, London
Health Advisory Service 1986 Bridges Over Troubled Waters. HMSO, London
Hersov L, Bentovim A 1985 In-patient and day-hospital units. In: Rutter M, Hersov L (eds) Child and Adolescent Psychiatry: Modern Approaches. 2nd Ed. Blackwell Scientific, Oxford
Jones A 1984 Counselling Adolescents: School and After. Kogan Page, London
Laufer M A 1980 Which adolescents must be helped and by whom? Journal of Adolescence 3: 265–272
Linnihan P C 1977 Adolescent day treatment: a community alternative to institutionalization of the emotionally disturbed adolescent. Journal of the American Academy of Child Psychiatry 19: 160–171
Steinberg D (ed) 1986 The Adolescent Unit. Wiley, Chichester

22

Treatment interventions.
II. Methods

Most treatments used in adolescent psychiatry are psychological rather than physical or psychopharmacological. This chapter is not intended to provide an exhaustive description of available methods; since there are no treatments that are used only with adolescents, the intention is to indicate how treatments used with children or adults are modified.

Individual counselling

On the basis that some adolescent turmoil or distress is a result of confronting developmental tasks, simple counselling in which the counsellor takes a non-judgemental stance, clarifies problems, gives simple advice or comment, and reflects the adolescent's moods and words back to him without reference to a particular model of the mind, is widely employed. There is no doubt that many adolescents find this approach helpful but also no medical prerogative on its use. Indeed, it tends to be assumed that it is most useful with crises of personal development rather than disorder or personality problems. As such it is quite widely used by a variety of non-medical agencies (see Jones 1984, Newsome et al 1975).

Counsellors working with adolescents become used to the way in which they may start well in a genuinely shared enterprise but then stop coming and may let it be known that the whole operation is in their view, a waste of time. Whilst this is quite consonant with Coleman's (1980) thesis that adolescents concentrate on one developmental issue at a time in a focal way, it also puts the counsellor on the spot. If he is to be non-judgemental, in the time-honoured manner, he cannot insist on attendance. Indeed, if he does, the odds are that he will be confronted by a belligerent or stubbornly silent client. There are several observations to be made about such an impasse.

Firstly, it may be that the adolescent is right and counselling is bad for him or her. In Adams' (1961) study of counselling young offenders, those who were poorly motivated (among other things, see Ch. 8) were made worse.

Secondly, it is not easy to gauge the end-point of treatment. Contrary to older views, brief psychotherapeutic treatments with adults seem to be as, or more, effective than protracted ones (Luborsky et al 1975) and incremental effects of treatment continue after treatment has stopped (Wright et al 1976).

Thirdly, it is only too easy to assume that the adolescent understands the ground rules of counselling: that he is supposed to volunteer suitable information, refrain from prying into the therapist's private life, recognise this sort of confidential conversation as treatment and so forth. It is not clear that many adolescents given counselling do understand these rules; the others may vote with their feet.

Fourthly, it seems on anecdotal grounds to be useful for the counsellor to show concern and persistence. The refusal to attend may be part of "the characteristic adolescent proposition that the adult is useless . . .one of the most potent of the disturbed adolescent's methods of checking whether the adult world is safe enough to challenge" (Steinberg 1983).

Individual psychotherapy

The boundary between counselling and psychotherapy is hard to define. The historical development of individual psychotherapy from psychoanalysis means that psychotherapy rests upon a model of mind which emphasises unconscious processes, though it is well recognised that the conceptualisation of these differs according to various schools of thought. Great weight is placed upon the relationship between patient and therapist, particularly in terms of transference. The therapist draws upon such ideas in order to make comments which link emotions, attitudes and behaviour in the therapeutic session to past experiences or present modes of thinking and feeling. Through an improved understanding in the context of a close relationship with the therapist, the adolescent patient is able to adopt more flexible and productive strategies in personal development and coping, freeing him from self-defeating and distressing symptoms. In order to facilitate this process, the therapist uses components of counselling: provision of a confidential and regular session, facilitation of the patient's communication and self-disclosure, and presentation of the therapist as a safe, interested and benign person, but goes beyond these provisions to make clarifications, confrontations and interpretations. These may, with advantage, be couched in terms of "dilemmas, traps and snags" (Ryle 1979).

The adolescent's capacity to participate in such an activity varies. Young teenagers commonly have difficulty in establishing a channel of communication with the therapist, finding play techniques too childish but not yet having acquired a ready facility with abstract conceptual thought, and restricted by the way in which the language of childhood (beyond which they may not have moved very far) serves the communication of information and simple ideas rather than feelings. Their sense of self may well be comparatively undifferentiated (Mullener & Laird 1971), impairing their capacity to reflect introspectively about their state of mind. Fears of passivity and dependency can lead to privacy and concealment of material from the therapist, particularly if there is a muddle about his role and intentions, especially as an agent of the parents (Wilson & Hersov 1985). As many authorities have emphasised, the natural tendency is for adolescents to attempt to discharge unpleasant affect by action rather than by using reflective verbalisation to share it with an adult.

Without the knowledge of what the components of effective psychotherapy are, it is impossible to be prescriptive as to how such problems might be overcome. One sensible suggestion, based on anecdotal experience, is not to be too ambitious. The impact of quite simple observations about an adolescent's feelings can quite often be seen to be dramatic. Sensitive observations about how he presents himself can be highly valued and the description of patterns of behaviour illuminate how he contributes to the traps he finds himself in. The tendency for young adolescents to externalise and blame others for their predicaments without reference to their own involvement is well recognised.

Many psychotherapy sessions with adolescents are typified by protracted silences in which it is clear that the teenager either does not know what to say, or, if there is something pressing, how to put it, or whether it is safe to try to do so. The therapist's response is helped by knowledge of their home or school life, obtained directly from parents or indirectly through a clinical colleague who meets with them regularly. There may be value in arranging experiences with others which can be reviewed in therapy: in a comparison of the styles of two psychotherapists, Ricks (1974) found that the therapist who was firm and direct in his handling of adolescents and arranged a number of group activities for them outside sessions, material from which was examined in therapy, obtained better results than a more reserved therapist who was mainly interested in depressive or anxious affect displayed during a session.

Some teenagers, perhaps mainly boys, become overwhelmed by the sexual overtones of a private meeting with another person in a situation where powerful feelings are discussed. Whereas the therapist may feel gratified by the introduction of sexual material into the sessions, there is a danger that the teenager may find this exciting in its own right and the proceedings take on a masturbatory flavour. Conversely, sexual feelings towards a therapist can inhibit any disclosure by a young teenager who has come to assume that the therapist knows what he is thinking.

The therapist who believes that adolescence is a time of fervent emotional turmoil may be disappointed by the vague, dull manner of some adolescents caught in the "doldrums" of adolescence. Misguided attempts to penetrate apparent emotional flatness can be seen as unwelcome prying by the teenager and result in withdrawal. The unwary therapist may try to enliven matters by provocation with equally negative results.

The use of therapist self-disclosure with adolescents has been advocated by Weiner & King (1977) as enlivening discussion and making it less impersonal. The risk is that the therapist's own feelings (which are quite likely to be intense and intrusive) may escape appropriate control and mask his sensitivity to the adolescent, or confuse the aim of therapy by stimulating in the therapist an inappropriate excitement or identification.

The indications for individual psychotherapy with adolescents can only be established by consensus, there being no outcome studies of scientific acceptability with this age group which examine an effect for psychotherapy according to diagnosis. Although there are grounds for thinking that individual psychotherapy may be helpful for some antisocial adolescents (see Ch. 8), most authorities assume that the indications are "mild to

moderate" emotional disorders and mixed emotional and behavioural disorders, excluding organic conditions, schizophrenia,
autism, severe deprivation, and serious conduct disorder (Wilson
& Hersov 1985). Denial of personal problems and poor impulse
control are also contra-indications, whereas an impression that
intrapsychic elements are particularly significant in aetiology is
an argument in favour of a psychotherapeutic approach. The
adolescent considered should be capable of a reflective attitude
and able to tolerate a reasonable amount of frustration whilst the
parents of younger teenagers must support the idea of their son
or daughter confiding privately in an unrelated adult.

Group psychotherapy

Adolescents, it is often said, form groups naturally and it would
seem only sensible to exploit this in group approaches to treatment. The kinds of therapeutic group activity employed with
adolescents form a continuum. At one end are the simple shared
activities and commentary about here-and-now interpersonal
issues used with severely disordered in-patients by Steinberg and
his colleagues (1978) and in some intermediate treatment activities. An intermediate position is exemplified by discussion groups
in schools organised by Kolvin's team (1981) which relied upon
conversational exchanges and included discussion of issues arising
from outside and inside the group. At the other end is the more
traditional reliance upon verbal material, with an emphasis on
reflection and a focus on such issues as working through and the
relationship of the group to the therapist, familiar in adult group
psychotherapy. This approach applies more to out-patient groups
and is described in texts such as that by Yalom (1975). Criteria
for entry to a group, its duration and general mode of functioning
will depend on whether it is a way of structuring a treatment
milieu (as in adolescent units) or a psychotherapy facility for
selected individuals, particularly out-patients. In the latter
instance, the principles familiar in general adult psychotherapy
apply: a balance of diagnoses, maturity levels and, possibly, sexes
needs to be considered in order to facilitate verbal and reflective
functioning. The progress of treatment follows the general course
of orientation, conflict and cohesive collaboration outlined by
Yalom (1975). On the other hand, groups set up as a way of
structuring milieu are usually unselective, more active and take

a view of group tasks which uses a developmental metaphor such as that of Erikson for assessing the group's maturity and progress (see Steinberg 1983).

There exist various accounts of the type of group psychotherapy which relies on words (e.g. Berkowitz 1972, Bruce 1978, Evans 1982). These concur in an emphasis on helping adolescents help each other, using their own resources as well as having their own needs met. The emphasis is very much on the here-and-now and on interpersonal interaction. Limits need to be set on disruptive or dangerous behaviour, particularly since a recurring theme is the acceptance or otherwise of authority in the person of the therapist. Facilitating an adolescent group extends beyond clarifying group process; it also requires some knowledge of child management in dealing with confrontation and challenge. Nonverbal behaviour tends to be unsophisticated, whether in anger or affection, so that competition to sit near the therapist, studied inattentiveness, or storming out are all frequent communications, and silences a common issue.

Various authorities (e.g. Maclennan & Felsenfeld 1968) have commented upon dynamic themes which are persistently encountered in adolescent groups and which obstruct progress. These include:

— scapegoating (which can be violent)

— domination of the group by one talkative individual

— rivalry with the therapist

— exceptional reticence and uneasiness about self-disclosure

— setting up sub-groups to defuse tension;

— limit-testing by confrontation with the therapist.

It is usually sufficient to draw attention to the process and label it. This has the effect of reframing and is preferable to attempts to meet the behaviour head-on, which often fail.

Outcome evaluation of group psychotherapy for adolescents is exceptionally sparse and most studies have investigated effects on educational problems, a curious choice of variable by ordinary clinical standards. The most important study of general relevance to psychiatry is the assessment of therapeutic discussion groups in Newcastle secondary schools by Kolvin et al (1981). During one school term, single-sex groups of about five 11–12-year-olds met for ten 30–60 minute sessions with a specially recruited, trained and supervised social worker. A variety of outcome measures were used: clinical state, self-report on the Junior Eysenck Personality Inventory, parents' and teachers' reports, academic performance, sociometry and attitudes to school and others. These were deployed at termination, 18-month and 3-year follow-ups. Compared with controls, significant improvements were found in all areas assessed, some remarkably persistent or continuing to improve after therapy had stopped. Peer relationships, teacher and parental reports showed improvement compared with controls at the 3-year follow-up. The therapist's judgement of change correlated well with objective measures, but no evidence emerged to link group process (as measured by indices of cohesiveness and openness of discussion) with improvement. Curiously enough, and contrary to received wisdom, only a modest effect was demonstrated for social isolation, less than the results of behaviour modification programmes carried out in the classroom.

Family therapy

Treatment of the pattern of relationships within the family by meeting with the family as a whole has been the most important therapeutic development in adolescent psychiatry over the last two decades. What is meant by 'family' is sometimes blurred over, with the result that two variants result: treatment of the relationship system which operates between the identified adolescent patient and his or her parents with the exclusion of siblings is one; the treatment of an entire household the other. In the last instance, grandparents may be included if they live with the adolescent. In either variant, a parent's sexual partner who lives in but is unrelated to the adolescent may be included. "Family" is shorthand for a number of natural groups involved in child-care responsibilities.

The concept of a system of family relationships is central and family therapists will use concepts derived from systems theory in their formulation of a problem. Hill (1986) supplies a brief glossary and summary of the theory.

Family therapy as a whole is a rather heterogeneous field. Given the intent to approach the presenting clinical problem as a manifestation of family system dysfunction (or, at least, believing that change in the system would assist problem resolution), and that a whole family interview will be the key method of appraisal and arena for intervention, then various styles of thinking can operate. Within the UK, the following modes can be observed:

— family interviews within which therapists facilitate communication and demonstrate empathy in a supportive, counselling stance which commonly draws on notions of family development

— a psychotherapeutic approach using an interpretative style with the use of ideas derived from transgenerational concepts (Lieberman 1980), myths (Byng-Hall 1973), projection and insight

— structural family therapy and its immediate derivatives which emphasise ideas such as boundaries, hierarchies, distancing and roles, and pay tribute to the lead given by Minuchin (e.g. 1974)

— strategic therapy using manipulative techniques such as paradoxical injunctions, ordeals or lengthy prescriptions. The original leaders in the field are well represented by Haley (1980) whose book *Leaving Home* is of great relevance to family therapy with families containing older adolescents. The work of the Milan Group (Selvini-Palazzoli et al 1978) has been very influential in the UK.

— behavioural approaches which embed behavioural interventions within a family though not always with a view to changing the system, symptomatic change in one individual being the primary aim in the most rigorous studies (e.g. Patterson 1971, 1982)

In practice, borrowing ideas from a number of schools of thought results in a "goulash" approach being commonly employed and an eclectic tradition is evident within British family therapy (Bentovim et al 1982). Given that there is very little hard evidence for the relative superiority of any one approach, this is unsurprising. The one study with families containing adolescents as identified patients that did assess the relative merits of behavioural, psychodynamic and placebo family therapies and found benefit superior to placebo only for a behavioural approach (Alexander & Parsons 1973) is not usually taken as utterly definitive owing to the junior status of the therapists, particularly in terms of psychodynamic sophistication.

The involvement of adolescents in family therapy is often an all-or-nothing affair. Particularly when the index patient is prepubertal, an older brother or sister may decide to opt out and not attend at all, not deigning to become involved with such child-like matters. If older siblings can be persuaded to attend, they often throw themselves into the process and prove valuable allies to the therapist by revealing perceived hypocrisy, blurting out family secrets, and teasing parental power. Not becoming involved in family therapy may be a statement about wanting to leave the family altogether, or at least to be seen as a potentially separate part of it, capable of leaving on one's own terms. For such reasons, some practitioners arrange to see adolescents separately as well as in a whole-family interview as a way of acknowledging their partial separateness.

Family therapy's position as a widely practised intervention rests almost entirely upon faith, there being hardly any evaluative studies of outcome to demonstrate scientifically any benefit over placebo. General anecdotal experience suggests that it is useful for the common out-patient problems to do with compliance, control and courtesy within families but there is nothing to justify its whole-hearted adoption by a psychiatric service as a sole treatment method. I have elsewhere (Hill 1986) suggested that, on first principles, there would be grounds for considering family therapy in the following circumstances:

— when the presenting clinical problem is a relationship difficulty between family members

— difficulties in separating from parents

— loss of one parent's authority over the adolescent (where this is potentially regainable)

— vicarious gratification for a parent through the deviant behaviour of a son or daughter

— obvious anomalous interpersonal perceptions or communication abnormalities within the family associated with scapegoating, or extremes of interpersonal distancing with enmeshment or disengagement

— when it has previously been found that improvement in one family member is associated with deterioration in another

— as part of the treatment of schizophrenia when family interviews are held with the aim of reducing high levels of expressed emotion (see Leff et al 1982)

— when treatment will only be accepted as a member of a family group

— as a treatment of last resort.

Behaviour therapy

Techniques that rely upon exposure to reduce anxiety are applicable to adolescents, with modifications appropriate to their individual level of maturation. For instance, flooding is rarely used with prepubertal children but becomes increasingly applicable with progression through the teenage years, as does desensitisation in imagination, a technique which makes conceptual and imaginative demands beyond the capacity of children. Adolescents vary in the amount of in-vivo homework they will undertake for an exposure programme but can usually be encouraged to use diaries, fear thermometers and other records. How far one can use parents as therapeutic allies depends to a large extent upon whether autonomy is a heavily loaded issue for the adolescent in question, since parental pressure to approach a feared situation or the help parents can give in a response prevention programme for obsessional states can easily be resisted out of a general wish to shrug off authority. Their authority as parents and their active involvement with a treatment plan are indistinguishable stances to a teenager who is preoccupied with adolescent individuation and concerned to fight free of parental control.

The way in which developmental issues can interfere with implementing treatment prescriptions is echoed in the difficulty some teenagers, particularly boys, have in learning to relax as a component of a desensitisation, graded exposure or anxiety management programme, should they construe this as a passive response. Preferring to see themselves as active, they may find working with a relaxometer as a biofeedback device more appealing than more traditional relaxation regimes, partly because it emphasises an idea of active control over the body, partly because it appeals to those who like gadgets. It can also be practised in privacy without the need for a therapist to be present.

Operant schemes which use charts and points to increase compliance with parental demands are disdained by most adolescents and are replaced by reciprocal contracting between parents and adolescent as a widely applicable method of containing unacceptable behaviour (Stuart 1971). The therapist acts as referee while helping adolescent and parents to draw up an agreement in which the demands of the adolescent (usually for greater freedom) and parents (often for unquestioning obedience) can be balanced. The trick is to ensure that the demands are expressed positively: to do something rather than to stop doing something, and to restrain the parents from unreasonably autocratic positions. Much of the work is in clarifying demands to make sure that they are understood (and incapable of being misunderstood) by all and in checking that the proposed arrangement is seen as fair. A useful approach is to start with items that are not too contentious, on the principle that success breeds success and will ease a tense recriminatory family atmosphere. The therapist is actually more than referee, of course, and is actively teaching communication, explaining about normal adolescent development, modelling negotiation, and demonstrating something about family systems.

More extensive operant schemes using tokens and specified rewards which can be purchased by fixed numbers of tokens in a formal economy have been used in a number of residential programmes for aggressive and antisocial adolescents following the pioneering work at Achievement Place (see Ch. 8). Moss & Mann (1980) and Bedford and Tennent (1981) provide accounts of such schemes in hospital settings which can also use systematic time-out, an option not easily available to parents at home. One well-recognised difficulty with such schemes is the difficulty in transferring acquired behaviours and expectations to the outside world where contingencies are less consistent and may be less benign. Accommodating to "the fact that life is unjust" (Gagnon & Davidson 1976) when faced with an outside world wherein there are factors such as widespread unemployment, inconsistent parents and lack of leisure opportunities is not easy for the individual following discharge from hospital.

Cognitive behaviour therapy in adult psychiatry terms becomes increasingly feasible during adolescence. Cognitive interventions in childhood are somewhat different, both in the problems that are addressed and the style of intervention used. From personal experience it appears as if young children lack a sufficient reflective capacity and are too field-dependent in their thinking for cognitive treatments employed for anxiety or depression with adult patients to work well in real life, though special techniques for children (particularly hyperactive children) have a place. These tend to be of either the self-instructional or the social problem-solving type and employed alongside other behavioural techniques such as contingency management (see Kendall 1984, Pellegrini 1985). Adolescents can certainly use such approaches, suitably adapted, with good effect in antisocial behaviours where impulsivity is prominent (Nilans & Israel 1981, Snyder & White 1979). This is interestingly different in emphasis from the applications of cognitive behaviour therapy in adult psychiatry which are typically concerned with anxiety, depression and ruminations. On personal anecdotal grounds, there would seem to be value in using covert self-evaluation and self-instruction for adolescents with low self-esteem, and self-monitoring in a variety of conditions associated with anxiety or shame. Obviously there are a host of less specific variables involved in a cognitive therapy approach: encouragement of self-disclosure, support, empathy, verbal discussion of painful topics, advice, counselling, praise for mastery and so on. Together with the fact that cognitive interventions are usually carried out alongside or following other measures, it would be wise to consider cognitive approaches as components of a treatment package rather than standing alone.

Social skills training

There is some overlap between cognitive approaches and training in social skills, whether by modelling, self-instruction or coaching. In general, such training takes place in groups which may, quite explicitly, include a component devoted to discussion of social problem-solving (Sarason & Sarason 1981). There is a little evidence that this cognitive component may be significant in its own right, being superior to behavioural measures alone in Kaplan's (1982) study of assertion therapy with students.

Most social skills groups place considerable weight on rehearsing socially difficult situations in role-play with accompanying discussion and homework. Spence (1983), for example, argues that modelling alone provides insufficient impetus for the learning of new responses though it can facilitate existing responses and advocates a package (Spence 1980) of games, video-feedback, and discussion to augment modelling demonstrations. However, as she points out, there is very little evidence indeed as to the relative efficacy of each component and a dearth of outcome studies on clinical populations. Most studies have been carried out on socially isolated, friendless or rejected children and adolescents yet, as Kolvin and his colleagues (1981) showed, improvement can follow interventions such as classroom management programmes which would appear to have little obvious relevance at first sight. Nevertheless, most adolescent psychiatric services include a social skills training group in their intervention repertoire and personal observation suggests that this is a valuable, enjoyable asset for unassertive, victimised and gauche teenagers.

Activity therapies

Through a variety of creative activities, adolescents can learn about themselves by allowing themselves freedom to reveal aspects of their self in art, drama, and play. Such activities can serve the ordinary developmental needs of the mind when pursued at home, school or club. For some adolescents who are denied sufficient opportunity or whose mental habitude is excessively constraining, an opportunity to create and play can be therapeutic. Adolescents in in-patient units who may be residential patients for months will need creative opportunities as part of the milieu in which they live, "discovering aptitudes that are genuinely their own" (to adapt Merry's (1986) Phrase).

Art therapy offers a space and medium together with a relationship within which a disturbed adolescent can experiment and express feelings in images, communicating to themselves and others the otherwise inexpressible. A number of techniques and approaches can be used to facilitate this: group or individual, structured or unstructured. Most art therapists associated with adolescent psychiatric patients work in in-patient units though there is every reason to believe that they could with advantage operate in out-patient settings. There is an obvious parallel with music therapy and an overlap with occupational therapy (Bell 1977) though occupational therapists use a wider variety of practical techniques both to assist self-exploration through creativity and to teach life skills.

Psychodrama or drama therapy uses a number of games and

techniques to facilitate the expression and clarification of feelings. Through sculpting and role-play, the adolescent can learn how he is seen by others, and by the empty chair technique coupled with role reversal, the differing expectations of family members can be explored. Usually conducted as a group activity, psychodrama can easily be made available in out-patient settings (Holmes 1984).

Evaluation of creative therapies in terms of effectiveness in their own right is hardly ever performed. Usually they are adjuncts to other treatment interventions, particularly by enriching an in-patient treatment milieu. The evidence for the usefulness of such approaches rests upon common sense and unstructured clinical experience.

Pharmacological and physical treatments

There is no reason not to use psychotropic medication with adolescents according to the indications established in child and adult psychiatry generally. A common mistake is to use doses that are insufficient; teenagers can and should take adult doses. Unfortunately, the low prevalence of use of medication in child psychiatry means that child and adolescent psychiatrists are not always as well-informed about the role of psychotropic medication in children's and young adolescent's disorders as they might be. The reviews by Greenhill (1985) and Taylor (1985) complement each other and are required reading, though their bias is towards children rather than adolescents.

The use of diets, electro-convulsive therapy, and the various alarms associated with the treatment of enuresis or high psychophysiological arousal, similarly stem from principles established in child or adult psychiatry respectively; there are no techniques specific to adolescence, though some consideration should be given to how the developmental status of the patient will affect compliance. For instance, oligo-antigenic or exclusion diets may prohibit certain fast foods and cause embarrassment to a teenager who eats out with friends. The type of enuresis alarm which has sensors embedded in a small perineal sanitary towel worn inside underpants is often unwelcome to a boy who is touchy about his developing masculinity; he would probably be less offended by the old-fashioned bell-and-pad apparatus.

Consultation

A prominent component of the work of an adolescent psychiatrist is consultation with other agencies and workers involved with adolescents. In such an activity, the psychiatrist discusses a case or a situation with a professional who is already concerned and who has a problem with management. The psychiatrist does not take over clinical management responsibilities; the case remains with the consultee. The approach was first articulated in detail by Caplan (1964, 1970) under the title of "mental health consultation" though there are now a variety of derivatives: behavioural consultation, referral consultation, consultation with schools etc.

Within such a framework a number of general principles are recognised:

— the consultant discusses the problem with the consultee but does not monitor progress as in supervision; the consultee is free to disregard the outcome of a consultation

— the skills possessed by the consultee are paramount and formulation of the problem remains essentially in those terms

— the extremes of over-didactic advice and bland sanction of the status quo are avoided, while the consultant encourages the consultee to reconsider or reframe the problem and assess the way in which their own assumptions, stereotypes and role position within their own organisation might be inhibiting the best use of their skills.

Three areas of concern may be discussed with the consultee: their client, their personal feelings, and their work setting (including their colleagues). It is a general assumption within consultative work that the consultee will have sufficient knowledge and skills but cannot employ them effectively because of such elements as mistaken assumptions, lack of confidence, overinvolvement, or too narrow a focus. Quite commonly, issues arise which are to do with the consultee's position within an organisation, so that a discussion of work relationships becomes relevant. A decision needs to be taken at that point as to who should be involved in the consultation, the individual consultee alone or the consultee together with key colleagues.

Steinberg & Yule (1985) point out that consultation may also be employed as a teaching exercise within a training programme or as a skill-building exercise. The distinction from ordinary tuition or from supervision lies in the freedom of the consultee to ignore the content of the consultation. This seems to parallel the use of a clinical workshop such as a family therapy workshop which may be consulted by a professional as if it were a book: collecting insights or ideas which there is no obligation to use if they are judged inapplicable or redundant.

The traps in consultation are well recognised. The consultee is not a patient and should receive neither unconditional support nor psychotherapy, nor should the consultant merely inform the consultee that he or she is anxious about the problem. The consultant must respect the consultee's skills without regressing into spurious egalitarianism. The consultant must not impose a particular perspective (such as a psychoanalytic view) upon the consultee but should continue to stick with the consultee's perception of the problem. If the organisation or network within which the consultee works becomes the topic of concern in a consultation it is often unwise to continue without involving senior staff (see Skynner 1974 for an informative tale about offering a consultation to a school and Steinberg & Yule 1985, for a short account of how consultation might progress).

It is quite often assumed that disturbed adolescents have a particularly disruptive effect upon the institutions and professionals involved in their care and treatment. Their difficulties, their attitudes to authority, and the questions they raise themselves can lead the unwary among the staff into identifications which they would ordinarily refrain from. Consultation would appear to be a sensible provision and a use of psychiatric or other expertise that might ultimately have preventative potential. Unfortunately this method has not, by and large, been evaluated by the usual scientific standards, though there are a number of anecdotal reports which suggest that, once consultees get used to the stance of the consultant, they find it useful. Whether their adolescent clients benefit is less clear and most studies ignore this. Kolvin et al (1981) provide an exception in showing modest improvement in antisocial behaviour following consultation to the teachers of difficult adolescents, but otherwise the field, as is so often the case in adolescent psychiatry, is scientifically unexplored.

Adolescent Psychiatry

REFERENCES

Adams S 1961 The PICO project. In: Johnstone N et al (eds) The Sociology of Punishment and Conviction. Wiley, New York

Alexander J F, Parsons B 1973 Short-term behavioral intervention with delinquent families: impact on family process and recidivism. Journal of Abnormal Psychology 81: 219–225

Bedford A P, Tennent T G 1981 Behavioural training with disturbed adolescents. Association for Child Psychology and Psychiatry News 7: 6–12

Bell V 1977 Occupational therapy with young disturbed adolescents. British Journal of Occupational Therapy 5: 116–117

Bentovim A, Gorell Barnes G, Cooklin A (eds) 1982 Family Therapy. Academic Press, London

Berkowitz I H 1972 Adolescents Grow in Groups. Butterworths, London

Bruce T 1978 Group work with adolescents. Journal of Adolescence 1: 47–54

Byng-Hall J 1973 Family myths used as defence in conjoint family therapy. British Journal of Medical Psychology 46: 239–250

Caplan G 1964 Principles of Preventive Psychiatry. Tavistock, London

Caplan G 1970 The Theory and Practice of Mental Health Consultations. Tavistock, London

Coleman J C 1980 The Nature of Adolescence. Methuen, London

Evans J 1982 Adolescent and Pre-adolescent Psychiatry. Academic Press, London

Gagnon J H Davidson G C 1976 Asylums, the token economies, and the metrics of mental life. Behavior Therapy 7: 528–534

Greenhill L 1985 Pediatric psychopharmacology. In: Shaffer D, Ehrhardt A, Greenhill L (eds) The Clinical Guide to Child Psychiatry. Free Press/Collier Macmillan, London

Haley J 1980 Leaving Home. McGraw Hill, New York

Hill P 1986 Family therapy. In: Hill P, Murray R, Thorley A (eds.) Essentials of Postgraduate Psychiatry 2nd edn. Grune and Stratton, London

Holmes P 1984 Boundaries or chaos: an outpatient psychodrama group for adolescents. Journal of Adolescence 7: 387–400

Jones A 1984. Counselling Adolescents: School and After. Kogan Page, London

Kaplan D A 1982 Behavioral, cognition and behavioral-cognitive approaches to group assertion training. Cognitive Therapy Research 6: 301–304

Kendall P C 1984 Cognitive-behavioural self-control therapy for children. Journal of Child Psychology and Psychiatry 25: 173–179

Kolvin I, Garside R F, Nicol A R, Macmillan A, Wolstenholme F, Leitch I M 1981 Help Starts Here: The Maladjusted Child in the Ordinary School. Tavistock, London

Leff J, Kuipers L, Berkowitz R, Eberlein-Vries R, Sturgeon D 1982 A controlled trial of social intervention in the families of schizophrenic patients. British Journal of Psychiatry 141: 121–134

Lieberman S 1980 Transgenerational Family Therapy. Croom Helm, London

Luborsky L, Singer B, Luborsky L 1975 Comparative studies of psychotherapies. Archives of General Psychiatry 32: 995–1008

Maclennan B W, Felsenfeld N 1968 Group Counseling and Psychotherapy with Adolescents. Columbia University Press, New York

Merry J 1986 Art in the education of the disturbed adolescent. In: Steinberg D (ed) The Adolescent Unit. Wiley, Chichester

Minuchin S 1974 Families and Family Therapy. Tavistock, London

Moss G R, Mann A 1980 Behavioral approaches in adolescent psychiatry. In: Sholevar G P, Bauson R M, Blinder B J (eds) Emotional Disorders in Children and Adolescents. MTP Press, Lancaster

Mullener N, Laird J D 1971 Some developmental changes in the organisation of self-evaluations. Developmental Psychology 5: 233–236

Newsome A, Thorne B J, Wyld K L 1975 Student Counselling in Practice. University of London Press, London

Nilans T H, Israel A C 1981 Towards maintenance and generalization of behavior change: teaching children self regulation and self-instructional skills. Cognitive Therapy Research 5: 189–195

Patterson G 1971 Families: Applications of Social Learning to Family Life. Research Press, Champaign, Ill.

Patterson G 1982 Coercive Family Process. Castalia, Eugene, Oregon

Pellegrini D S 1985 Training in social problem-solving. In: Rutter M, Hersov L (eds) Child and Adolescent Psychiatry: Modern Approaches. 2nd Ed. Blackwell Scientific, Oxford

Ricks D F 1974 Supershrink. Methods of a therapist judged successful on the basis of adult outcomes of adolescent patients. In: Ricks D F, Thomas A, Roff M (eds) Life History Research in Psychopathology. Vol. 3. University of Minnesota Press, Minneapolis

Ryle A 1979 The focus in brief interpretive psychotherapy: dilemmas, traps and snags as target problems. British Journal of Psychiatry 134: 46–54

Sarason I G, Sarason B R 1981 Teaching cognitive and social skills to high school students. Journal of Counselling and Clinical Psychology 49: 908–918

Selvini-Palazzoli M, Boscolo L, Cecchin G, Prata G 1978 Paradox and Counter-paradox. Aronson, New York

Skynner A C R, 1974 An experiment in group consultation with the staff of a comprehensive school. Group Process 6: 99–114

Snyder J J, White M J 1979 The use of cognitive self-instruction in the treatment of behaviorally disturbed adolescents. Behavior Therapy 10: 227–235

Spence S H 1980 Social Skills Training with Children and Adolescents: A Counsellor's Manual. National Foundation for Educational Research, Windsor

Spence S H 1983 Teaching social skills to children. Journal of Child Psychology and Psychiatry 24: 621–627

Steinberg D 1983 The Clinical Psychiatry of Adolescence. Wiley, Chichester

Steinberg D, Yule W 1985 Consultative work. In: Rutter M, Hersov L (eds) Child and Adolescent Psychiatry: Modern Approaches. 2nd Ed. Blackwell Scientific, Oxford

Steinberg D, Merry J, Collins S 1978 The introduction of small group work to an adolescent unit. Journal of Adolescence 1: 331–344

Stuart R B 1971 Behavioral contracting with families of delinquents. Journal of Behavior Therapy and Experimental Psychiatry 2: 1–11

Taylor E 1985 Drug treatment In: Rutter M, Hersov L (eds) Child and Adolescent Psychiatry: Modern Approaches 2nd Ed. Blackwell Scientific, Oxford

Weiner M F, King J W 1977 Self-disclosure by the therapist to the adolescent patient. In: Feinstein S C, Giovacchini P L (eds) Adolescent Psychiatry: Developmental and Clinical Studies. Vol. 5. Aronson, New York

Wilson P, Hersov L 1985 Individual and group psychotherapy. In: Rutter M, Hersov L (Eds) Child and Adolescent Psychiatry: Modern Approaches. 2nd Ed. Blackwell Scientific, Oxford

Wright D M, Moelis I, Pollack L J 1976 The outcome of individual psychotherapy: increments at follow-up. Journal of Child Psychology and Psychiatry 17: 275–285

Yalom, I D 1975 The Theory and Practice of Group Psychotherapy. 2nd ed. Basic Books, New York

Index